Dental Management of the Child Patient

by
Hannelore Taschini Loevy, C. D., M. S., Ph. D.
Associate Professor of Pediatric Dentistry
College of Dentistry
University of Illinois
Chicago

Quintessence Publishing Co., Inc.   1981
Chicago, Berlin, Rio de Janeiro, Tokyo

© 1981 by Quintessence Publishing Co., Inc., Chicago, Illinois.
All rights reserved.

This book or any part thereof must not be reproduced by any means or in any
form without the written permission of the publisher.

Lithography: Time Scan, Leinfelden.
Composition: Adolph Fürst & Sohn GmbH & Co., Berlin
Printing: Kupijai & Prochnow, Berlin
Binding: J. Godry, Berlin

Printed in Germany

ISBN: 0-931386-40-3

Dedication

To my daughters Thea Clara and Luciana,
who have spent their lives trying to teach me
to understand children.

Introduction

The aim of this book is to provide factual information to the dental practitioner concerning management of the child patient so that the dental treatment of the child can best be accomplished by means of careful examination, appropriate treatment, and sound preventive measures. It emphasizes the child as an individual with special problems which require attention, careful evaluation and proper management. It is hoped that this book will also be useful to the general practitioner and to dental students. No attempt has been made to be all things to all people, but I hope it will find enough use so that a second edition can be more inclusive and complete. Some repetition is unavoidable, but an attempt has been made to keep it at a minimum, while trying at the same time to make each chapter a separate entity.

Acknowledgements

Many colleagues and friends have made the preparation of the book possible. I am particularly grateful to Drs. A.F. Goldberg, S.W. Shore, and J.G. Crawford for their valuable suggestions and encouragement from the beginning of the preparation of the manuscript. Many persons graciously gave permission for the use of their tables and photographs and these have been acknowledged throughout the text. I also express special thanks to the Library staff of the American Dental Association, in particular to Mrs. Ruth Schultz and Miss Mildred Blackburn, for their invaluable help in locating reading material. Thanks are also due to Drs. J.C. Kusek, E.B. Weiss, I.M. Rosenthal and A.J. Steffek for their willingness to read and correct parts of the manuscript. The secretarial assistance of Mrs. Isobelle M. McKinnon and Mrs. Rita Munday must also be acknowledged, as well as the help of Mr. Peter Sielaff and Miss Tomoko Tsuchiya in the production of the book. To Miss Aletha Kowitz a very special thanks for her help in providing information and editing the text and to Mrs. Ethel G. Rosenthal for her help. I also must thank Mr. H. Koehler and Mr. H.W. Haase for having suggested the idea of a book to me and for their encouragement during its preparation. Thanks are also due to my many students who helped me over the years with their questions. Finally, a special acknowledgement to my husband and my daughter, Luciana, who have been patient and understanding during the preparation of the book.

Contents

Contents

Chapter 1

The Child in the Dental Office

In 1875 a *Dental Cosmos* article by E. H. Raymond[14] encouraged dentists to treat children and suggested ways to minimize management problems. We have been treating young patients successfully at least since that time; some dentists with more success than others. The basic idea was restated by Olsen in 1964: "The objective of caring for the young child should be accomplishment of the maximum amount of work in the minimum time with the least degree of discomfort[13]."

A visit to a dental office may cause emotional stress in most patients, adults and children alike. Anxiety and fear of pain have been recognized by dentists as major factors in the reluctance of patients of all ages to accept dental treatment. For the young child, this stress is aggravated by a natural and normal fear of the unknown, coupled with past experiences, many of them unpleasant, of other medical specialties. The reaction of the child who is not yet fully able to express his fears verbally or even to hide his feelings can be – and many times is – one of loud protest. This is particularly true if the youngster has learned by experience that a good protest, in the form of a tantrum, can give him control and help him to avoid unpleasant situations.

Unless the child and the dentist have a good relationship, the many treatment needs that may develop over time will not be met fully and effectively. Patient cooperation in adjusting to stressful situations is greatly diminished in a situation of unresolved or suppressed resentment. When trust and respect are lacking in any part of the patient-dentist-parent team (Fig. 1-1), results can be disastrous.

When the pediatric patient manifests apprehension and reluctance, it is important to ascertain the reasons for this behavior so that the best method of overcoming resistance may be chosen. Any of many different factors, alone or in combination, may cause anxiety in the child. Some of these factors depend on the patient's personality and background, the dentist's personality and experience, the chronological and psychological age of the patient, the child-parent relationship, the parental relationship to dentistry, and prior experience at other medical and dental offices. A healthy, normal child who is easily handled and usually cooperative will be a difficult child when ill or when he has spent a sleepless night with a toothache. Moreover, he can be restless, fretful, and nervous when feverish.

The child in the dental office

When a child comes to the dental office for the first time, two major causes for anxiety are present: fear of the unknown and fear of physical discomfort. Fear dictates responses that vary in different individuals. Some psychologists feel that interference in the oral

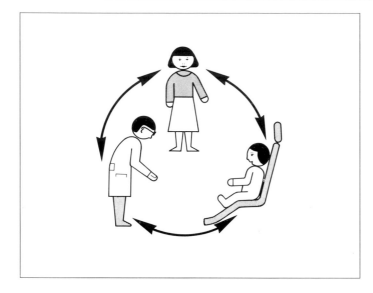

Fig. 1-1   Patient – dentist – parent team.

cavity will stimulate fears associated with the "primary pleasure zone", as the mouth plays an important role in taste, touch, and recognition in infancy. It must not be forgotten, however, that children react negatively to any procedure that is potentially damaging to any part of the body[11].

Fear of the unknown is a normal reaction. Furthermore, children have been exposed many times to stories about the dental office, in which adults and other children have described real or imaginary sufferings; these are then enlarged by the child's own imagination. Explanations, which depend on the child's age and understanding, need to be formulated clearly. In no case should the explanation be deceptive, particularly if pain may be involved. Once a child has been deceived, he will have little or no confidence in future statements, and regaining his trust becomes a major task.

The choice of appropriate words is important. Each new state of treatment should be explained and a routine of "tell, show, and do" should be established. As the child is unfamiliar with every kind of new dental pro-cedure, a running account of what is being done and the purpose of a newly introduced instrument will diminish much of the anxiety. Usually each dentist develops his own vocabulary for his instruments, to make the procedure understandable to a child. An explorer may be called a "counting instrument", a saliva ejector can be compared to a vacuum cleaner, and so on.

Fear is also dissipated when children contribute actively to the treatment by holding saliva ejectors or prophylaxis paste containers (when feasible). Children's cooperation should be praised to them and to their parents.

Evaluation of crying is a very effective means of ascertaining the type of behavior to expect. Elsbach[3] has described four characteristic types of crying: the frightened cry, the obstinate cry, the compensatory cry, and the hurt cry. The sound of each of these cries is different. The ability to differentiate between them is of great value in the management of the child as a patient.

The *frightened cry* expresses the child's real fear of the new unknown situation or the threatening procedure, usually through an abundance of tears. The most important thing is to attract the child's attention, so that appropriate explanations can be presented. This expression of lack of confidence can be handled best by gentle firmness.

The *obstinate cry* is a form of tantrum. The child is loud but usually has no tears. Many children who display this form of behavior are accustomed to getting their way through tantrums. Mild restraint and firmness may be necessary to obtain willingness to listen and to establish a dialogue.

The *compensatory cry,* according to Elsbach, is a noise to drown the sound of the dental drill. The sound of the drill apparently causes much discomfort to some children. This behavior, however, does not interfere with the delivery of good dental care, and the noise does not have to be curtailed. Gentle discussion with the child will usually reduce the problem after a few visits.

The *hurt cry* may not be loud, but is usually tearful and is associated with pain. The reason for the pain must be found and properly handled.

Abnormal and inordinate resistance to treatment by a child requires further evaluation of the underlying disturbance. Occasionally, consultation with the child's physician may be indicated.

Education and training of parents is an important factor in a child's treatment. Parents should not be permitted to associate dentistry with a form of punishment, and also should not bribe the child or make unattainable promises. As the child will cooperate willingly only when he fully trusts the dentist, there must be parental trust if a successful relationship is to develop.

Emotional development of the normal child

Knowledge of the normal psychological development of children is unquestionably of paramount importance in the evaluation of possible communication problems that may arise during treatment and especially during the first visits of a child to a new office and a new health professional. Critical periods of child development have been recognized for a long time. These developmental changes can affect the child's relationship to the dentist. As early environmental influences are important in the development of behavior of any individual, "typical behavior" for any given age varies greatly between individuals. Some characteristics, however, have been described for each age, because they are found in a large number of children. These developmental changes can be expressed as successions of adaptations which each individual must make.

The *one-year-old child* is usually friendly. He is social and is beginning to appreciate and recognize adult approval of his acts.

The *two-year-old child* has much more motor development. He is a social individual and usually able to express himself. The size of the vocabulary at this age varies greatly from a few to hundreds of words. The child is used to his home environment and does not like separation from his parents or other people on whom he is dependent. At about age 2½ a marked need for autonomy develops and this phase is recognized as the negativistic period. The child will resist authority and may have tantrums if he is challenged. The adult must show firmness. This period is known as the "terrible two's", and not infrequently the child will actually be doing what has been asked of him at the same time he is protesting.

The *three-year-old child* is a more secure and positive child. He no longer uses *"No"* as an answer for every request, but is willing to conform and please.

The *four-year-old child* is often a defiant and imaginative child. In fact, his energy and imagination are so intense that he is prone to exaggeration of imagination and acts. The adult must be firm when dealing with him.

The *five-year-old child* is usually a reliable and docile child. While he is very fond of his home environment, he does not fear short separations. He is pleasant and cooperative.

The *six-year-old child* is often difficult and his mood can change from moment to moment, from being a very loving child to having a tantrum. The child usually has acquired considerable independence from his mother by this age.

Each child's emotional and mental status develops through a series of steps. In early childhood, there is usually complete dependence on the mother. Until the age of three or four, when the child first starts major activities outside the home, such as nursery school, the mother is closely inter-related to the child.

By the time the child reaches age 4, he will begin to test authority and try to increase his independence. This is also a time when children in our culture usually start taking part in structured activities outside the home, e.g., nursery school. The child therefore becomes more accustomed to being separated from the mother. During this period of "resistance" the child may become difficult to manage. Resistance may increase considerably if the child is accustomed to obtaining advantage in the home through this behavior. For such children, the presence of the parents in the operatory is contraindicated. It is important at this age to distinguish resistance or authority testing from actual separation fear. In some instances, and in some cultures, a four-year-old may still be very dependent on the mother. A four-year-old child also has a very vivid imagination and

the potential danger of separation anxiety should be recognized.

Developmental stages do not necessarily parallel chronological age, but depend on environmental factors and family relationships. Some psychologists believe that the affection shown by a child reflects the treatment he has received. It should be remembered that a child learns through experience. If angry and excessive outbursts have achieved the desired objectives, they may become an integral and important part of his behavior.

Parental attitudes vary greatly in a wide range from overprotection to complete rejection. Parental attitudes are reflected in the child. Children of overindulgent parents may be hostile, and children of overauthoritative parents may be difficult to reason with and withdrawn.

In addition to the obvious developmental landmarks, certain behavior problems have their origins in familial background; their analysis can be helpful in improving communication with the young patient. Children who have been mistreated because their parents are alcoholics or those who are used to severe physical punishment often react badly to any authority symbol, especially adults. They may have deep emotional problems that can be reached only with understanding, goodwill, and after careful evaluation.

Children from large families may have different problems. They may be inhibited because they are always compared to others who do better; the oldest child may always be expected to set an example. A child who has always been repressed needs confidence, while the child who reacts by seeking refuge in early childhood behavior to avoid responsibility needs understanding and goodwill.

The parent in the dental office

Do parents play a significant role in good behavior management? Is their presence in the operatory acceptable or even advisable? Does the child need support? If so, how much and why? Is the parental influence advantageous and supportive? These and similar questions have been discussed in the dental literature since Jordon wrote of them in 1925[9]. Professionals differ concerning the advantages or disadvantages of parental presence in the operatory. Several authors have evaluated the benefits and disadvantages as well as parental anxiety *per se,* and its influence on the child's fear of dental treatment. In addition to fear of the unknown, there is also fear of separation from the parent. This fear can be extremely traumatic, especially in the young, dependent child. At any age, parental misinformation and anxiety may create a very real fear in the child, which hinders good communication between dentist and child.

Effective patient management requires parental cooperation and understanding. Moreover, the assistance of parents is essential in follow-up and success of treatment. Parents generally are concerned and willing to cooperate once the problems are made clear to them.

Dietary problems sometimes are the result of overindulgence. The parents must understand the damage to dental health of excessive sugar intake. Proper oral hygiene also has to be explained; that of many parents needs improvement. A discussion of the problem usually will be effective. Parents who are kept informed of the progress of treatment by the dentist usually stay interested and will try to cooperate.

The manner in which a child copes with his anxiety in the dental situation depends on several factors. If a child is reared with a fear of dentistry, his attitude toward dentistry is negative and little parental cooperation can

be expected. Johnson and Baldwin[8] and Wright and Alpern[17] found that the mother's anxieties toward the dental situation affect the child's behavior independently of the nature of the procedure. As parental apprehension is relayed to the child, a parent in the office cannot be helpful under these conditions.

Many pedodontists prefer that the parent remain in the reception area, away from the treatment area. Some dentists are not comfortable with the parent in the operatory, and that in itself can affect the child's behavior. In some very young children, however, separation anxiety is such that the parent's emotional support is advantageous, at least during the initial visits, and the parent may be asked to come to the operatory. Frankl *et al.*[5] compared a group of children with the mother present or absent during dental treatment. They found that the presence of a passive, observing mother was beneficial, particularly to the child under age five. Much has been published about feelings of security and insecurity in the child in new, strange environments. While long periods of separation seem to have deleterious effects on psychological development, short separations do not appear to cause significant damage[15] and depend on the type of person "substituting" for the parent, the language being used, and the type of restrictions placed after separation from the parent.

When a parent is permitted to accompany the child into the operatory he must not interfere with the work or the dentist's communication with the patient. Parents should not hold the child's hands or talk or explain treatment plans. Dialogue should be strictly between the child and the dentist. The parent should not be permitted to converse with the staff during treatment. Such conversation diverts attention that rightfully belongs to the child. Neither should a parent be permitted to express his feelings about a particular instrument or procedure, or convey such feelings through facial expressions or movement. If the child does not cooperate, the major reason for parental presence is lost, and it is better to request that the parent leave the operatory. Sometimes the small child will learn from this that cooperative behavior is the prerequisite to parental presence. Most children already attending a formal school program do not require the presence of the parent, as they have learned to stand on their own. Ethnic backgrounds, however, play a role in this situation, as some cultures have different customs and family relationships and these factors should be taken into consideration by the dentist.

In a study in which parents were given the option of remaining in the operatory, many parents preferred to remain for the first few visits. As familiarity with treatment increased, the need for the presence of the parent decreased. In this study[16] the presence of the parents was not associated with increased negative response by the children.

It is important that the parent knows beforehand whether he will stay in the waiting room or be in the operatory, so that any promises made are kept. It helps if the mother does not promise to remain during treatment without first consulting the dentist, since this interferes with the child's trust.

Scheduling should be such that the child is not kept waiting in the reception area but is given prompt attention. Neither should there be lingering or excessively long goodbyes or other delaying tactics when the patient leaves for the operatory.

Behavior management

Because patient cooperation is essential to delivery of high quality dentistry to every child or adult, the first aim of the dentist is to alter negative behavior and develop an effective dentist-child relationship.

Patient behavior management and behavior modification techniques are indispensable aids in the effective management of the child. It is not realistic to expect a patient to delight in the idea of dental or any other medical treatment. Behavior is acquired through learning but specific goals must be established before any program is initiated. These goals must be progressive and reasonable and in accord with the age and health of the child.

The most common methods of behavior modification involve use of reinforcement techniques. Positive behavior is always reinforced by praise. Initially praise may be frequent, and can be given even if the behavior is not completely satisfactory until the desired goals are attained. It is helpful to praise a child for at least some positive contribution to the dental visit. Children, like adults, enjoy praise and this is one means of reinforcement of positive accomplishment.

The adamant child may need more drastic control. He should be handled alone because in this case the parent is usually of no assistance. A firm attitude by the dentist is usually enough. Simply saying, "In my office, I tell *you* what is going to be done", or, "In my office, we do not like screams", is usually enough to demonstrate command and can obtain cooperation. Occasionally it is necessary to resort to stronger measures to establish communication. A frantic child is unable to comprehend orders because he is screaming so loudly that he is unable to hear them. The restraining technique usually known as "hand over mouth exercise" (HOME)[10] consists of placing the hand gently but firmly over the child's mouth. The child is told, in a quiet, slow voice, that when he is willing to cooperate, the hand will be removed. It is important not to raise the voice, so that the child has to stop screaming to hear the dentist. Once the noise has stopped and the child has agreed to cooperate, the hand is removed immediately. If the problem starts again, the hand is placed over the mouth again and removed when the child indicates by head movement that he will cooperate. The process may have to be repeated a few times, but the child retains control of the situation at all times. When the child cooperates, he should be complimented, and the reasons for each of the dental procedures explained. Many dentists have opposed this technique, considering the possibilities of frightening the patient. It is a drastic and extreme procedure which should be used only if patient cooperation cannot be obtained in a less drastic manner. In 1967, a questionnaire circulated by the Association of Pedodontic Diplomates indicated that among the 95% who responded, 75% had used the method[2]. The treatment should never be used in anger, and is contraindicated in physically disabled, medically compromised, and mentally retarded patients. Restraints should not be used as a punishment but only as a means of getting the attention of the child so that a dialogue may be established.

The personality of the dentist also plays a part in behavior management. The dentist who does not like children or is afraid of them will not be able to communicate with young patients. A child can sense insecurity and will react, usually in an antagonistic manner. Use of "baby talk" is an inept way of communicating with children because they are fully aware that this is not natural. Children, even very young ones, expect pleasant, professional, friendly behavior which is not patronizing or insulting to their intelligence.

The handicapped child

Environmental and genetic factors, acting prenatally or postnatally, can produce a handicapped individual with mental or organic problems or both. With advances in general medical care, life expectancy of the handicapped patient has increased greatly and adequate dental care must be provided. Because many patients with major disabilities are unable to take proper care of their teeth and are unable to cope with artificial prostheses, it is important for them to maintain a healthy natural dentition to the greatest extent possible.

In the past, great emphasis was placed on institutionalizing many handicapped children at a very early age. Today, wherever and whenever possible, emphasis is placed on proper home care. While a small percentage of handicapped patients require hospitals or other specialized treatment centers, many patients with handicaps can be treated in the private office. Parental cooperation is essential in the treatment of these children since some will require a considerable amount of assistance for oral hygiene and diet control, and need frequent, regular check-up visits as preventive measures. Preventive dentistry is of great importance since it will reduce treatment required by children who cannot cooperate and may be unable to wear dentures. Unfortunately, parents are often so involved with the handicapped child's major medical and social problems that they give little attention to the oral structures. A large percentage of handicapped patients are only brought for dental care in crisis or emergency situations[12].

Children may be handicapped by:

1. Major organic disease
2. Mental subnormality
3. Emotional disturbance

As dental treatment of the handicapped patient concerns not only the dental problem but also the management of the patient, it is essential to understand the psychological composition of the individual problem. Some of the behavioral and psychological

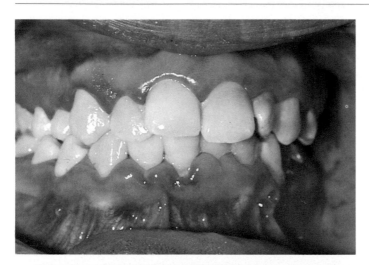

Fig. 1-2   Gingival inflammation in patient with Down syndrome.

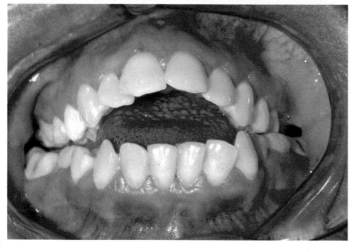

Fig. 1-3   Malocclusion in patient with Down syndrome.

problems experienced by handicapped patients can be related to parental reactions such as over protection associated with parental guilt feelings. The parental attitude is particularly critical to the development of adequate normalizing mechanisms.

The establishment of good communication and rapport is an important aspect in the treatment of the handicapped patient. Inadequacies in perception, language, or mobility may create high levels of anxiety; an adequate social and family history is required for proper evaluation of internal stresses that may interfere with the establishment of a positive relationship between patient and dentist. In some cases of extreme mental retardation or psychological problems, this relationship cannot be attained.

Several dental problems are closely related to specific handicaps. Patients with *Down syndrome* often show periodontal disease (Fig. 1-2) and malocclusion (Figs. 1-3 and 1-4). Prolonged use of certain drugs in the control of specific handicaps also may affect oral structures. The use of phenytoin may pro-

Fig. 1-4   Malocclusion in patient with Down syndrome. Lateral view of patient in Fig. 1-3.

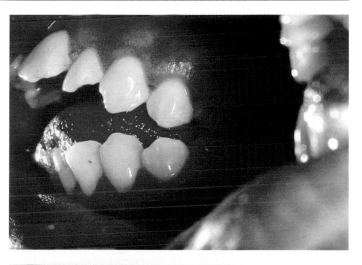

Fig. 1-5   Gingival hyperplasia in patient taking phenytoin.

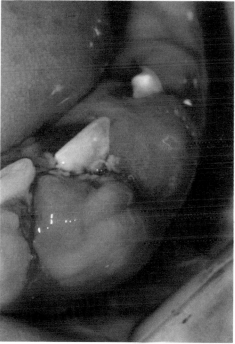

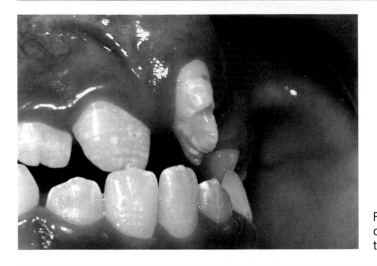

Fig.1-6   Malocclusion in patient with cleft palate. Note hypoplasia of tooth 8.

duce gingival hyperplasia (Fig. 1-5). Certain immuno-suppressive drugs used in the treatment of blood disorders may cause oral lesions.

In *cleft palate* patients, a large number of psychological problems are associated with the visible orofacial abnormalities and the patient's inability to camouflage them. These patients usually react very intensely to any treatment in the oral cavity (Fig.1-6).

Cerebral palsy is manifested by spasticity, athetosis rigidity, ataxia, tremor, or a combination of these. The lack of muscular coordination makes it very difficult or impossible for the patient to perform an adequate oral hygiene regimen and complicates chewing and swallowing procedures. Tongue and cheek movements may be abnormal and a high incidence of malocclusion is seen. Bruxism is a common problem. The physical disability in patients with cerebral palsy varies greatly, from complete helplessness to minor disability. The patient's ability to co-operate will determine the measures necessary to permit treatment in the dental office. Because of the frequency of involuntary movement of these patients, certain adaptations have to take place to allow proper treatment. It is unreasonable to expect that

a spastic child, unable to control his neuro-muscular functions, can keep his mouth open for long periods of time. In these patients, biteblocks or mouth props are essential. The reason for their use, however, has to be explained to the patient. The intensity and frequency of involuntary movements tend to increase under stress and in the effort to cooperate, so biteblocks of appropriate size should be used[1]. The head should be supported to avoid interference of the patient's involuntary movements. Premedication with an antianxiety drug such as diazepam can be helpful in some instances.

The *blind child* has learned to substitute hearing and feeling for seeing. He must be approached cautiously so that he may know the dentist is present by voice and physical contact without being startled. While he is unable to see the instruments, he can and should become acquainted with them by touch. Voice control is very important. The dentist should speak slowly and, above all, take nothing for granted and use a "show, tell, and do" technique.

The *deaf child* understands and learns through visual perception and the gradual adaptation of past experiences. It is part of the "normalization" process in dealing with

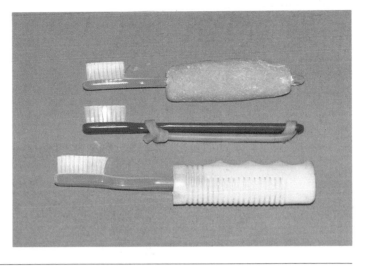

Fig. 1-7 Modified toothbrush handle to facilitate easier grasp for handicapped patients.

these patients to talk to them since many have learned to understand a great part of what is being said even if they are not yet formally trained in lip reading. The patient definitely understands pleasant smiles of approval.

If the blind patient is also deaf, his contact is only through touch and all explanations have to be based on this sense. The age of the patient will determine whether he can be treated in the office or if he should be treated in a hospital setting.

The *retarded patient* has problems of understanding and interpretation. Retarded patients usually suffer great separation anxiety because of the extra attention they are accustomed to receive from their parents. Often it is advisable to have the parent in the dental operatory as he or she is well acquainted with the moods of the patient and can contribute to a better dentist-patient relationship.

Many such patients are hypermobile and have a short attention span. Therefore extraneous environmental stimulants should be kept to a minimum. Instrumentation and explanations must be presented in an easy and simple manner. As the execution of simple tasks is difficult for many retarded pa-

tients, verbal compliments are very helpful and warranted. Management requires an adequate number of appointments to allow the dentist to reassure the patient and thus to reduce anxiety and tension. Premedication may be helpful but gradual conditioning and teaching through sound pedodontic patient management practice can reduce the need for drugs[6]. A detailed medical history is very important, and consultation with the patient's physician often is necessary. If drugs are to be used, the dentist must familiarize himself with the patient's drug regimen and the side effects and interactions of these medications.

The course of treatment is planned according to the findings at the first office consultation. With few exceptions, detailed evaluations of the hard and soft mouth structures are made in the office and the appropriate radiographs are taken. Those patients whose cooperation is so poor that adequate clinical and radiographic examination is impossible should be treated under general anesthesia.

Oral hygiene instructions are particularly important to reduce the incidence of oral disease in the handicapped patient. The American Dental Association publishes a pamphlet ("Caring") for parent orientation in preventive dentistry for the handicapped child. Poor oral hygiene in these patients is usually a consequence of the difficulty the patient has in cleaning his own teeth and his dependency on other individuals to perform this task. In many types of handicaps, muscular tonus and type of saliva also may interfere with the efficiency of oral hygiene. Several types of oral hygiene devices have been designed to aid the patient in becoming more self-sufficient. When neuromuscular coordination and intelligence permit, a modification of the oral hygiene aids will permit better patient cooperation. Regular toothbrushes can be adapted for the handicapped patient by simple and inexpensive modification of the handle (Fig. 1-7). If the patient is not able to grasp a normal toothbrush properly, an increase in size or weight of the handle may be necessary. Rubber tubing placed at the end of the toothbrush can then be slipped over the hand of the patient for easier grasping. A bicycle handlebar grip filled with plaster or acrylic can be inserted over a toothbrush handle; the increased weight and size make it easier for the handicapped patient to manipulate the brush[4]. Special metal tubing may be used to increase the length of the toothbrush. Studies have also shown that electric toothbrushes can be effective in some types of handicapping conditions[7].

Table 1-1 **Handicaps, their oral manifestations, and possible modifications of treatment**

TYPE OF HANDICAP	PATHOLOGY/ETIOLOGY	ORAL MANIFESTATIONS	TREATMENT MODIFICATION

Cerebral palsy
Disorder involving motor function.
Other handicaps often associated:
Mental retardation
Convulsions
Sensory problems
	Types:
	Spasticity: injury to motor cortex (extreme motor stiffness and hyperactivity)
	Athetosis: injury to basal ganglia or extrapyramidal tract (lack of voluntary muscle control and increased purposeless movements such as facial grimaces)
	Ataxia: injury in cerebellum (problem in balance and equilibrium)
	Rigidity: lesion of basal ganglia (problems of muscle movement)
	Tremor: lesion of basal ganglia (constant quivering of certain muscles)
		Enamel hypoplasia
		Malocclusion (associated with abnormal muscle activity)
		Gingival hyperplasia (in cases of phenytoin administration)
		Fractured teeth (associated with trauma)
		Bruxism
		Open bite
			Mouth props and biteblocks to aid mouth opening
			Restraints
			Premedication for muscle relaxation
			General anesthesia for extensive treatment
			Careful evaluation of tooth brushing:
			  electric toothbrush
			  modification of toothbrush
			  parental instruction in toothbrushing
			  diet evaluation and consultation

Cystic fibrosis	Hereditary generalized dysfunction with progressive chronic pulmonary and pancreatic disease	Intrinsic stains of teeth due to medication (tetracyclines) Viscous and ropy saliva Enlarged salivary glands	No inhalation agents Evaluation of diet with patient's physician Short life expectancy prognosis may affect treatment plan Avoid loss of salt by avoiding excessive perspiration

Table 1-1 **Handicaps, their oral manifestations, and possible modifications of treatment** (continued)

TYPE OF HANDICAP	PATHOLOGY/ETIOLOGY	ORAL MANIFESTATIONS	TREATMENT MODIFICATION
Diabetes mellitus	Impaired carbohydrate metabolism due to low production of insulin	High susceptibility to infection Increased incidence of periodontal disease	Antibiotic premedication for extractions Careful attention to avoid interference of dental appointment with medication schedule Emergency: hypoglycemia – give sugar
Down syndrome Trisomy 21	Genetic disorder with increased chromosomal material Frequently associated heart abnormalities, mental retardation	Protruding tongue Missing and malformed teeth Underdeveloped midface Malocclusion and open bite Increased periodontal disease Poor oral hygiene Low caries incidence	Preventive techniques to improve oral hygiene and decrease periodontal disease Patients frequently are docile and affectionate with short attention span Orthodontic and prosthetic prognosis generally poor Antibiotic coverage indicated in case of heart disease
Emotional disorders	Neurotic disorders Psychotic disorders Autism	Varied (can be self-inflicted)	Consultation with physician for drug therapy Extreme cases may require general anesthesia
Epilepsy (chronic with recurrent convulsions)	Grand mal generalized convulsions with tonic and clonic muscle spasm Petit mal transient loss of consciousness	Gingival hyperplasia partially associated with medication (phenytoin) Tooth fractures and trauma to hard and soft oral structures during seizures	Highly controlled oral hygiene to decrease phenytoin hyperplasia Emergency: control of seizure

Table 1-1 **Handicaps, their oral manifestations, and possible modifications of treatment** (continued)

TYPE OF HANDICAP	PATHOLOGY/ETIOLOGY	ORAL MANIFESTATIONS	TREATMENT MODIFICATION
Glycogen storage diseases (several types of glycogenoses)	Abnormal synthesis or degradation of glycogen with consequent utilization problems	Bleeding complications possible Abnormal tooth eruption pattern in some forms	Appointment schedule should not interfere with meal times- avoid hypoglycemia Consult physician for drug interaction
Heart diseases	Congenital or postnatally acquired heart defects Rheumatic fever	Transient bacteremia can cause bacterial endocarditis	Antibiotic coverage if danger of bacteremia exists Careful endodontics to avoid bacteremia – no instrumentation beyond tooth apex
Hemorrhagic diseases	Defects in coagulating mechanisms from various causes		Consultation with hematologist for packing therapy in cases of extraction No tissue damage if at all possible Occasionally systemic therapy may be necessary See page 88
Leukemia	Synthesis of abnormal leukocytes, often with reduced platelet count	Infections Hemorrhage Gingivitis	Consultation with hematologist for treatment during remission Coverage for infections See page 172
Mental Retardation	Genetic, prenatal perinatal and postnatal factors I.Q. 70-85 = borderline I.Q. 55-70 = mild I.Q. 40-55 = moderate I.Q. 25-40 = severe I.Q. 0-25 = profound	Tooth anomalies Enamel hypoplasias in many cases Malocclusion associated with abnormal muscle physiology Poor oral hygiene	Preventive techniques to improve oral hygiene Sedation or restraint necessary in some cases but verbal communication can be successful

Table 1-1 **Handicaps, their oral manifestations, and possible modifications of treatment** (continued)

TYPE OF HANDICAP	PATHOLOGY/ETIOLOGY	ORAL MANIFESTATIONS	TREATMENT MODIFICATION
Renal diseases	Loss of function of the kidney glomerulus from inflammation, degeneration or malformation	Susceptibility to infection Intrinsic tooth stains due to medication (tetracyclines)	Consultation with physician if patient is using steroid therapy for increased medication during stressful situations Antibiotic premedication before extraction
Respiratory diseases	*Asthma:* bronchial spasm common *Bronchiectasis:* bronchial dilation often with secondary infection	Intrinsic tooth stains due to medication (tetracyclines)	Great care with anesthesia, especially general anesthesia Careful evaluation of medications for possible drug interaction If steroids are being used, consult physician for increased medication during stress
Sensory disorders Blindness Deafness	Genetic, prenatal, perinatal and postnatal factors	Dental anomalies and occasional hypoplasia	Attention and removal of hearing aid may be indicated Communication can be obtained through non-affected senses Increased use of touch as means of communication
Sickle cell disease	Genetic disorder of hemoglobin *Homozygote:* disease present *Heterozygote:* trait	Prone to infection and thrombi Often over protected children	Avoid vasoconstrictors in anesthetic solution Care with general anesthesia and inhalation anesthesia in the office No "HOME"

References

1. Campbell, O.:
Dental treatment of the cerebral palsied child.
J. New Jersey Dent. Soc. 37:197-201, 1966.

2. Craig, W.:
Hand over mouth technique, J. Dent. Child.
38:387-389, 1971.

3. Elsbach, H.G.:
Crying as a diagnostic tool. J. Dent. Child. 30:13-16,
1963.

4. Ettinger, R.L. and J.R. Pinkham:
Dental care for the homebound – assessment and
hygiene. Aust. Dent. J. 22:77-82, 1977.

5. Frankl, S.N., F.R. Shiere and H.R. Fogels:
Should the parent be with the child in the dental
operatory? J. Dent. Child. 29:150-163, 1962.

6. Green, A. and M. Mendelsohn:
Premedication necessary for handicapped children? J. Dent. Child. 27:40-45, 1960.

7. Green, A. L., S. Rosenstein, A. Parks and
A.K. Kutscher:
The electric toothbrush as an adjunct in main-
taining oral hygiene in handicapped patients.
J. Dent. Child. 29:169-171, 1962.

8. Johnson, R. and D.C. Baldwin, Jr.:
Maternal anxiety and child behavior J. Dent. Child.
36:87-92, 1969.

9. Jordon, M.E.:
Operative dentistry for children. Brooklyn, Dental
Items of Interest, 1925.

10. Levitas, T.C.:
HOME – Hand over mouth exercise. J. Dent. Child.
41:178-182, 1974.

11. Lewis, H.W.:
The unconscious castrative significance of tooth
extraction. J. Dent. Child. 24:3-16, 1957.

12. Nowak, A.J.:
The role of dentistry in the normalization of the
mentally retarded person. J. Dent. Child. 41:456-
460, 1974.

13. Olsen, N.H.:
Behavior control of the child dental patient. J. Amer.
Dent. Assoc. 68:873-877, 1964.

14. Raymond, E.H.:
Children as patients. Dent. Cosmos 17:54-56, 1875.

15. Robertson, J. and J. Robertson:
Young children in brief separation: a fresh look.
Psychoanalytic Study of the Child. 16:264-315,
1971.

16. Venham, L.L., D. Bengston and M. Cipes:
Parent's presence and the child's response to
dental stress. J. Dent. Child. 45:213-217, 1978.

17. Wright, G.Z. and D.G. Alpern:
Variables influencing children's cooperative behavior at the first dental visit. J. Dent. Child. 38:124-128,
1971.

Chapter 2

Clinical Examination in Pedodontics

The purposes of the child's initial visit to the dentist are establishment of an accurate diagnosis through a careful and thorough examination and development of a proper treatment plan. However, the initial visit to the dentist also may be for treatment of an emergency caused by pain or trauma or it may be the first visit to any dentist. Not infrequently, a "first visit" is in fact a visit to a new dentist's office. Sometimes the first dentist seen simply was unable to handle the child and to provide services.

Several preliminary pieces of information are essential before the patient is actually seen and examined by the dentist. The name of the patient, age, date of birth, address, telephone number, name and occupation of the parent or guardian, and billing address are requested routinely in each dental office. Additional information helpful in dentistry for children is the name and age of siblings and the nickname of the child. Knowledge of pets, if any, in the home may be interesting information that can be useful as an "ice-breaker" in the dentist's first conversation with the child.

Detailed past medical and dental histories are essential to avoid unnecessary problems during the progress of dental treatment. The name and telephone number of the child's pediatrician, as well as the date of the last medical examination should be obtained. This information is particularly relevant in handicapped children or children taking medication. In either case, consultation with the child's physician before initiation of treatment or during subsequent dental visits is advisable. Whether the child has been seen previously by another dentist is pertinent information, especially if the prior experiences were not pleasant.

Diagnosis requires critical and careful evaluation of facts and a good past history of the family and of the patient from both the medical and dental points of view. In cases of an emergency visit, care is usually limited to the more immediate examination of the region causing the emergency, but a knowledge of past medical history is essential nonetheless. In a routine follow-up examination it is only necessary to note changes in previously recorded data.

In addition to a history and clinical examination, there are several other important tools in pedodontic diagnosis. These include radiographs, dental casts and, often, photographs. Additional useful information, especially of handicapped patients, includes speech evaluation and diet analysis.

Most offices have printed forms available so that many items of information can be provided by the parents at the time of the initial examination. This form can be completed either by the parent alone or with the help of the dental assistant, and should include the following:

Vital statistics: Name, date of birth and age, place of birth, address, telephone, name of parents or guardian, occupation and marital status of the parents and information about persons with whom the child is presently living, if not with parents. The place of birth is of interest in cases of evaluation of possible fluorosis. In a child, the date of birth is more specific than age because a large number of physical and emotional changes can take place during a very short period of time. The family status can yield information regarding the child's home environment and this may be reflected in his behavior patterns.

Past medical history of the patient and his family

Information should be available about the health conditions of the patient and his family, particularly with regard to

organs:

heart
kidneys
lungs
endocrine glands (this includes questioning about diabetes)
liver

conditions:

allergies to foods and medications
bleeding disorder, any blood dyscrasias
anemias (including sickle cell anemia)
rheumatic fever
central nervous system problems (including seizures and other nervous disorders)
arthritis
asthma
hepatitis
hearing problems
learning problems
mental retardation
nutritional problems
psychiatric problems.

It should be noted specifically if the child has ever been hospitalized. The age of hospitali-

zation is of concern as the separation from the family might have been psychologically traumatic and could have predisposed the patient to an unfavorable reaction to dental procedures and equipment. For a child, a record of conditions at birth may be important because a child's prematurity or very low birth weight may provide some insight into developmental patterns. Evaluation of the growth pattern, however, should also take into consideration familial tendencies.

Clinical examination of the patient

General evaluation of the patient

General physical characteristics, height, weight and skin appearance

When the child enters the office, one notices whether the child is tall or short and under- or overweight. Gross deviations from the norms must be evaluated further. Face, arms and hands may sometimes show skin changes due to certain pathologic conditions, metabolic deficiencies, or allergies.

Gait

A seriously abnormal gait requires further evaluation of general health of the patient. The unsteady walk of a child suffering from a debilitating condition or from a developmental handicap is to be specially noted if present.

Temperature

If a deviation from norm is suspected, temperature changes should be investigated further, to assure appropriate handling of the condition and possible referral to the physician.

Head and neck examination

The size of the child's head may be abnormal from early or late suture closing due to genetic and familial factors or hydrocephalus. Abnormal hair quantity and texture may indicate genetic problems (e. g., ectodermal dysplasia) or nutritional (protein) deficiencies. Abnormalities of the position and shape of eyes and ears should be observed and evaluated. Enlargements of the neck and facial asymmetry should be noted and the etiology established.

Examination of the oral cavity

Breath

Bad breath can result from local factors (food retention, local pathological conditions) or systemic factors (gastrointestinal and oropharyngeal disturbances, acidosis, or general pathological states including some febrile conditions).

Salivary glands

Unilateral or bilateral swelling or tenderness of the parotid glands may be present. The areas above the submaxillary and sublingual glands should also be observed for detection of abnormal size.

Lips and lip tonus

Ulcerations and crusts of the lip commissures may be caused by nutritional imbalance, but the most common lesion of this area is herpes simplex. Evaluation of the lip posture at rest and during speech is important in the determination of possible musculature inadequacies and lip and tongue influences on occlusion. An abnormal median superior labial frenum can account for an abnormally large diastema of the maxillary incisors and the need for future surgery may be evaluated.

Oral mucosa, tongue and sublingual area

Lesions and color changes of the oral mucosa need careful evaluation. The papilla at the orifice of the parotid gland may be inflamed, indicating some pathologic change

of the gland. Small blue-white spots (Koplik's spots) on the oral mucosa of the cheek region may indicate the initial stages of measles. Changes in color or desquamation of the tongue may be evidence of nutritional imbalance or febrile states. Ranulae are due to swelling, and retention of fluid in the salivary glands is caused by obstructions of the ducts of the submaxillary or sublingual glands. An abnormally short lingual frenum may interfere with normal tongue movement leading to development of speech defects (ankyloglossia). Overdevelopment of the lingual musculature resulting in macroglossia is often found in Down syndrome and cretinism, and may interfere with tooth position. Oral habits of abnormal tongue function (tongue thrusting) also may interfere with tooth position.

Palate and pharynx

The consistency of the palate should be investigated to rule out submucosal clefts. Large tonsils are often indicative of frequent upper respiratory disorders and may be responsible for development of mouth breathing habits.

Gingiva and mucosa

The gingival color and consistency and the possible presence of fistulae should be evaluated carefully. Recurrent aphthae requiring palliative treatment may also be present. Any major color changes of the mucosal regions must be investigated further to rule out systemic disorders and neoplasms (Fig. 2-1). The most frequent cause of inflammation of the gingivae is poor oral hygiene (Fig. 2-2), but gingival swelling may be a response to certain drugs (Fig. 2-3). Periodontal disease is often seen in patients with Down syndrome (see Fig. 1-2) but may also be present in some nutritional deficiencies. Fistulous tracts (Fig. 2-4) usually indicate pathology of the teeth of the region. Severe swelling (Fig. 2-5) caused by an abscessed

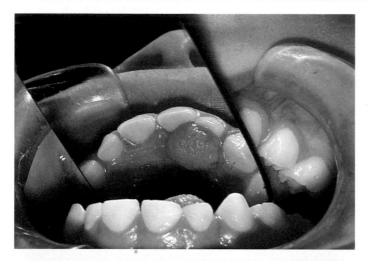

Fig. 2-1   Papilloma in 3-year-old boy requiring surgery.

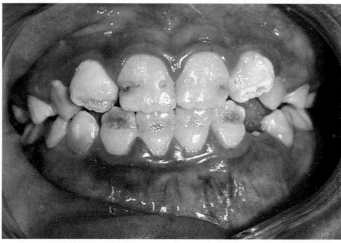

Fig. 2-2   Gingivitis in patient with poor oral hygiene; also note hypoplasia of the enamel secondary to illness during infancy.

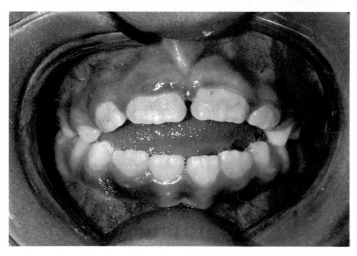

Fig. 2-3   Gingivitis in patient taking phenytoin.

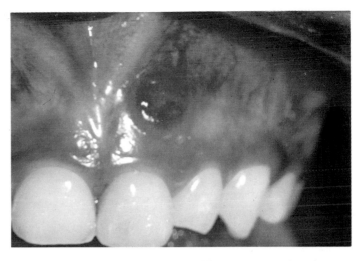

Fig. 2-4 Fistulous tract associated with pulp pathology of tooth F.

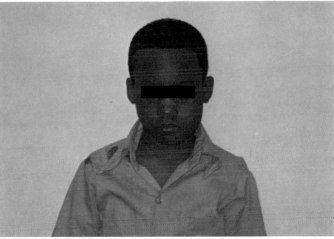

Fig. 2-5 Severe swelling associated with pulp pathology of tooth 14.

tooth may require antibiotic therapy. Drainage should be established through the pulp chamber if possible. Warm saline rinses may be helpful and aid drainage. After the acute symptoms have subsided, the tooth either can be treated or extracted.

Examination of the teeth

The number, size, color and shape of teeth are evaluated. Spacing between primary teeth is normal and desirable, as the anterior permanent teeth will require more space.

A complete lack of diastema between anterior primary teeth may indicate future crowding of the permanent teeth. A notation to this effect is very important.

Since the introduction of computer systems, tooth charting systems have had to be adapted to new standards of nomenclature as the older charting systems utilizing one digit Roman and Arabic numbers and quadrant indication is not suitable to computer application.

The Fédération Dentaire Internationale has recommended a system in which the quadrants are numbered from 1 to 4 for the permanent dentition and 5 to 8 for the primary dentition. The teeth are numbered 1 to 8 for the permanent dentition and 1 to 5 for the primary dentition starting at midline (Table 2-1).

Table 2-1 **FDI tooth numbering system**

Permanent dentition

Right	Left	
18-17-16-15-14-13-12-11	21-22-23-24-25-26-27-28	Maxillary
48-47-46-45-44-43-42-41	31-32-33-34-35-36-37-38	Mandibular

Primary dentition

Right	Left	
55-54-53-52-51	61-62-63-64-65	Maxillary
85-84-83-82-81	71-72-73-74-75	Mandibular

In speaking, the digits should be pronounced separately so that the permanent upper right canine is one-three, not thirteen. Another frequently used system of tooth designation, used throughout this book, numbers each permanent tooth from 1 to 32 starting at the maxillary right third molar and ending at the mandibular right third molar. Primary teeth are designated by letters A to T also according to location (Table 2-2).

Table 2-2 **Army tooth numbering system**

Permanent dentition

Right	Left	
1- 2- 3- 4- 5- 6- 7- 8	9-10-11-12-13-14-15-16	Maxillary
32-31-30-29-28-27-26-25	24-23-22-21-20-19-18-17	Mandibular

Primary dentition

Right	Left	
A-B-C-D-E	F-G-H-I-J	Maxillary
T-S-R-Q-P	O-N-M-L-K	Mandibular

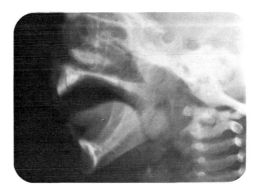

Fig. 2-6 Radiograph of a 6-month-old patient with ectodermal dysplasia. Note that no tooth buds are present in the jaws with exception of the incisors (Courtesy of Dr. I. M. Rosenthal).

In addition to the obvious examination for the presence of decay and restorations, attention should be given to abnormalities in the number of the teeth and the size, shape, and position of individual teeth. In the mixed dentition it is essential to locate the position of an unerupted canine for early detection of abnormally located permanent canines. Judicious extraction of primary teeth may avoid impaction. The observation of supernumerary or missing teeth is important, especially in the permanent dentition in which there can be an abnormal eruption pattern of the normal teeth. Ectodermal dysplasia is of genetic origin and is characterized by the absence of all or most teeth (oligodontia and anodontia, Fig. 2-6). Color changes of teeth may result from general systemic causes (e.g., porphyria or erythroblastosis fetalis, see Fig. 5-25) or extrinsic causes such as chromogenic bacteria (see Fig. 5-24). Jaw relation analysis will demonstrate the possible presence of anterior or posterior cross bites as well as other types of malocclusion (see Chapter 9). The path of closure should be noted carefully to diagnose midline shifts during closure.

Complete charting must include the recording of the conditions existing before initiation of treatment. Thus the chart will include existing restorations and will describe all that is to be done, including proposed restorations. Many types of charts and forms are available commercially for graphic recording and are selected according to personal preference.

Oral habits

Open bites may be caused by oral habits such as thumbsucking. Knowledge of habits such as this is important in the establishment of the etiology of some tooth malpositioning and should be investigated. Continuous obstruction of airways results in mouth-breathing and may alter facial appearance and occlusion. Counselling may help in discontinuing deleterious habits depending, of course, on the age and cooperation of the patient.

Radiographic examination of the patient

A high quality radiographic survey of a child's dentition will provide some of the most valuable information needed for the diagnosis

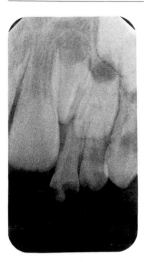

Fig. 2-7 Supernumerary lateral incisors in the primary and permanent dentition; 7-year-old boy.

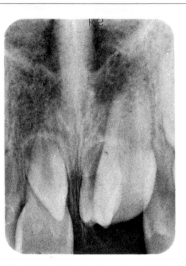

Fig. 2-8 Mesiodens interfering with the eruption of tooth 9; 10-year-old boy.

of dental and systemic problems and treatment planning. The number of radiographs necessary varies according to age and level of cooperation of the patient[2, 3, 5].

In a very young child, sometimes it is difficult to obtain acceptable intraoral radiographs of high quality at the first visit, but often it is possible to complete the survey with good radiographs made later. Taking the radiographs at different visits when the child is more cooperative has some advantages, as dangers of cumulative doses of ionizing radiation can be reduced in this way. Development of high-speed film and the panoramic technique also have been helpful in reducing radiation dosage[7]. Intraoral (perapical, occlusal, bitewing) or extra-oral (lateral jaw, panoramic, cephalometric) radiographs have specific uses in pedodontic oral diagnosis. Successful radiographic interpretation requires precise technique, use of good development procedures, and good film[6]. Periapical intraoral radiographs are the choice for the evaluation of a specific tooth or specific region. They are used in the de-

tection of dental caries, root and periapical pathology, bone abnormalities, presence of foreign bodies such as retained roots, and the presence of supernumerary teeth (Figs. 2-7 and 2-8). Periapical films can be used not only to determine the position of such abnormalities but also for an approximation of the size and shape of developing teeth for the study of arch length and space loss in the mixed dentition. Periapical films also are suitable for the evaluation of pathologic changes of teeth and jaws in traumatic injuries and in the evaluation of resorption patterns and patterns of development of permanent teeth.

Bitewing radiographs are used specifically for the detection of interproximal caries (Fig. 2-9a and b) and especially for detection of incipient lesions. These radiographs are also useful in the identification, localization, and estimation of size of pulp horns and chambers and their relation to the position of the carious lesion. Conditions affecting the alveolar bone also will be demonstrated in bitewing films (Figs. 2-10 to 2-15).

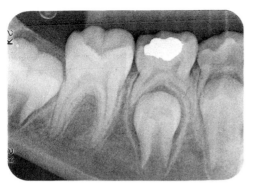

Figure 2-9a

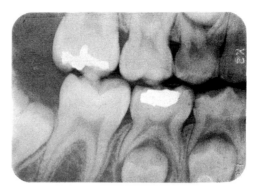

Figure 2-9b

Fig. 2-9a and b   Periapical radiograph and bitewing radiograph of the same patient demonstrating interproximal caries on the bitewing radiograph, not visible on the periapical film.

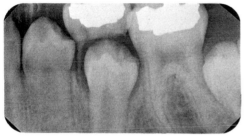

Figure 2-10a

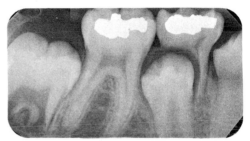

Figure 2-10b

Fig. 2-10a and b   Abnormal resorption pattern of teeth S and L with long roots that will have to be removed carefully; 9-year-old girl.

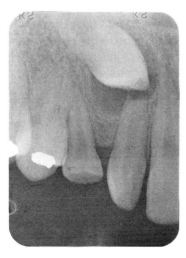

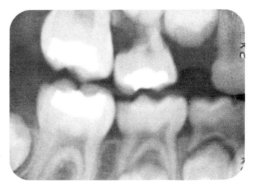

Fig. 2-11   Abnormal root resorption of tooth 7 due to abnormal eruption pattern of tooth 6; 9-year-old boy.

Fig. 2-12   Abnormal resorption of tooth J due to the eruption pattern of tooth 14; 8-year-old boy.

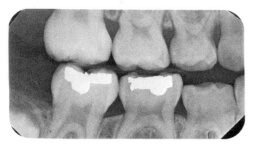

Figure 2-13a

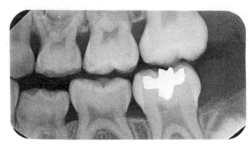

Figure 2-13b

Fig. 2-13a and b   Bitewing radiographs of an 8-year-old girl showing ankylosed first primary molars.

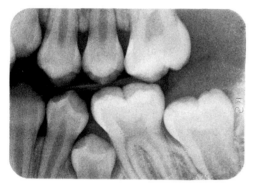

Fig. 2-14 Bitewing radiograph demonstrating lack of space for eruption of tooth 20 because of premature loss of tooth K.

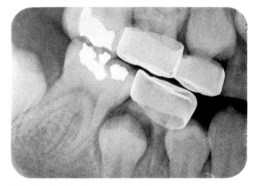

Fig. 2-15 Bitewing radiograph showing improperly contoured stainless steel crowns. Note that the crown placed on tooth T is interfering with the eruption of tooth 28.

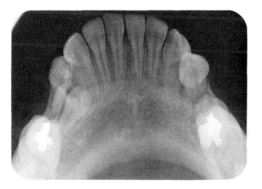

Fig. 2-16 Occlusal radiograph showing supernumerary premolar.

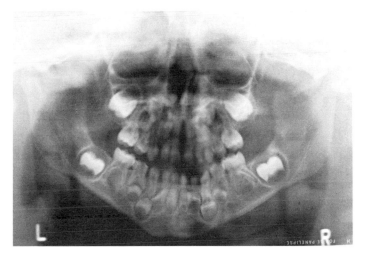

Fig. 2-17   Panoramic radiograph of a 3.5-year-old girl.

Occlusal films may be used for the evaluation of dental caries of the anterior maxillary and mandibular region in very young children by folding the film (Fig. 2-16)[8]. The technique of placing a film anteriorly and holding the film on the occlusal plane can also be done with one folded occlusal film. In older children, occlusal films are used for the evaluation of tooth relationships, supernumerary teeth, and determination of midline pathology of the soft tissues, salivary glands, and bone fractures.

Development of panoramic radiography has provided a helpful tool for evaluation of growth and development in the young child who is not able to cooperate or cannot tolerate intraoral radiography techniques. It is an important tool in the evaluation of normal dental development (Figs. 2-17 to 2-22). It is a very useful tool in those patients who, because of pathologic conditions, cannot open their mouths and cannot tolerate the pressure of intraoral films. This method is used in the study of condylar pathology and in detection of pathology in jaw regions away from the teeth (Fig. 2-23).

Dental caries and tooth position can be detected with the panoramic technique but this method does not give a reliable evaluation of the extent of the lesion or the amount of crowding in the arch. It is a separate tool, and not meant to substitute for intraoral periapical radiography. Where intraoral radiography is not possible, lateral jaw radiographs can be used for the detection of bone pathology, and for radiographic surveys[4]. This technique has largely been replaced by panoramic radiography techniques, but is still used in orthodontic diagnosis by some professionals[1]. It is a very useful adjunct in diagnosis of pathological processes that cannot be evaluated fully with regular intraoral and panoramic techniques.

Cephalometric radiography is intended to assist in the evaluation of the growth and development pattern of the child by use of extraoral radiographs and comparison with standard measures. In cephalometric radiography, the head of the patient is positioned in a special device which allows later duplicate repositioning. This special device includes ear and nose pieces which correctly orient the head of the patient. Measurements are made of angles and distances on the radiographs, using specific cranial landmarks. The data are compared to previous data for the same patient. Average values of growth and development are available in

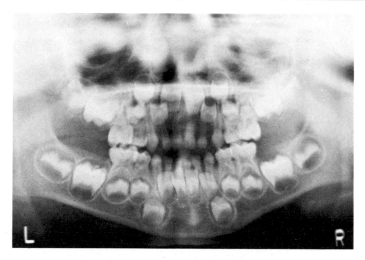

Fig. 2-18 Panoramic radiograph of a 5-year-old boy. Note the further development of permanent teeth and the development of the second permanent molars. The permanent molars have not started eruption.

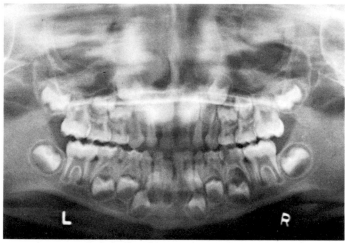

Fig. 2-19 Panoramic radiograph of a 6-year-old boy. The first permanent molars have erupted and reached the occlusal plane.

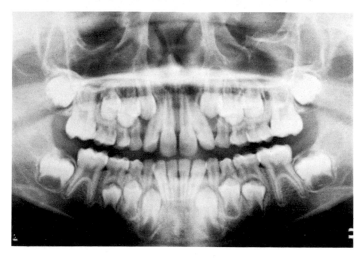

Fig. 2-20 Panoramic radiograph of an 8-year-old boy. The anlagen of the third molars can be detected in the mandible.

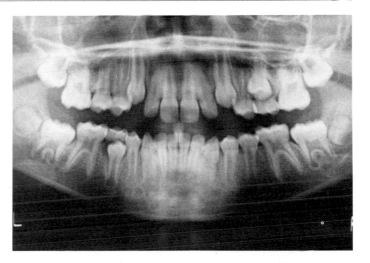

Fig. 2-21   Panoramic radiograph of a 9-year-old girl. Note the supernumerary tooth in the lower premolar region.

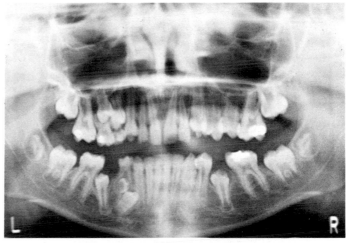

Fig. 2-22   Panoramic radiograph of an 11-year-old boy. This is the same patient as in Fig. 2-20, three years later.

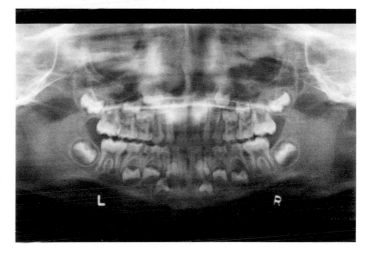

Fig. 2-23   Panoramic radiograph of a 12-year-old girl with juvenile rheumatoid arthritis. Note the pathologic appearance of the head of the condyle of the mandible.

published tables and are used for comparison (see page 79 for a discussion of cephalometry).

The number of radiographs in a pedodontic survey depends on the cooperation and the age of the patient and the number of teeth present. The use of mechanical film holders can facilitate the positioning of the films and of the cones for appropriate beam direction. For the handicapped patient who cannot tolerate intraoral films, extraoral radiography is utilized.

References

1. Aduss, H. and S. Pruzansky:
   Orthodontic diagnosis, *in* Oral diagnosis and treatment planning. L. Cohen (Ed.). Springfield, IL, Thomas 1973.

2. Beaver, H. A.:
   Radiographic technics for the young child in your practice. J. Mich. Dent. Assoc. *54*:282-287, 1972.

3. Feasby, W. H.:
   Number and types of films necessary for a satisfactory radiological survey for children. J. Dent. Child. *27*:91-96, 1960.

4. Groper, J. M., K. Nishimine and C. C. O'Grady:
   A simplified radiographic technique for difficult patients. J. Dent. Child. *32*:269-270, 1965.

5. Khanna, S. L. and T. J. Harrop:
   A five-film oral radiographic survey of children. J. Dent. Child. *40*:42-48, 1973.

6. McRae, P. D., A. Bodnarchuk, C. R. Castaldi and W. A. Zacherl:
   Detection of congenital dental anomalies. How many films? J. Dent. Child. *35*:107-114, 1968.

7. Mitchell, L. D.:
   Panoramic roentgenograph. A clinical evaluation. J. Amer. Dent. Assoc. *66*:777-786, 1963.

8. Silha, R. E.:
   The versatile occlusal dental x-ray film. Part III. Dent. Radiog. Photog. *39(2)*:40-43, 1966.

9. Starkey, P.:
   Bitewing radiographic technique for the young child. Dent. Dig. *73*:488-491, 1967.

Chapter 3

Facial Growth and Development

Prenatal development

Growth and development of the face

Prenatal and postnatal factors influence the growth of bone which is a dynamic and ever changing tissue. External and internal form and architecture are inherited to some extent but are greatly affected by environmental factors. Normal facial skeletal growth is dependent on synchronous coordinated activities. It is dependent on:

1. endochondral growth at the base of the skull at sphenooccipital and sphenoethmoidal junctions as well as at the mandibular condyle,
2. appositional growth and surface remodeling resorption (endosteal and periosteal), and
3. sutural growth at various bone levels.

We have learned about the different aspects of craniofacial growth from various human and animal studies in which implants and markers were used. A review of the details of facial growth and development and the various hypotheses of etiological mechanisms involved in this growth was prepared by Enlow[12]. To summarize, different parts of the head grow at different rates. The growth of the brain case follows neural growth and starts and is completed early in life. The face however, closely follows the body pattern. This difference in growth pattern has allowed researchers to use the relatively stable cranial base as a reference point for the evaluation of changes taking place in facial growth.

Growth processes in general depend on the increase in size of the bone itself, with accompanying remodeling. If a structure such as the face is analyzed, there is also a "carrying" growth due to a displacement of the bone with growth of the components of the structure[13]. Thus facial growth has to be visualized not only by the size of the enlargement of individual bones, but also by a continuous displacement of the individual landmarks caused by intervening growth processes of each part. Serial growth changes of relative components or individual bones can be studied by the use of metallic implants[5]. Therefore the commonly cited "forward and downward" growth of the face as visualized by the superimposition of serial cephalometric tracings on Sella-Nasion is in reality a summation of multidirectional growth of many structures.

Ossification of bones of the skull and maxillofacial complex begins between the 6th and 8th week of intrauterine life. Because of the difficulty of establishing precise age and genetic variations among specimens, different dates for time of appearance of ossification centers of different bones have been given by different investigators. The maxilla, palatine, nasal, lacrimal, frontal, zygomatic and vomer bones have an intramembranous type of ossification. The ethmoidal bone is of the endochondrial type having cartilaginous anlage. The temporal, sphenoid, and occipital bones have an endochondrial ossification

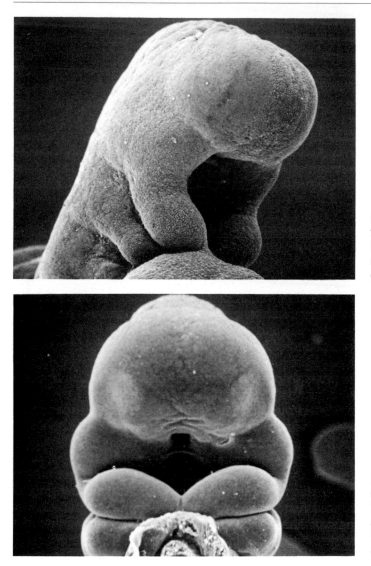

Fig. 3-1 Lateral stereoscan electron micrograph of a 16-day-old ferret in utero showing frontonasal and mandibular processes and stomatodeum (Courtesy of Dr. A. J. Steffek).

Fig. 3-2 Frontal stereoscan electron micrograph of an 18-day-old ferret in utero showing frontonasal process and developing mandibular process below the stomatodeum (Courtesy of Dr. A. J. Steffek).

in some parts and intramembranous development in others. The midsagittal axis of the cranial base of the young fetus is cartilaginous. With growth and development, the cartilaginous tissue ossifies, but synchondroses of cartilage are retained; these allow for elongation of the cranial base during the prenatal and early postnatal life. The first of these synchondroses usually is fused at birth but the other two continue during

postnatal life. Most bones of the fetal skull begin remodeling at the time they reach some morphological development (about the 14th week of prenatal development). There is a relation between bone remodeling and soft tissue development. The orbital roof grows superiorly at the time of fast growth of the eye bulbs. During the period of relative slowing of growth of the eye bulb, there is an increase in the growth rate of the

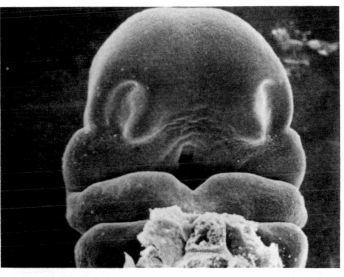

Fig. 3-3 Frontal stereoscan electron micrograph of a 19-day-old ferret in utero showing development of olfactory placodes and maxillary processes (Courtesy of Dr. A. J. Steffek).

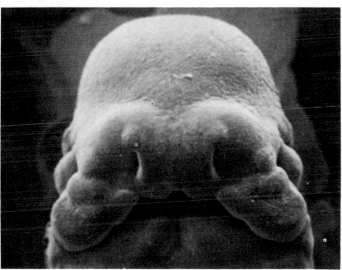

Fig. 3-4 Frontal stereoscan electron micrograph of a 22-day-old ferret in utero showing further development of the maxillary processes and olfactory pits (Courtesy of Dr. A. J. Steffek).

frontal lobes. A this time too, there is reversal of growth of the orbital roof to accommodate this soft tissue growth[13].

Formation of the face and primary palate

At the end of the first and the beginning of the second intrauterine month, the primordia of the face consist of five facial processes which surround the *stomatodeum,* or entrance into the primary oral cavity (Figs. 3-1 and 3-2). Above the stomatodeum is a large prominence called the *nasofrontal process.* On each side of this process are thickened oval epithelial areas, the *olfactory placodes*

(Fig. 3-3). Below the oral orifice, which at this stage is still covered by a thin epithelial membrane (the buccopharyngeal membrane), is the first branchial or mandibular arch (Fig. 3-4). The lateral boundaries of the oral opening form prominences called the *maxillary processes.* The two maxillary processes are separated from the nasofrontal process by a shallow groove. About the 5th or 6th week of intrauterine development, the buccopharyngeal membrane ruptures and the oral cavity then continues into the pharynx.

Differential growth at the beginning of the second month leads to progressive formation of a prominence of the nasofrontal process. At the same time the mesoderm around the nasal placode grows faster than that underlying the placode itself and thus the oval placode area sinks in forming the *olfactory pit,* and the *medial nasal process* can be distinguished. The inferior region of the medial nasal process is known as the *globular process.* As differential growth continues, the developing maxillary process extends towards the midline, reaching the *lateral nasal processes* which have been growing at a slower rate.

As a result of differential growth of these facial processes, the horizontal area formed by the fusion of the medial nasal process with the lateral nasal process forms the primary palate by the end of the 6th week of intrauterine life. This region differentiates into the upper lip and the anterior portion of the maxillary alveolar process. During the 7th and 8th weeks, differential growth of the median nasal process and lateral nasal process is responsible for the development of the bridge of the nose. Meanwhile the eyes become more anteriorly positioned in the facial region, and the outer ear develops in a more posterior area through the fusion of several small tubercles. By the end of the 2nd month, the mandibular region is fairly well developed. Mandibular growth lags during later embryonic life, and relative micrognathia is common at birth.

The tongue develops from contributions of the first three branchial arches. Three swellings arise on the internal surface of the mandibular arch, two lateral or *lingual swellings* and one central and caudal, the *tuberculum impar.* The base of the tongue develops from a more caudal swelling originating from the second and third branchial arches; this difference in origin explains the different innervation of the various parts of the tongue, the anterior part being innervated by the trigeminal nerve and the posterior part by the glossopharyngeal nerve. The fusion of the tongue processes takes place about the 6th week of embryonic development. At the time of fusion of the different components the tongue is a compact body occupying the oral cavity and separating the two lateral maxillary processes.

Formation of the secondary palate

Accelerated vertical growth of the maxillary and medial nasal processes takes place before the formation of the secondary palate. At this stage, the roof of the oral cavity is incomplete. About the second month of intrauterine life, the vertically oriented palatine processes enlarge and subsequently become horizontal. The fusion of the palatine processes with each other and with the nasal septum forms the secondary palate. At approximately 7 weeks of intrauterine development the palatine processes developing internally at the side of the tongue translocate into a horizontal position above the tongue. When they have become horizontal, the palatine shelves fuse; the epithelial rests at the site of the fusion disappear soon after, and the secondary palate not only closes the communication between the nasal and oral cavities and

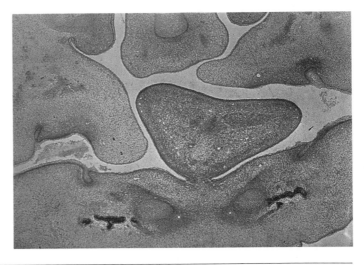

Fig. 3-5 Frontal section through the head of a pig embryo showing one palatine process in vertical position and one horizontal above the tongue, in close proximity to the nasal process.

forms the hard palate, but also forms the soft palate (Fig. 3-5).

The developing bony palate is separated from the lip and cheek by a shallow groove. This groove gives origin to the dental and vestibular epithelial laminae. Separation of the latter results in the oral vestibule interrupted at the level of the midline and of the future primary first molars by connecting folds. The alveolar ridge develops caudally and appears at the midline between the lip and the palate.

Tooth formation

About the 6th week of embryonic development, the dental lamina develops and ectodermal thickening occurs in which ectoderm grows inwards into the mesenchymal area to form the jaws. The furrow separating the future lips and the fibrous cheeks from the area of the jaws also develops at this time. A 2-month-old embryo shows ten distinct round enlargements on each jaw. These enlargements stimulate mesenchymal proliferations in the 20 distinct regions and are the first primordia of tooth development. The tooth germs are formed by the proliferation of an ectodermal

and mesenchymal component. During later fetal development, the dental lamina initiates the proliferation of the primordia of the permanent teeth. These primordia develop lingual to the corresponding primary tooth germs. In addition, the dental lamina extends posteriorly to form the primordia of the permanent molars. Each area of dental lamina proliferation passes through several distinct phases of growth and differentiation which ultimately give rise to a distinct tooth.

At first, the tooth germ is bud-shaped but later in development, through differential growth it will acquire a bell shape (Figs. 3-6 and 3-7). The epithelial component of this bell-shaped tooth germ gives rise to the enamel whereas the mesenchyme within the concavity of the bell forms the pulp and the dentin. The mesenchyme around the bell gives rise to the cementum, the periodontal ligament, and some sections of alveolar bone. The different parts of this structure have been named the *enamel organ,* which is the ectodermal condensation, the *dental papilla,* which results in the dental pulp and dentin, and the enveloping *dental sac,* which results in the periodontium (Fig. 3-8). All of these different parts develop

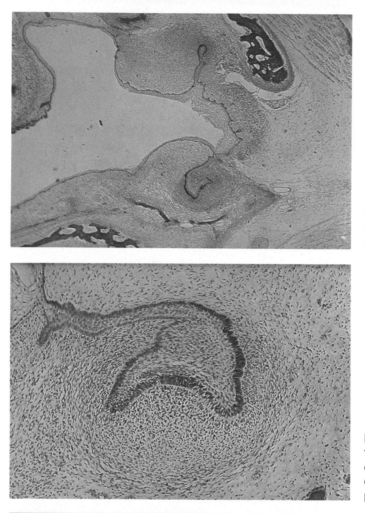

Fig. 3-6 Frontal section through a pig fetal head showing dental lamina and developing tooth bud.

Fig. 3-7 Higher magnification of tooth development showing enamel organ and connective tissue condensation that will form the dental papilla and dental sac.

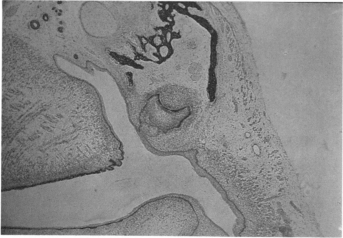

Fig. 3-8 Primary tooth germ showing enamel organ, dental papilla and dental sac.

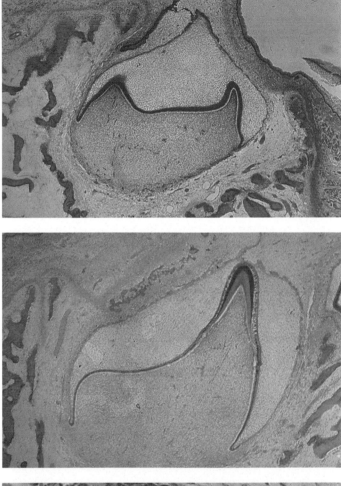

Fig. 3-9 Advanced stage of tooth development showing dental sac enclosing the developing tooth.

Fig. 3-10 More advanced stage of tooth development showing the deposition of first layers of enamel and dentin matrix. The different cell types of the enamel organ can be seen.

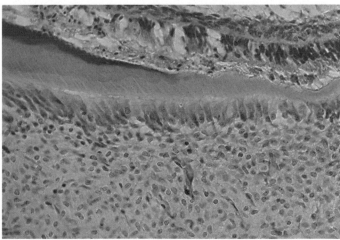

Fig. 3-11 Higher magnification of the developing hard tissues of the tooth showing developing dentin, odontoblasts, ameloblasts and enamel matrix.

through a mechanism of interdependent inductive forces in which development of each part is necessary for the development of the others (Fig. 3-9).

The enamel organ consists of three types of cells: an external layer of short epithelium-like cells, *the outer enamel epithelium;* an internal layer of taller prismatic cells, the *inner enamel epithelium;* and a group of cells which occupy the space between the inner and outer enamel epithelium, the *stellate reticulum,* so named because of their shape. The area of transition between the inner and outer epithelium is the *cervical loop.* By the time the enamel organ has differentiated into the bell stage, the columnar cells of the inner enamel epithelium have differentiated into tall cells (about 40μ in height) which later will become the ameloblasts. A new cell layer of low squamous cells, several layers thick, can now be distinguished between the inner enamel epithelium and the stellate reticulum and is called the *stratum intermedium* (Fig. 3-10). Toward the end of the bell stage, the enamel organ assumes a characteristic shape that will function as the template of the shape of the different teeth. The basement membrane separating the pre-ameloblasts from the underlying condensed mesenchymal tissue determines the outline of the dentinoenamel junction for each tooth. Differentiation of pre-ameloblasts is more advanced in the areas corresponding to the future incisal edges and cusps, but the areas of the cervical loops develop later. This differentiation of the pre-ameloblasts stimulates differentiation of tall columnar cells (odontoblasts) in the mesenchyme and it is these cells that are responsible for the formation of dentin (Fig. 3-11).

After the first layer of dentin is laid down in the area of the tooth growth center, the ameloblasts in that area produce short processes called Tomes' processes. These processes, which are continuously laid down,

form the enamel rods. The intercellular substance between the Tomes' processes differentiate later into the interprismatic substance of the enamel. As ameloblasts and odontoblasts continue to form enamel matrix and predentin, they recede from the dentinoenamel junction, and mineralization occurs. The mineralization of the enamel matrix is incomplete at this time, containing 25 to 30% mineral salts. The functional life of the ameloblasts varies but is longest at the cusp tips and shortest at the cervical region. After the enamel matrix is formed to complete thickness, it undergoes further mineralization with a final mineral content of about 96% in mature enamel. This maturation process starts at the incisal edges and cusp tips and proceeds towards the cervical region.

After enamel formation reaches its cervical limit, the future cementoenamel junction, the outer enamel epithelium and the inner enamel epithelium form *Hertwig's epithelial sheath.* Root development is preceded by lengthening of Hertwig's epithelial sheath which is involved in the induction of odontoblastic differentiation which in turn is essential for dentin formation. The ameloblasts cease to be columnar after the full thickness of enamel is attained, and together with the outer enamel epithelium, form a protective layer for the enamel, the *reduced enamel epithelium.* After eruption, the reduced enamel epithelium results in the epithelial attachment.

As dentin formation continues, odontoblasts recede, leaving part of their cytoplasm embedded within the calcified dentin. These odontoblastic processes are embedded in the dentinal tubules. After the formation of dentin has started, the mesenchyme of the dental papilla may be considered to be the dental pulp. It is a well vascularized connective tissue containing many lymph vessels and some nerves as well as some fibroblasts, collagen fibers, and macrophages. The pulp also contains the nuclei and the perinuclear cytoplasm of the odontoblasts. Formation of dentin continues in a more or less regular manner even after tooth eruption. With normal aging, maturation of the pulp tissue takes place with an increase in collagen fibers and decrease in cellularity.

Development of periodontal tissues

The dental follicle, which surrounds the enamel organ, is responsible for the development of the cementum, periodontal membrane, and alveolar bone. After the Hertwig's sheath has induced the differentiation of odontoblasts and dentin formation, it degenerates. The connective tissue of the dental sac then comes into contact with the surface of the dentin and some of the mesenchyme cells differentiate into cementoblasts and are involved in cementum formation. Sparse remnants of Hertwig's sheath sometimes can be found in the periodontal membrane, in which case they are called epithelial rests of Malassez. At the time of the disintegration of Hertwig's epithelial sheath, the connective tissue cells of the dental follicle adjacent to the dentin differentiate into the cementoblasts.

Cementoid substance is laid down on the outside of the previous layer and the older layer calcifies, forming cementum. (A healthy tooth always has a layer of cementoid as cementum formation is a continuous process throughout the life of the tooth.) While cementum formation is taking place, collagenous fibers are also differentiating and becoming embedded in the cementum. These fibers form the periodontal membrane and function as an attachment of the tooth to the surrounding alveolar bone which is being developed simultaneously.

Before tooth eruption, the collagen fibers can be found loose around the tooth and within the bony crypt which is holding the tooth. As the tooth erupts, the different fiber bundles extend from the cementum to the bone and gingiva surrounding the root. The fully mature periodontal ligament consists of dense collagen fiber bundles and areas of loose connective tissue containing blood vessels, lymphatics, nervous tissue, and connective tissue cells such as fibroblasts and macrophages.

Growth of the upper face

The growth of the upper face is dependent on the skeletal growth of several different bones. According to Sicher[42] this growth is dependent on 3 sutures on each side: the frontomaxillary, the zygomaticomaxillary, and the pterygomaxillary sutures. The downward shift of the hard palate with increased size of the nasal cavity is associated with resorption on its nasal surface and apposition on its oral surface and is related to the growth of the nasal septum. The upper facial skeleton enlarges because of the increase of the size of orbits and development of the maxillary, frontal, and ethmoidal sinuses.

The maxillary complex moves downward and forward. This growth is accompanied by eruption of the teeth and alveolar bone apposition which contributes to an increase of height and width of the middle facial skeleton.

The transverse growth at the median palate suture which is concurrent with the growth in other areas of the face is correlated with the downward relocation of the maxillary complex (Fig. 3-12).

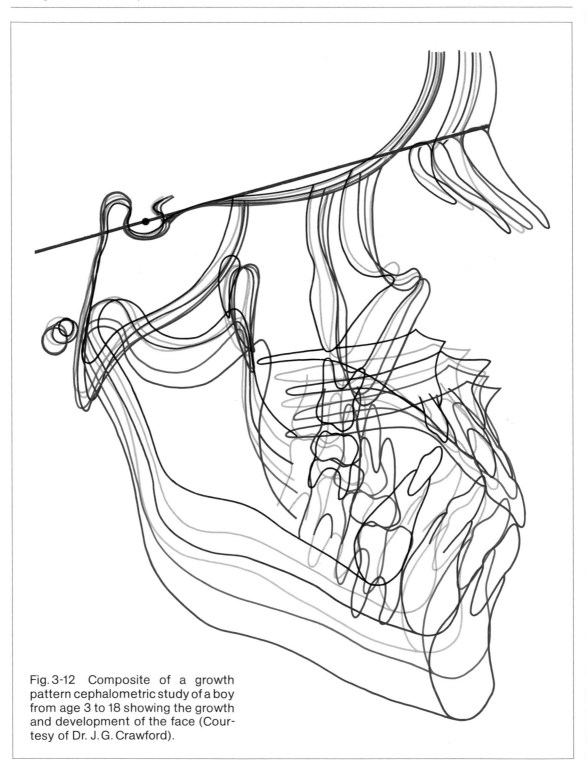

Fig. 3-12 Composite of a growth pattern cephalometric study of a boy from age 3 to 18 showing the growth and development of the face (Courtesy of Dr. J. G. Crawford).

Mandibular growth

Mandibular growth takes place through endochondral growth at the condyle and the remodeling and appositional growth of various mandibular surfaces. The growth of the condyle and ramus is in a superior lateral and posterior direction, but since the condyle articulates with the temporal bone at the mandibular fossa, the final result is a downward and forward positioning of the mandible. The appositional and resorptive growth differs in the different surfaces of the mandible. The posterior border of the ramus is a particularly active site of bone apposition while the anterior border is a site of active bone resorption. This type of growth permits the placement and eruption of permanent molars.

Growth of the mandible is dependent on its major components, the *corpus* and the *ramus,* and there is a range of functional and anatomical variations in the relationship of these parts. The corpus of the mandible is continuously elongating with a remodeling of the ramus into the corpus to allow for such elongation. The ramus, on the other hand, relocates posteriorly and increases its longitudinal dimensions at the time of the horizontal growth of the middle cranial fossa and pharynx. With growth of the nasomaxillary complex there is also lengthening of the mandible to accommodate the erupting teeth. These changes permit a harmonious development of the maxillofacial complex and mandible.

Tooth eruption pattern and chronology

The time and eruption sequence of primary and permanent teeth have been investigated in many groups of children of different nationalities, races, and socioeconomic backgrounds. The aims of these studies were evaluation and comparison of chronological and physiological development of the child as well as understanding of the factors involved in tooth eruption. Some of these studies were longitudinal and evaluated the same children over several years, while other studies were cross-sectional and evaluated large groups of known chronological ages.

It has been demonstrated repeatedly that chronology of tooth eruption varies among different populations[16]. It has also been demonstrated that socioeconomic conditions and nutritional factors as well as the general physiologic state of the individual influence the eruption rate[16]. Local conditions such as premature loss of a primary tooth, malocclusion, and trauma also will alter the eruption pattern. Systemic conditions such as certain syndromes (cleidocranial dysotosis, osteopetrosis, hypopituitarism, hypothyroidism, avitaminosis A or D, vitamin D resistant rickets, Fanconi syndrome, Down syndrome, acrocephalosyndactyly and epidermolysis bullosa[31]) delay tooth eruption. Eruption also may be retarded by interference of a supernumerary tooth or the development of a cyst or simply by its malposition in the jaw. Conditions such as hypergonadism and adrenocortical tumors, among others, may accelerate tooth eruption.

Sex and racial differences seem to play a role in tooth eruption but some of the studies involving different racial groups do not take into consideration the physiological and nutritional differences of these groups[16, 33]. Infante[25] indicates in his studies of the eruption pattern of the primary dentition of white and black children in Michigan that boys in both groups showed earlier tooth eruption in the early stages of eruption while girls showed an earlier eruption time after 15 months of age (Fig. 3-13).

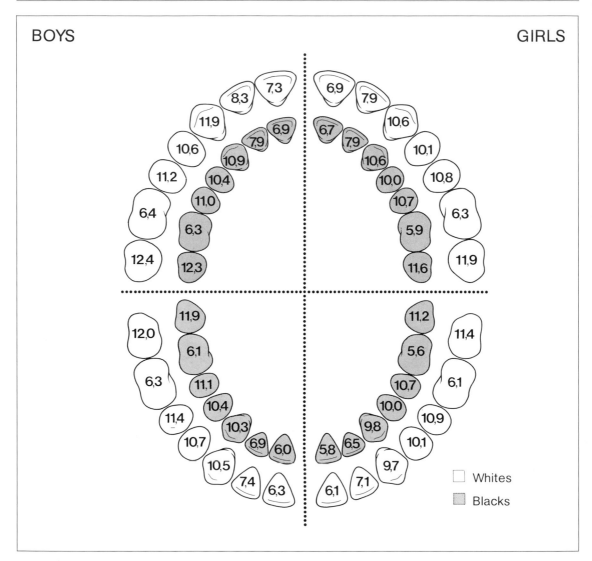

Fig. 3-13   Eruption time (in years) of permanent teeth in relation to sex and race (modified from Garn).

According to Infante and Owen[27] timing of primary tooth eruption is related to general somatic growth and possibly nutritional status. Eruption of the primary teeth usually starts around the 6th month and is completed around the second birthday. Eruption rates vary greatly in different groups and the tables available reflect only the average eruption age for the area in which they were studied. The most widely used table on tooth eruption chronology is based on histologic and radiographic findings of jaws of 25 children by Logan and Kronfeld in 1935 and modified by Schour and Massler in 1940[34]. A detailed chart has been prepared by Gustafson and Koch[18] (Fig. 3-14) after study-

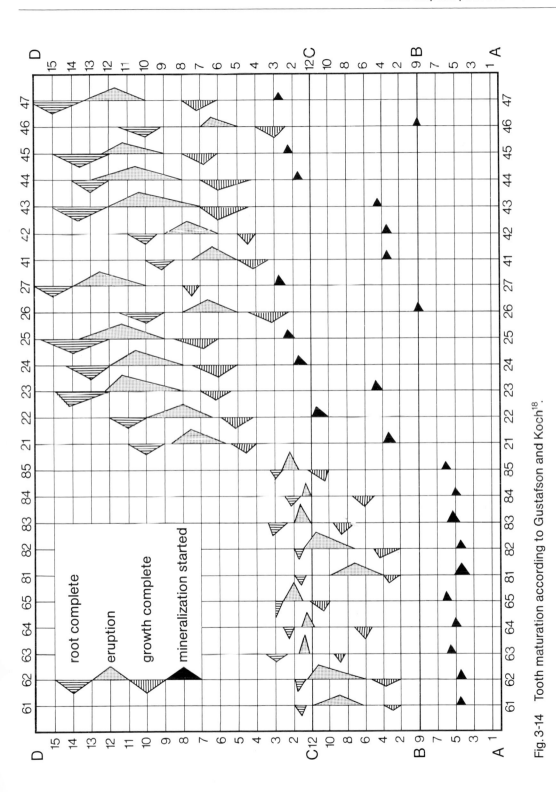

Fig.3-14   Tooth maturation according to Gustafson and Koch[18].

ing the tooth eruption pattern of white children. A study of white children in Finland gives a mean time of 7.1 ± 1.9 months for the first primary tooth eruption (mandibular central incisor) and 27.1 ± 4.2 months for the completion of the eruption of all primary teeth[35]. For Japanese children, Sato and Ogiwara[39] give a slightly later age. According to Trupkin[47] eruption of primary teeth is delayed in children who weigh less than 5 pounds (2,500 grams) at birth. He found further, that the weight at the time of the first tooth eruption of these children of low birth weight was similar to the weight of the normal birth weight group. There is a wide variability in the chronology of tooth eruption, and small variations from the available charts should be considered normal.

Tooth eruption

The process of tooth eruption is not fully understood despite numerous studies and theories which have been presented over the years[41]. Soon after radiographic evidence of root formation can be detected, movement towards occlusion of the developing tooth can be seen. Studies indicate that the apical region of the root remains stationary while the root elongates in the eruptive direction of the tooth[11]. After the first stage of slow tooth eruption with increased root length, there is a period of rapid eruption caused by a more rapid movement than root formation. After the teeth occlude there is an apparent cessation of eruption while the roots complete development. Slow eruption continues because of increased development of alveolar bone to accommodate the growing root. According to Darling and Levers[11] another short active phase of eruption in the occlusal direction can be noticed in permanent teeth about the time of root completion.

Eruption of primary teeth is asymptomatic in most children, although increased salivation and drooling may be noticed, and some children may be restless. While most investigators consider systemic disturbances and respiratory and alimentary diseases coincidental, some believe that tooth eruption may be considered a stress which lowers body resistance[15]. Minor gingival inflammation may be present during eruption but surgical exposure of the tooth is seldom indicated.

Occasionally a small *eruption cyst* with fluid accumulation may develop in the area of tooth eruption. This is most frequent in posterior regions of the mouth. An eruption cyst is a small swelling of reddish-blue color and variable size, associated either with primary or permanent teeth. Fluctuation cannot always be demonstrated and is dependent on the amount of gingival tissue covering the erupting tooth. The eruption cyst is seldom painful but a few instances of pain and tenderness due to a superimposed infection have been reported[40]. Treatment is not usually required and the tooth will erupt through the area within a few days.

Occasionally teeth are present at birth or soon thereafter (see chapter 5). If these teeth are very mobile and constitute an aspiration danger, or where the teeth interfere with proper nursing, they should be removed. It is interesting to note that some reports indicate that a type of formation resembling dwarfed roots may be found in some cases of early removal of these neonatal and natal teeth. Removal of the natal or neonatal tooth crown but not all of the tooth-forming material may explain this condition[6]. However, if possible the tooth should be maintained if it is a regular primary tooth and not a supernumerary.

Eruption sequence

Calcification of primary teeth usually begins about the 4th to 6th month *in utero* and considerable calcification takes place before birth. Some calcification of the primary teeth and most of the calcification of permanent teeth occurs after birth. In general, the crowns of the primary teeth are partially formed at birth. The first permanent molars begin calcification at birth or shortly thereafter. Often poor calcification may reflect nutritional and health problems at the time of development.

The most frequent order of eruption for the primary dentition of both jaws is: central incisor, lateral incisor, first molar, canine, and second molar, but other patterns of eruption have been found. In 20% of Nystrom's sample of white children in Finland[35], the eruption sequence was: lateral incisor, central incisor, first molar, canine, second molar. Ando[2] reports 65 different combinations of eruption sequence. Eruption of permanent teeth was delayed in a group of institutionalized Japanese children with cerebral palsy but these children were also found to weigh considerably less than normal Japanese children of the same age[29].

The first permanent teeth to erupt are the mandibular first molars (at about 6 years of age). These are followed by the maxillary permanent first molars and mandibular central incisors.

Because correct timing for orthodontic therapy is an important factor in the success of treatment, many studies have attempted to predict the relationships between age, tooth emergence, skeletal age, morphological conditions of the child, and possible circumpubertal growth spurts. The results vary according to different investigators, but most reports indicate that dental age is not closely related to skeletal age. Tooth emergence under normal conditions is dependent on root formation and appears to take place when at least one-half of the root has formed[17]. For this reason, hand and wrist radiographs are better indicators of circumpubertal growth than dental age.

Many factors affect eruption. When premolar development was studied in a group of patients in whom a primary molar had been removed (using the opposite side of the jaw as control), primary tooth extraction caused an initial spurt in eruption regardless of stage of development. However, extraction before the premolar crown was complete frequently was followed by a slower eruption on this side than the opposite one. Premolar eruption is delayed in children who have lost primary molars at the age of 4 or 5, but may be accelerated in patients who lost the primary molars at the age of 8, 9, or 10[2, 36]. In cases of extensive bone necrosis caused by periapical involvement, a marked acceleration in eruption is found when there is crown formation with very little root development (Fig. 3-15a to c). In a small sample of children who had prematurely lost a primary central incisor because of trauma or infection, Korf[30] noticed that there was a delay in eruption time of the succedaneous permanent central incisors in nine of ten cases.

Root resorption

After complete eruption, each primary tooth goes through a series of stages of progressive root resorption. Resorption usually starts at the root apex with the presence of large multinucleated osteoclast-like cells at the resorption site (Fig. 3-16). Resorption also may start in the area of the bifurcation of the molars; it continues until the tooth exfoliates.

Root resorption timing has been studied in different healthy populations and time tables of initiation, velocity and duration of the process have been established. Normally, the rate accelerates during the initial phases

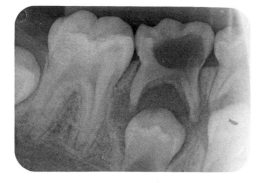

Fig. 3-15a to c   Accelerated tooth eruption after removal of infected primary molar. Note the small amount of root present in the erupted premolar.

Figure 3-15a

Figure 3-15b

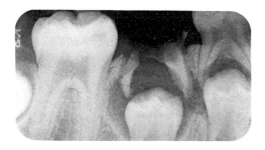

Figure 3-15c

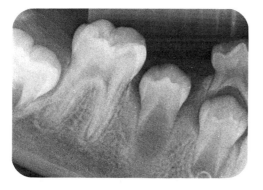

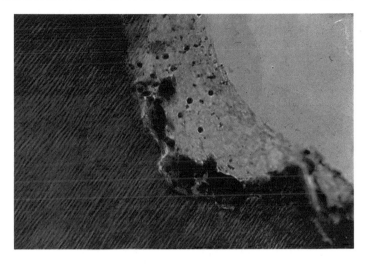

Fig. 3-16 Root surface of primary human tooth showing area of root resorption with multinucleated cells.

Figure 3-17a

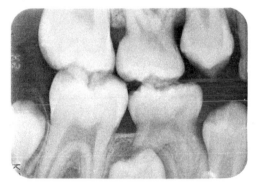

Figure 3-17b

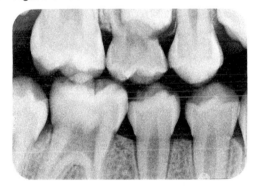

Figure 3-17c

Fig. 3-17a to c Atypical root resorption.

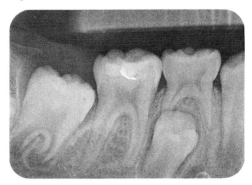

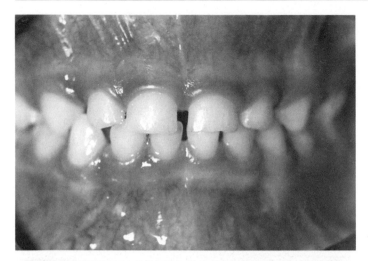

Fig. 3-18   Normal spacing in primary dentition.

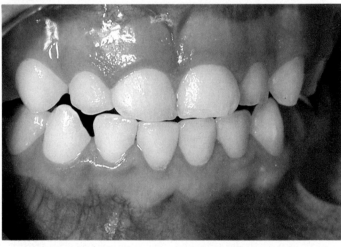

Fig. 3-19   Lack of spacing in primary dentition.

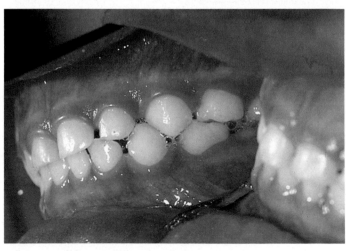

Fig. 3-20   Primate space.

of apical resorption, decreases during the 2nd and 3rd quarter of the process, and accelerates again just prior to exfoliation. Pathologic tooth conditions such as dental caries may accelerate root resorption.

A good correlation between the amount of root resorption of primary teeth and the stages of development of their successors has been demonstrated[10]; however, the presence of a permanent successor tooth is not necessary for the resorption of the primary tooth. Primary molars were found to be retained for a longer period in some studies of agenesis of permanent teeth; other studies have shown that root resorption occurred without regard to the presence of a permanent tooth[50]. The resorption of the roots of primary molars may show an atypical pattern (Fig. 3-17 a to c) caused by the abnormal position of the premolars. Such atypical pattern can lead to abnormal exfoliation, root fracture, and fragmentation with retention of the fragment, and abnormal position or eruption of the premolar.

Arch development

Two types of dental arches can be distinguished after eruption of the primary teeth has occurred. Either diastemas may be present creating a spaced type of primary dentition (Fig. 3-18) or the primary dentition is of the closed type without diastemas (Fig. 3-19). Diastemas between the primary maxillary lateral incisor and the primary maxillary canine and between the primary mandibular canines and the primary first molar are called primate space because they are also present in primates other than humans (Fig. 3-20).

Occlusion in the primary dentition is classified according to the relation between the primary second molars and the primary canines. The relation between the molars may be:

1. *Flush terminal plane:* The distal surfaces of the mandibular and maxillary primary second molars are in the same vertical plane. When there is space between the teeth, the maxillary canines occlude in the space between the mandibular canine and the primary first molar (primate space).

2. *Distal step:* The distal surfaces of the mandibular second molar are distal to the distal surfaces of the maxillary second molar, and the canines are in an end-to-end relation.

3. *Mesial step:* The distal surfaces of the mandibular second molar are mesial to the distal surface of the maxillary second molar, and the mandibular canines are in a mesial relation to the maxillary canines.

The crowns of the permanent central incisors develop lingually to the roots of their primary predecessors, with the lateral incisors lingual to their neighboring teeth. The amount of space provided in the anterior segment of the child's dental arch is insufficient because the permanent teeth are larger than their predecessors. Often the normally occurring diastema and primate space are inadequate. Some of the space required is derived from the labially directed eruption pattern of the permanent teeth leading to a more anterior position of the crowns and a greater axial inclination than the primary teeth. This is particularly evident in the maxilla. The gradual alignment of the permanent teeth after eruption was recognized by Broadbent[7] who described the "ugly duckling" stage of tooth eruption in the 7 to 8-year-old child with large teeth in a fan-shaped orientation. Frequently the anterior teeth will profit from the space available in the premolar region after the loss of the primary molars which are replaced by premolars which have a smaller mesiodistal width.

Interarch occlusal relationship

Developmental changes of interarch occlusal relationship are of clinical importance in the primary and mixed dentitions. Understanding the developing molar occlusion is basic to diagnosis, prevention, and treatment of occlusal problems.

The anteroposterior relationship of the dental units is determined according to the relationship between canines and first permanent molars. The relationships of the distal surfaces of the primary second molars, or terminal plane, have been studied by several investigators. The change from a flush terminal plane to a mesial step permits the first permanent molars to occlude in an Angle Class I relationship (see page 69). Persistence of the flush terminal plane will produce a "cusp to cusp" relationship of the permanent first molars which may become either a Class I or Class II molar relationship. A distal step is consistent with establishment of an Angle Class II occlusion.

Infante[26] reported a decrease in distal step with increased age in a sample of 2 to 5-year-old children and concluded that a distal terminal plane in a very young child would not necessarily lead to Class II occlusion. Baume[4] described an early mesial shift in which the mandibular primate space distal to the mandibular primary canine closed with eruption of the first permanent molars. Crawford[9] suggested that acceleration of mandibular growth in comparison to the maxilla could also lead to mesial shift and favorable interarch relationship.

Placement of primary teeth in the jaws varies with the width of the jaws, but the incisors are often crowded in the prenatal period. An increase in size of the anterior parts of the jaws takes place during the first year of life[38]. During later development, the permanent anterior teeth are positioned lingually and apically to their predecessors. This relationship leads to inclination of the permanent teeth after eruption, and a gradual increase in protrusion (depending on the concurrent skeletal growth and the location of the apical base as well as the development of the midface and mandible).

Once the primary molars have erupted, the primary dental arches do not increase in width but some vertical growth occurs through further alveolar development. Anteroposterior growth takes place to accommodate the permanent molars in the retromolar space (Fig. 3-21a and b).

Malocclusion

While malocclusion in some patients may be attributed to local environmental factors such as the condylar anomalies developing in cases of rheumatoid arthritis or trauma, the pattern of malocclusion can be found very early in the child's development when bony discrepancies exist.

Malocclusion may be present because of:

1. inadequate tooth positioning in arches and bony bases that are themselves normally related to each other,
2. inadequate dental arches in bony bases that are themselves normally related to each other, or
3. unfavorable skeletal morphology leading to an inadequate tooth relation.

As in every other area of medicine and dentistry, progress in methods of classification and treatment of malocclusion have not been even and orderly. Since the initial attempts of Fox in 1803[14] to classify irregularities of tooth position based primarily on the relation of the anterior teeth, many investigators have attempted to evaluate human occlusion and to find the etiological factors leading to malocclusions. It is not possible here to consider more than the most important contributions to this question.

Fig. 3-21a and b Panoramic radiographs of a 3.5 and a 6-year-old child showing development of the retromandibular region and positioning of the molar teeth.

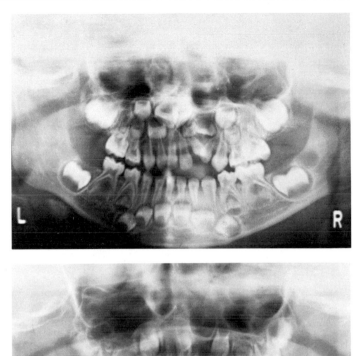

Figure 3-21a

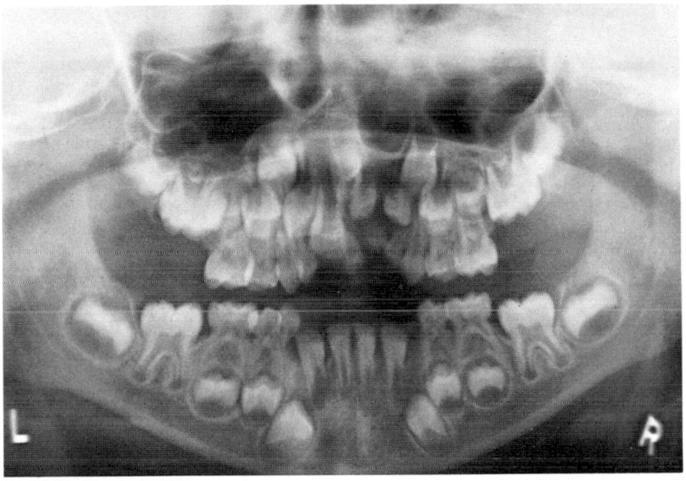

Figure 3-21b

In 1898, E. H. Angle introduced a classification of malocclusion which was published in the March-April 1899 issue of Dental Cosmos and is regarded as a milestone in modern orthodontic diagnosis. Angle attached great importance to the maxillary permanent first molars and his classification is based on the relation of the mandibular permanent first molars to the maxillary permanent first molar, e.g., correct (Class I), backward (Class II), forward (Class III) (Fig. 3-22).

Angle's Classification is:

Class I – the first mandibular permanent molars are one-half cusp mesial in relation to the maxillary first molar. The malocclusion is almost exclusively dental.
Class II – the first mandibular permanent molars are distalized by at least one-half cusp in relation to the maxillary first molars and two divisions require consideration:
Division 1 – protrusion of the maxillary incisors, usually with overjet,

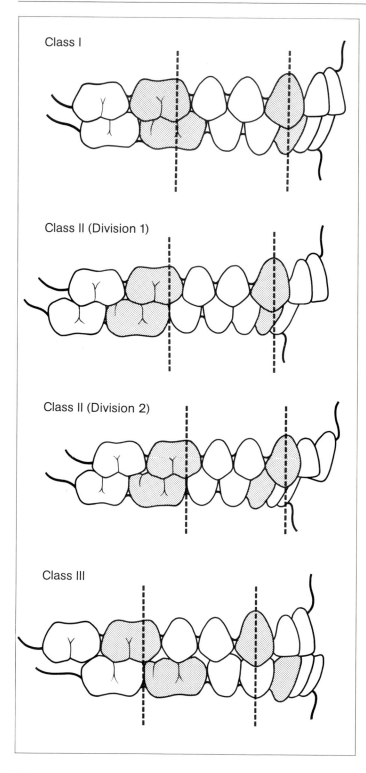

Class I

Class II (Division 1)

Class II (Division 2)

Class III

Fig. 3-22 Interarch relationship according to the classification of Angle (Courtesy of D.E. Wilkins, Clinical practice of dental hygiene, Philadelphia, 1971, Lee & Febiger).

Division 2 – retrusion of the maxillary incisors, usually associated with overbite, *Class III* – the mandibular permanent first molars are mesial in relationship to the maxillary molars, and usually the mandibular incisors are anterior to the maxillary counterparts.

As was pointed out by Angle and his group, this classification can be used only if the arch has lost no teeth and the molars have not drifted. If drift has occurred the diagnosis should be made by imagining the position that the molars occupied before any drift took place[3].

Angle's classification is a convenient starting point in diagnosis. Its function today is only to evaluate those anomalies of occlusion which are on the horizontal plane, and it must be remembered that the maxillary permanent first molars are not fixed points in the skull and that the relation of the arches to the skull also must be considered.

In 1922, Simon[43] published "A system of diagnosis of dental anomalies" in which he used anthropological landmarks of the head to evaluate tooth position in relation to several planes:

the *Frankfort plane* passing through the lowest border of the bony orbit and the upper border of the external auditory meatus,
the *midsagital plane* which divides the skull into two halves, and
the *orbital plane* which is perpendicular to the Frankfort plane and passes through the lowest point of the border of the bony orbit (orbitale). Simon believed that the orbital plane also passes just distal to the tip of the maxillary canines, but this is not always so. In Simon's system, a plane establishes each spatial dimension and anomalies can be related in space.

While some of the theories of Simon were not completely correct, the concept of relating teeth to other head structures proved valid and provided a strong incentive for the advancement of the concepts of occlusion. They led to further studies of the relation of the teeth, jaws, and the craniofacial complex. In recent years greater emphasis has been placed on the spatial relation of the dental structures and the craniofacial complex. Thus a diagnostic system based on fundamental skeletal relation has been substituted for one based entirely on interdental features.

Genetics of occlusion

Genetic factors play a role in determining morphology of the craniofacial complex. However, the genetic influence is very difficult to ascertain, since there are so many different factors involved. Population, family, and twin studies indicate that genetics play a role in craniofacial development. The role of the environment also must be taken into consideration. How strongly the hereditary or environmental factors act upon development has been a matter of controversy for many years; an extensive literature has developed. Numerous examples of syndromes and diseases of genetic origin which affect the growth and development of the craniofacial complex are known.

Because several structures are involved in craniofacial development and each component may be under separate genetic influence, the total evaluation of a large region is of little practical use. When small areas have been considered separately it has been possible to demonstrate some genetic influence on the development of the craniofacial complex[21]. Early investigators had already observed that hereditary factors in members of the same family are independent for the maxilla and mandible. More recent studies have shown that various parts of the mandible are under different developmental controls, some of which are genetic and others environmental. According to Watnick[48], the variability of gonial angle and antigonial notch areas is predominantly determined environmentally while the lateral surface of the transverse and frontal curvature of the mandible are predominantly controlled genetically.

A number of studies evaluating similarities of type of occlusion in several family members have been reported. Stein, Kelley, and Wood[44] studied families of college students with and without malocclusion and concluded that there was a greater similarity between siblings than between unrelated individuals of the same age. They also found a high correlation between measurements of fathers and daughters. A family resemblance for mandibular shape was also reported.

Support for the concept of a possible genetic component of malocclusion is presented in the many reports of families with specific types of malocclusion. Studies such as that of several generations of the Habsburg family demonstrate the well known prognathic mandible and prominent lower lip[22]. Harris and his collaborators[20] have extensively studied possible genetic factors involved in Class II division I malocclusion. Their studies seem to favor a polygenic inheritance pattern. Stiles and Luke[45] reported a dominant inheritance pattern in a black family showing mandibular prognathism, but Suzuki[46] could not demonstrate this type of inheritance in his sample of 243 Japanese families. He did find, however, that prognathism occurred in other members of the family in 34% of his cases.

Obvious differences among the features of the facial complex and various interracial characteristics which are influenced by heredity have been studied by comparison of facial structures in different populations[37]. Significant differences in mean values and standard deviations for cephalometric measures of Chinese and whites[8] and blacks and whites[1] have been demonstrated.

Similarities between monozygotic and dizygotic twins also have been studied and reported repeatedly[23]. Figure 3-23 illustrates the malocclusion of a set of triplets, 2 monozygotic and the third dizygotic. The two identical members have a similar type of occlusion which is quite different from that of the third triplet.

Iwagaki[28] also studied a Japanese sample and concluded that mandibular prognathism was transmitted as an autosomal recessive trait. Kraus et al.[32] concluded that mandibular prognathism was inherited as an autosomal dominant in some populations and in others as an autosomal recessive trait.

Defects of facial bones associated with maxillary hypoplasia and depressed nasal bridge have been described in Down syndrome and anhidrotic ectodermal dysplasia. In mandibular facial dysostosis (Treacher Collins syndrome) the characteristic appearance of the face is associated with a hypoplasia or even absence of zygomatic bones and deficient midface development.

Special breeding studies in experimental animals to obtain specific skeletal changes are also known and the development of malocclusion in sheep has been studied extensively in New Zealand[10].

Other oral abnormalities in which genetic factors have been extensively studied include tooth size and shape and diastemas. Hereditary factors in true medial diastema of the maxilla have been reported in many studies. Weninger's study[49] of 24 families suggested an autosomal dominant inheritance.

Fig. 3-23 Triplets, 2 monozygotic. Note the similarity of malocclusion of the two monozygotic twins compared to the dizygotic brother.

Chapter 4

Developmental Abnormalities of Head and Jaw

Morphological anomalies present at birth are called congenital malformations or birth defects and can be either of genetic or environmental origin or a combination of both. If the defect is of genetic origin, it may be transmitted from one generation to the next and on to future offspring, and is therefore a heritable defect. An environmental defect is the result of a non-heritable cause, e.g., a chemical that can alter human systems. Some birth defects, genetic or environmental, although present at birth may not be detected until later in life.

Some of the more common human dental genetic problems are described here, emphasis being placed on those conditions encountered in pedodontics.

The rapid advances of genetics since the nineteen-fifties has had a major effect on our understanding, prevention and treatment of genetically determined diseases. Interest and knowledge in the field of human genetics have been increasing because the subject is relevant to every specialty in medical practice.

Understanding these principles will help to explain the familial aspects of health and disease, susceptibility to certain diseases, and response to such treatment as is available. Familiarity with genetic principles can give the dentist a scientific rationale for better management of the families in which genetic diseases occur. The decrease in other medical conditions such as communicable diseases has permitted more atten-tion to be focused on less common genetic disorders.

Specificity of genetic information depends on the type of message transmitted through deoxyribonucleic acid (DNA) and ribonucleic acid (RNA). Mutations alter the genetic code by substituting different nucleotide sequences or changing the type of nucleotide. An example of a disease in which a single mutation has altered the biochemical pathway and synthesis is sickle cell anemia. In this disease the patient produces sickle cell hemoglobin, which contains valine in-stead of the glutamic acid of normal adult hemoglobin.

While chromosomes were recognized as carriers of genetic information and "genes" by Boveri[2] in 1903, it was not until 1956 that Tjio and Levan[30] established that 46 chromosomes were the normal comple-ment in humans. These include 22 pairs of autosomes and one pair of sex chromosomes (XX for females, XY for males) Figure 4-1). The medical importance of chromosome abnormalities was demon-strated in 1959 by Lejeune et al.[17] who showed that trisomy of chromosome 21 was responsible for Down syndrome. Since that time a growing number of specific diseases and malformations have been associated with syndromes caused by chromosome abnormalities of either the autosomes or the sex chromosomes.

Chromosome analysis is carried out through evaluation of a karyotype. A karyotype is a

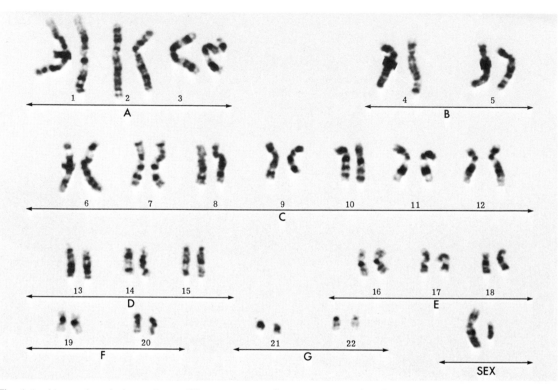

Fig. 4-1   Normal male karyotype. Chromosomes 3 are an example of metacentric chromosomes, chromosomes 4 of submetacentric, and chromosomes 21 of acrocentric chromosomes.

conventional arrangement of chromosomes according to specific parameters of shape and size (Fig. 4-1). The analysis is performed by study of the chromosomes obtained from cells from peripheral blood or from skin biopsy. These cells are cultured and treated chemically to isolate a large number of cells in the process of mitosis. The cells are photographed, the photographs are enlarged, and the individual chromosomes cut out and arranged to produce the karyotype. Chromosomal abnormalities can be of structure, number, or both.

A chromosome consists of 2 chromatids attached at the centromere. *Metacentric chromosomes* have the centromere located in the center. If the centromere is located off center dividing the chromosome into a long arm designated 'q' and a short arm designated 'p', the chromosome is called a *submetacentric chromosome.* An *acrocentric chromosome* has its centromere close to the extremity of the chromosome. Chromosomes 3 are an example of metacentric, chromosomes 4 of submetacentric, and chromosomes 21 of acrocentric chromosomes (Fig. 4-1).

Many diseases of genetic basis can affect

the oral cavity and the oral structures. Diseases that are controlled by genetic factors may be classified into four groups:

Group I: Diseases with Mendelian patterns of inheritance

This group includes those diseases which are caused by a single mutant gene inherited from one parent and acting as a dominant gene, or a pair of genes inherited from both parents in which the inheritance pathway is recessive.

If a condition is controlled by a *dominant gene* all offspring receiving the affected gene will exhibit the condition. If human families were very large, half of the offspring would be affected. However, as families are usually small this is not obvious and only a few individuals are affected in each generation. Dominance can be recognized by the fact that only one affected parent can give rise to an affected child. The normal child will have received the normal allele of the affected parent and will not show or transmit the condition to any offspring. In dominant pattern inheritance there should be no significant difference in the number of males and females affected. A dominant condition may also appear sporadically because of a chance mutation in the gametes of one of the parents. While the parents of such a child have no greater chance of having a second child with the condition than other normal couples of the same age, the affected child will have a 50% chance of having affected offspring. The expression of an abnormal gene may be affected by several conditions including the normal allele which is the normal gene located at the same place on the nonaffected chromosome of the pair. Conditions which are inherited through auto-

somal dominant mechanisms include cleidocranial dysostosis, achondroplasia, Marfan syndrome, and dentinogenesis imperfecta.

While a disorder that involves a single gene theoretically does have an abnormal chromosome this abnormality cannot be detected by the chromosome analysis techniques available at present. Those conditions categorized as chromosome disorders must have numerous genes involved to have sufficient abnormal genetic material to be detected by present methods.

When the condition is transmitted through *recessive genes,* two normal parents, each being heterozygous for the gene, may have an affected child. Recognition of the heterozygocity of the parents is complicated in practice as many matings of heterozygotes may result only in normal offspring. The expression of a recessive trait requires the presence of two essentially identical genes, one from each parent. In many diseases of recessive inheritance, consanguinity can be demonstrated. Hurler syndrome, hypophosphatasia, and Papillon-LeFèvre syndrome are examples of diseases transmitted through autosomal recessive pattern of inheritance.

When each member of a couple is a carrier of the recessive gene there is one chance in four for a pregnancy to result in an abnormal child and one in two for the children to be carriers. It is important to emphasize that each time the carrier parents have a child they will have one chance in four of an abnormal child and this probability holds for each subsequent child. Each pregnancy must be considered individually and not as a part of a total. The same independence of pregnancies applies to dominant genes. This explains why in a family in which one parent is affected by an autosomal dominant condition, the number of affected children may range from none to all. For the same reason in autosomal recessive inheritance no affected member may be found in several generations.

Sex-linked inheritance involves the X and Y chromosomes. A *dominant* trait that is sex linked to the X chromosome will show up in all children to whom the affected X chromosome is transmitted (very few genes are known to be located on the Y chromosome). A *recessive* trait sex linked to the X chromosome is not transmitted through the father to a son since only the Y chromosome is transmitted from the father to the son. Daughters will be carriers because they have inherited the affected X chromosome from the father. These heterozygotes will then transmit the affected X chromosome to half of their sons who will be affected and to half of their daughters who again will be carriers. The disease will be expressed only in the homozygous female when X chromosomes from both parents are affected. Examples of sex linked dominant diseases include orofacial digital syndrome (fatal in males), and vitamin D resistant rickets. Examples of sex-linked recessive conditions include pseudohypoparathyroidism, type A hemophilia, and Duchenne's muscular dystrophy[23].

Group II – Developmental anomalies of multifactorial origin

This group includes those diseases which are known to occur in certain groups and families but in which the inheritance pattern does not follow simple Mendelian rules. Many genes with additive effects are presumed to be involved and no clearly defined ratios can be applied. This group includes common birth defects such as hydrocephalus, spina bifida, and cleft lip and palate.

Cleft lip and cleft palate are common congenital defects affecting the maxillofacial complex. It is estimated that one in every 700 live births in the U.S. has a cleft lip or cleft palate or both. Orofacial clefts are the second most common malformation reported and represent approximately 13% of all reported anomalies[13]. Data differ among studies because of variations of population groups and accuracy of reporting. The incidence of this malformation is somewhat higher in Japanese and lower in Blacks than in Caucasians[13]. As the malformations are extremely disfiguring and affect function, there have been many studies of etiology and therapy (surgical, prosthetic, and functional). Many multidisciplinary teams concerned with treatment and rehabilitation of cleft lip and cleft palate patients have been assembled. While some genetic influence seems to be a part of the etiology of clefts, environmental factors are also important. Cleft palate has been produced in the offspring of many types of mammals by administration of teratogenic agents during pregnancy[19] and some medications have been considered to be involved in cleft palate formation in humans[15]. A large number of syndromes involving clefts of the lip and palate as one of the stigmata have been described[25]. The majority of cases of cleft lip and/or cleft palate probably have a multifactorial etiology with multiple genes and multiple environmental factors interacting, but some seem to be associated with only one abnormal gene[3] (Fig. 4-2). Clinically, the extent of the facial cleft may vary greatly, from minimal involvement of the uvula only to extensive involvement of both lip and palate.

Family studies conducted in Denmark indicate that families with a history of isolated cleft palate do not have a higher incidence of cleft lip (with or without cleft palate), but do have a higher occurrence of cleft palate alone among other members of the family. The same is true for cleft lip with or without cleft palate, indicating that cleft lip with or

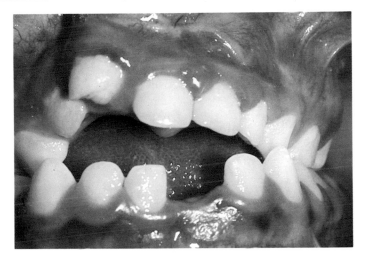

Fig. 4-2 Occlusion of a patient with cleft lip and palate showing tooth malposition in the area of the cleft.

without cleft palate apparently is inherited differently from isolated cleft palate[10].

Sex differences also have been noted in the incidence of cleft lip and cleft palate. Cleft lip with or without cleft palate appears more often in males while cleft palate alone appears more frequently in females. Cleft lip may be bilateral or unilateral, and when unilateral is more frequent on the left side. According to Fogh-Andersen[10], 85% of bilateral and 70% of unilateral cleft lips are associated with cleft palate.

Group III – Diseases with genetic predisposition

This group includes those diseases probably evoked by exogenous factors, but in which a genetic predisposition plays a major role. Genetic factors in predisposition to dental caries have been demonstrated in rats[4], but further studies are required to establish the relation in humans.

Group IV – Chromosome abnormalities

One child in every 200 live births has a chromosomal abnormality. The incidence is considerably higher in stillbirths and spontaneous abortions.

Structural chromosome abnormalities are deletions, duplications, inversions, or translocations of parts of chromosomes. A *deletion* is the presence of an extra piece of a chromosome derived from the fragmentation of a chromatid or chromosome and resulting in the duplication of one or several genes of one chromosome. *Inversions* of chromosome segments are the result of fragmentation of a chromosome followed by reconstitution but with one of the arms inverted.

Chromosome breaks involving two non-homologous chromosomes followed by union of the pieces of the two different chromosomes can also occur; this process is known as *reciprocal translocation* (Fig. 4-3). Since the genetic material is rearranged on different chromosomes but not lost, the individual is phenotypically normal but may produce abnormal offspring through genetic

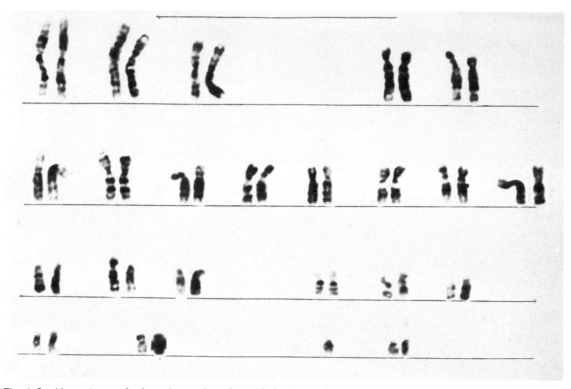

Fig. 4-3   Karyotype of a female carrier of a 14/21 balanced translocation. Note that one chromosome 14 has an additional amount of chromosomal material.

imbalance of some of the gametes. A gain of genetic material under these conditions is called *unbalanced translocation.* Individuals carrying this type of translocation have the same clinical signs as patients carrying extra chromosomes with extra genetic material.

Numerical chromosome abnormalities are usually caused by non-dysjunction, either during meiosis and gamete formation or during mitosis after formation of the zygote. It is an error which occurs during cell division in which the chromosomes are distributed unequally among the daughter cells. If a gamete with one extra chromosome is fer-

tilized, the resulting zygote will be *trisomic* for this chromosome. Two stem lines will be formed, if non-dysjunction occurs during mitosis at the level of the first cleavage, one with 45 chromosomes (monosomic) and one with 47 chromosomes (trisomic). If non-dysjunction occurs during cell division of the zygote, some cell lines may be normal with the normal 46 chromosomes. An individual with different lines of cells is called *mosaic.* If there is extra genetic material in some cell lines, the patient will show some signs of trisomy but in a milder degree than a person trisomic in all cells.

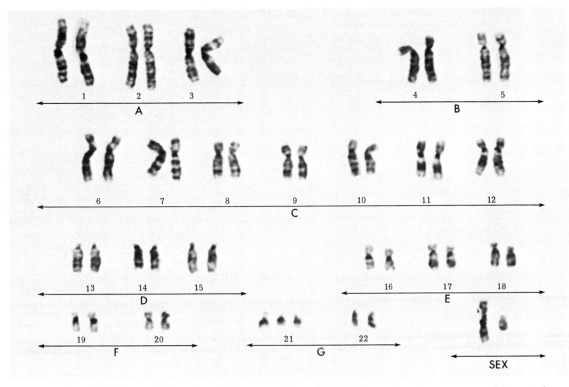

Fig. 4-4   Regular Trisomy 21 in a boy (Down syndrome). Note the extra chromosome 21 (arrow).

Factors which seem to predispose to chromosome aberrations include:

1. advanced maternal age,
2. radiation and cytotoxic drugs,
3. virus infection of the mother, and
4. certain autoimmune diseases.

Autosomal chromosome abnormalities

Many types of autosomal chromosome abnormalities have been described.
The most frequent are trisomies of certain chromosomes with the development of characteristic syndromes.
Down syndrome, one of the most frequent chromosomal aberrations, is characterized by the presence of 47 chromosomes including an extra small acrocentric chromosome 21 in the somatic cells (Fig. 4-4). The syndrome is characterized by mental retarda-

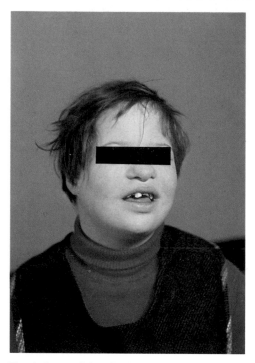 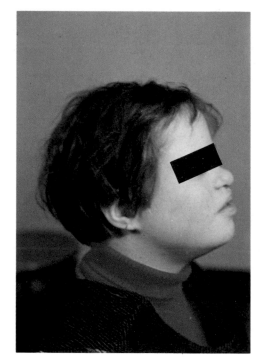

Fig. 4-5a and b   Patient with regular trisomy 21. Note the characteristic facial appearance with epicanthal fold, mongoloid slant, flat nose and protruding tongue.

tion, a peculiar facial appearance consisting of epicanthal folds, mongoloid slant of the eyes, and protruding tongue (Fig. 4-5a and b). These children manifest mental retardation, hypotonia, short broad hands and in many instances congenital heart defects. The incidence of the disease is about 1 in 600 live births. Lejeune *et al.* demonstrated in 1959[17] that the condition was caused by the extra chromosome 21. While the extra chromosome is found as a separate chromosome in all somatic cells in most cases of trisomy 21, examples of translocation and of mosaicism have been reported. Oral manifestations of trisomy 21 commonly include open mouth, tongue thrust beyond the lips, fissuring and furrowing of the tongue, and tooth abnormalities. Maxillary lateral incisors frequently are absent, and abnormal or absent teeth are common manifestations. Delayed tooth eruption pattern is also common. While the incidence of dental caries is not a major problem, the incidence of periodontal disease is high[5]. The high incidence of Class III malocclusion has been attributed to the relatively poor development of the midface.

Trisomy 18, also known as Edwards syndrome or trisomy E, was described by Edwards *et al.*[9] Incidence of 1 in 3000 births has been established for this syndrome and life expectancy is only a few months. The clinical signs include mental retardation, low birth weight, failure to thrive, abnormalities of the abdominal region, and abnormalities of the skull. Several cases of cleft lip with or without cleft palate have been described in

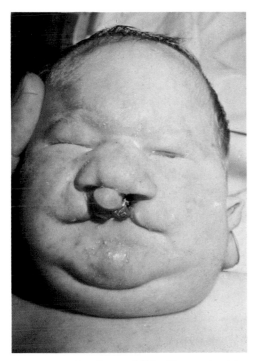

Fig. 4-6a   Newborn child with regular trisomy 13 (Courtesy of Dr. I. M. Rosenthal).

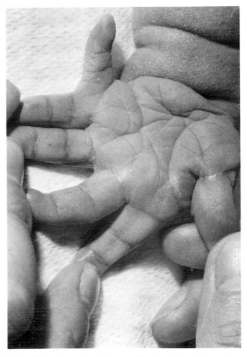

Fig. 4-6b   Hands of the patient showing the extra digit (Courtesy of Dr. I. M. Rosenthal).

cases of trisomy 18, as have malformed or micrognathic mandibles.

Trisomy 13, also known as Patau syndrome or trisomy D, was first reported by Patau *et al.* in 1960[26]. Patients usually show several malformations including microphthalmia or even absence of eyes, low set and deformed ears, deformities of the hands, and abnormalities of the circulatory system (Fig. 4-6a and b). There is usually evidence of generalized underdevelopment as well as mental retardation. High incidence of cleft lip with or without cleft palate has been associated with the syndrome. While life expectancy of patients with a complete trisomy 13 is low, partial trisomies and mosaics have been reported who have lived to their teens[21].

Trisomies of other autosomes have been described and analyzed but as no descriptions of major dental abnormalities have been included no discussion of these chromosomal aberrations is relevant here[18].

Sex chromosome abnormalities

Turner syndrome was described in 1938[31] as a condition showing sexual infantilism, cubitus valgus, webbed neck, short stature and primary amenorrhea in females (Fig. 4-7). In 1959, Ford *et al.*[11] demonstrated that patients with this condition had only 45 chromosomes, 44 autosomes, and one X chromosome. The other sex chromosome is absent (Fig. 4-8). Since that time, the characteristics of Turner syndrome have also been found in

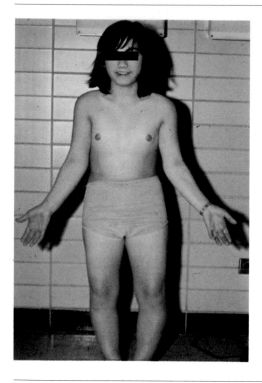

Fig. 4-7 Patient with Turner syndrome
(Courtesy of Dr. I. M. Rosenthal).

many mosaics (chromosome complement of 45X in some cells and 46XX in others). Still other patients have some 45X cells, some 46XX and some 47XXX cells. Oral findings in cases of Turner syndrome include high palatal vault and hypoplastic mandible[16]. Early tooth eruption has been reported repeatedly. Twins, one normal and the other with Turner syndrome have been studied[21], and the twin with Turner syndrome showed an earlier eruption pattern than her twin sister.

Klinefelter syndrome patients are phenotypical males with an extra X chromosome in addition to the normal XY sex chromosomal complement. The karyotype is 47XXY although some may be mosaic with a normal male cell line as well. Signs of this syndrome include impeded spermatogenesis, elevated urinary gonadotropins, and relatively underdeveloped secondary sex characteristics. Several recent reports associate tau-rodontism with an extra X chromosome, but more cases will have to be studied[29].

With further study, more conditions involving chromosome abnormalities are likely to be described, and some conditions in which only mosaicism or a partial chromosome abnormality is present also are likely to be found. Some of these conditions may have oral anomalies as part of the syndrome.

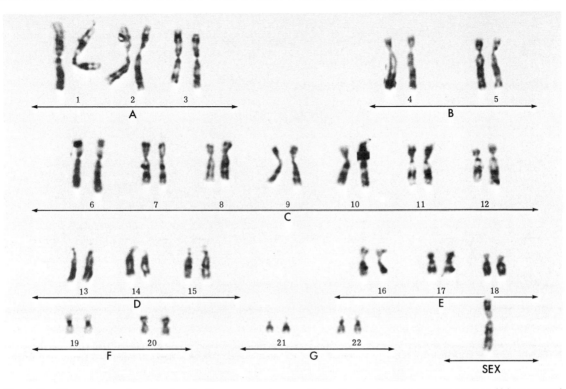

Fig. 4-8 Karyotype of patient with Turner syndrome. Note that only one chromosome X is present (arrow).

Inborn errors of metabolism

Many diseases caused by hereditary biochemical disorders disrupt normal functions. Garrod[12] studied four such diseases in 1908 and coined the term "inborn error of metabolism". Modern biochemical genetics has established the occurrence of hundreds, and new ones are being defined, investigated, and studied all the time.

A few such conditions will be discussed here because the dental aspects and treatment are important in pedodontics.

Glycogen storage disease

Different diseases have been identified in which there is a glycogen storage disorder because of an enzymatic defect in the synthesis pathway or because of glycogen breakdown. Among such diseases, Von Gierke, or Type I glycogen storage disease, is the most frequent. In this disease there is a glucose-6-phosphatase deficiency with deposition of massive amounts of glycogen in the liver. The glycogen cannot be mobilized from glucose-6-phosphate because of the enzyme defect. In the classic form, the patients fail to develop properly and are of short stature with a large protuberant abdomen. They are prone to hypoglycemia and feeding schedules must be carefully adjusted. In the past, life expectancy was short, but modern treatment with adequate control of hypoglycemic episodes has improved life expectancy. Tooth eruption patterns seem to be delayed in these patients[20].

Type II glycogen storage disease is caused by a faulty debranching enzyme. The accumulation of abnormally structured glycogen is significant and damaging but not of massive proportions.

Other types of glycogen storage disease occur but are rarer than Types I and II.

Galactosemia

Abnormally high concentrations of galactose in blood may result from either of two enzymatic defects. The most commonly occurring is an enzyme deficiency of galactose-1-phosphate uridyl transferase activity. In rare cases the missing enzyme is galactokinase. The clinically normal heterozygotes have approximately half the normal transferase activity. Patients homozygotic for the enzymatic defect appear normal at birth but show listlessness, feeding difficulties, vomiting with weight loss, and sometimes jaundice. If milk feeding is not interrupted, liver damage, lenticular cataracts, and mental retardation may develop. Substitution of a galactose-free diet results in cessation of galactosemia and galactosuria. If treatment is initiated at an early age, other abnormalities do not develop. Enamel hypoplasia has been demonstrated in patients with unrecognized galactosemia[1].

Phenylketonuria

Phenylketonuria is an inborn error of metabolism of the deoxylase enzyme which is responsible for oxidizing phenylalanine to tyrosine. In the normal individual, dietary phenylalanine is converted to tyrosine through hydroxylation with the help of phenylalanine hydroxylase. Recently another group of patients deficient in either dihydropteridine reductase (DHRR) or deficient synthesis of dihydrobiopterin have been identified. A deficiency of this enzyme leads to an accumulation of phenylalanine and phenylpyruvic acid. Metabolites which accumulate in the blood and cerebrospinal fluid are apparently involved in the mental deterioration, possibly by interference with myelinization. Melanin formation is also altered in this condition and manifests itself in hair and skin color alterations.

Patients with this disease have been reported to have increased caries rates, which may result from hypoplasias. Careful monitoring of dietary phenylalanine has permitted the development of patients without mental retardation, but the condition must be diagnosed before damage to brain tissues takes place.

Blood coagulation defects

Disorders of blood coagulation are important in pediatric dentistry. These disorders are the result of abnormalities of a group of plasma factors necessary for the formation of a firm clot. Hemophilia is the most important abnormality resulting from a congenital defect in plasma clotting factors. Hemophilia A is transmitted as an X-linked recessive trait and is caused by a deficiency in factor VIII. In patients with hemophilia A there is a difference in severity in different families depending on the degree of deficiency of factor VIII. Hemophilia B (Christmas disease) is also transmitted as an X-linked recessive trait and is associated with a deficiency of factor IX. The relative incidence of factor VIII to factor IX deficiency is 84:16.

The symptoms of hemophilia B are similar to those of hemophilia A. In hemophilia A, bleeding seldom occurs during the eruption of primary teeth. Significant bleeding may occur during eruption of permanent teeth.

Most of the dental care of such children can be accomplished by a proper preventive program. These patients should be examined at least 3 times annually in the dental office and proper prophylactic dental care given, including fluorides, pit and fissure sealants, and dietary counseling. The usual limitation of refined carbohydrates is of particular importance in patients with hemophilia. Through these methods there can be a marked reduction in the need for operative dentistry and tooth extractions.

Exfoliation of primary teeth may present problems, with development of bleeding. In most instances treatment with local pressure and powdered topical thrombin will arrest the bleeding. The use of a soft or liquid diet is also helpful. If severe bleeding occurs while the tooth is exfoliating (despite local measures) the tooth should be removed after replacement of the deficient factor. Hemostatic levels should be maintained for about 3 days. The site of exfoliation is usually shallow and healing occurs rapidly so that a prolonged period of replacement therapy is not required.

In routine dental procedures, local infiltration analgesia can be administered without replacement of the deficient factor. The pedodontist may prefer, however, to replace the missing factor if local anesthesia is to be used. Mandibular alveolar nerve block, however, is dangerous without provision of the deficient factor, and should not be attempted without replacement therapy. Ordinarily only a single replacement dose is required but additional medication should be administered if signs of bleeding or inflammation are noted at the time the level of the deficient factor is expected to become low[28].

Patients requiring dental extraction should be hospitalized. The deficient factor should be administered preoperatively and coagulation tests performed to assure that the concentration of the missing factor is adequate. Sutures may be placed if required, and the socket may be packed with gelatin sponge to which topical thrombin can be added. As in other forms of surgery, the deficient clotting factor should be supplied for about 7 days. The level of deficient factor should be above 10% of normal. Preliminary studies suggest that desmopressin (DDAVP, an antidiuretic compound) can raise factor VIII levels and may prove to be useful in the milder cases of factor VIII deficiency. Epsilon-aminocaproic acid also has been used in conjunction with replacement factor VIII for control of oral bleeding.

For the treatment of factor VIII deficiency, although fresh frozen plasma has been used, cryoprecipitate or commercial concentrates are presently employed. For factor IX deficiency, plasma concentrate or stored plasma can be utilized. The half life of factor VIII is 12 hours and that of factor IX 24 hours. In preparing a patient for dental surgery, a hematologist should be consulted. Salicylates should be avoided in patients with coagulation disorders because of interference with platelet factors[27].

Von Willebrand disease, a related abnormality, is transmitted as an autosomal dominant trait. Prolonged bleeding may occur after dental extraction and there may be considerable variation in severity of symptoms even among members of the same family; there is a diminished level of factor VIII as a result of failure of synthesis. Prolonged bleeding time is found in Von Willebrand disease. Defective platelet adhesiveness is present suggesting absence of a factor necessary for normal bleeding time. Treatment of the coagulation disorder in this condition can be accomplished by plasma infusion. Cryoprecipitate or fresh frozen plasma can be used.

A variety of other coagulation defects may occasionally be of concern to the pedodontist[8].

Unusual bleeding after dental procedures (extraction) should suggest the possibility of coagulation disorder and consultation with the hematologist should be requested.

Patients with hemophilia who have had multiple transfusions may be carriers of hepatitis associated antigen. The dentist should be aware of the potential hazard and should be sure that all instruments are sterilized properly after use. The dentist also should take proper preventive measures for his own protection.

Hypophosphatasia

Congenital absence of alkaline phosphatase is associated with a condition of skeletal inadequacy which histologically resembles rickets. The age of onset of the disease varies. In the very young patient it is fatal, but if onset is delayed, clinical symptoms may be mild. The findings are related to defective bone formation with increased decalcified osteoid. Long bones show typical rachitic changes and cranial sutures may calcify early with consequent intracranial pressure and brain damage. Premature loss of teeth with abnormal periodontal membranes is a common feature.

Acatalasia

Acatalasia is a rare condition which was first identified in Japan. Catalases are involved in the breakdown of hydrogen peroxide. In patients with congenital absence of catalase, hydrogen peroxide formed by oral bacteria is not broken down and results in ulcerations and tooth loss.

Syndromes

A syndrome is a set of symptoms present as a group which characterize a type of illness, the cause of which may not be well understood. It is usually assumed that the abnormal traits comprising the syndrome are transmitted to the offspring as a unit. In some cases, fundamental biochemical defects or major chromosomal abnormalities can be identified but in the majority of syndromes the etiological factors have not been elucidated. More study and better understanding will identify basic etiological factors for the various entities and possibly lead to management by counselling or therapy, or both. If the complications associated with a syndrome are known they can be monitored and preventive steps can be taken.

Cohen[6] classifies syndromes as follows:

A. Unknown genesis syndromes
   1. provisionally unique pattern syndrome
   2. repeated pattern syndrome

B. Known genesis syndromes

   1. pedigree syndrome
   2. chromosome syndrome
   3. biochemical defect syndrome
   4. environmentally induced syndrome

Other syndromes which may or may not involve oral structures have been studied and identified, but a complete review of the literature is impossible as new ones are being described each year. Several comprehensive surveys are available[14] and should be consulted if much information about a specific syndrome is needed. Only the more frequently occurring syndromes with face and head manifestations will be reviewed here (Table 4-1).

Table 4-1 **Common syndromes with head and neck manifestations**

ACROCEPHALOSYNDACTYLY
(Apert syndrome)

Transmission:

Sporadic, autosomal dominant in some families.

General manifestations:

Characteristic pointed skull with prominent steep forehead and flat occipital region. Irregular closure of the cranial sutures, particularly the coronal suture. Syndactyly varies. Other skeletal abnormalities.

Oral manifestations:

Cleft palate of the hard or soft palate may occur. Maxillary hypoplasia is common with accompanying relative mandibular prognathism.

ATAXIA-TELANGIECTASIA SYNDROME
(Louis-Bar syndrome)

Transmission:

Autosomal recessive.

General manifestations:

Short stature, cerebellar ataxia, slow speech, oculocutaneous telangiectasia of the butterfly area of the face, neck, and other parts of the body. Mental development reduced in older children. Frequent upper respiratory infections. Increased number of chromosomal breaks and rearrangements.

Oral manifestations:

Telangiectasia of the hard and soft palate in some cases.

CHONDROECTODERMAL DYSPLASIA
(Ellis-van Creveld syndrome)

Transmission:

Autosomal recessive.

General manifestations:

Bilateral manual polydactyly, acromelic dwarfism with chondrodysplasia of long bones, nail hypoplasia, cardiac defects.

Oral manifestations:

Absence of upper vestibule due to fusion of the middle part of the upper lip to maxillary gingival margin. Hypodontia and abnormal tooth shape. Natal teeth present in 25% of reported cases.

CLEIDOCRANIAL DYSOSTOSIS

Transmission:

Sporadic; autosomal dominant.

General manifestations:

Aplasia or hypoplasia of one or both clavicles. Delayed fontanelle ossification, increased frontal and parietal bossing. Short stature.

Oral manifestations:

High arched palate with clefting in some cases. Delayed or failure of tooth eruption with cyst formation in some cases. Supernumerary or unerupted teeth frequent. Delayed exfoliation of primary teeth may occur.

Table 4-1 **Common syndromes with head and neck manifestations** (continued)

ENCEPHALOFACIAL ANGIOMATOSIS
(Sturge-Weber syndrome)

Transmission:

Not fully understood.

General manifestations:

Venous angioma of the leptomeninges of the cerebral cortex with characteristic calcifications of brain tissue. Facial angioma lesions on the same side. Contralateral hemiplegia. Epileptic seizures. Mental retardation in some cases.

Oral manifestations:

Vascular hyperplasia of varied size of oral mucosa. Gingival hyperplasia and angiomatosis also associated with phenytoin hyperplasia in some cases.

EPIDERMOLYSIS BULLOSA DYSTROPHICA
(Goldscheider syndrome)

Transmission:

Autosomal recessive.

General manifestations:

Spontaneous formation of bullae filled with sterile fluid on arms and legs. Ruptured bullae result in raw, painful surfaces and scar formation. Dystrophic nails frequent. Eye and conjunctiva involvement frequent. Simple form (Weber-Cochrane syndrome) has been described without associated oral manifestations.

Oral manifestations:

Mucosal lesions of the tongue, lips, gingiva, and palate followed by scarring. Tooth abnormalities particularly enamel hypoplasia.

HEMIFACIAL MICROSOMIA

Transmission:

Not fully understood.

General manifestations:

Size reduction of the maxillary and zygomatic bones, muscular hypoplasia and malformation of external ear of affected side. Microphthalmia and coloboma of iris.

Oral manifestations:

Agenesis or aplasia of the ramus of mandible. Macrostomia in some cases. Teeth maloccluded on affected side.

CRANIOFACIAL DYSOSTOSIS
(Crouzon syndrome)

Transmission:

Autosomal dominant.

General manifestations:

Cranial dysostosis associated with exophthalmos. Hypertelorism. Mental deficiency in some cases. Other abnormalities in some cases.

Oral manifestations:

Maxillary hypoplasia with relative mandibular prognathism may cause crowding and unerupted teeth. High arched or cleft palate in some cases.

HYPERKERATOSIS PALMO-PLANTARIS
WITH PERIODONTAL DISEASE
(Papillon-LeFèvre syndrome)

Transmission:

Autosomal recessive.

Table 4-1 **Common syndromes with head and neck manifestations** (continued)

General manifestations:

Hyperkeratosis of the palms and soles.

Oral manifestations:

Hyperkeratosis with development of gingival inflammation and periodontal disease with exfoliation of primary teeth between 2 and 4 years of age and permanent teeth at young age.

HYPOHIDROTIC ECTODERMAL DYSPLASIA
(Anhidrotic ectodermal dysplasia)

Transmission:

X-linked recessive in most cases, some cases of autosomal dominant described.

General manifestations:

Usually manifested in males but some females reported. Carrier mothers sometimes exhibit minimal expressions with hypodontia or peg-shaped teeth. Characteristic facies with marked frontal bossing and depressed nasal bridge. Inability to sweat with hyperpyrexia caused by heat. Thin hair with eyebrows and eyelashes usually absent.

Oral manifestations:

Anodontia or severe hypodontia. Teeth present are often peg-shaped. Lips appear thick and exaggerated.

IDIOPATHIC GINGIVAL FIBROMATOSIS AND HYPERTRICHOSIS

Transmission:

Autosomal dominant.

General manifestations:

Facial appearance of the patient varies with amount of gingival hyperplasia present. Hypertrichosis of variable degrees.

Oral manifestations:

Gingival hyperplasia particularly in the anterior maxillary region (sometimes covering the teeth). Tissues composed of thick bundles of collagen fibers.

INCONTINENTIA PIGMENTI (Fig. 4-10)

Transmission:

Dominant sex linked (fatal in males).

General manifestations:

Bullous and varicose formations on skin of extremities. Pigmented areas present over the trunk and extremities. Mental retardation reported in some cases.

Oral manifestations:

Hypodontia and delayed tooth eruption. Peg-shaped teeth.

MANDIBULO FACIAL DYSOSTOSIS (Fig. 4-9)
(Treacher Collins syndrome)

Transmission:

Autosomal dominant.

General manifestations:

Characteristic bird face with downward sloping palpebral fissures (anti-mongolian slant). Poorly developed supraorbital ridges. Cheek areas depressed with underdevelopment of malar bone. Absence of zygomatic arches. Receding chin. Coloboma of the lower lid and iris. Deformed pinna.

Table 4-1 **Common syndromes with head and neck manifestations** (continued)

Oral manifestations:

Hypoplastic mandible with deficient ramus. Cleft palate frequent. Open bite or other malocclusion frequently associated with jaw abnormalities.

MARFAN SYNDROME (Fig. 4-11a and b)

Transmission:

Autosomal dominant.

General manifestations:

Long face with frontal bossing. Large ears, frequently with abnormal helix. Disproportionately long extremities. Pectus excavatum and carnictum. Arachnodactyly. Frequent aortic dilatation.

Oral manifestations:

Abnormally high palate or cleft palate. Malocclusion frequent.

MORQUIO-ULLRICH SYNDROME

Transmission:

Autosomal recessive.

General manifestations:

Skeletal abnormalities usually including spinal deformities. Markedly reduces skeletal growth. Chondroitin sulphate n-acetylhexosamine sulphate phosphatase deficiency.

Oral manifestations:

Enamel defects include pitting and flakiness of very thin enamel.

MUCOPOLYSACCHARIDOSIS I (Hurler syndrome, Fig. 4-12)

Transmission:

Autosomal recessive, X-linked recessive.

General manifestations:

Characteristic skeletal deformity. Small stature. Mental retardation. Corneal clouding. Deafness. Frequent upper respiratory problems with chronic rhinitis. Mucopolysaccharide metabolism disorder due to iduronadase deficiency with storage of large amounts of mucopolysaccharides. Several rarer types of mucopolysaccharides are known.

Oral manifestations:

Characteristic facial aspect with gingival hypertrophy particularly in the anterior maxillary region with associated tooth spacing. Macroglossia.

OROFACIAL DYSOSTOSIS

Transmission:

X-linked dominant, fatal in males.

General manifestations:

Midline pseudo upper cleft lip. Varied degree of alopecia. Thin nose with hypoplasia of the alar cartilages. Frontal bossing. Abnormal fingers (brachydactyly, syndactyly, clinodactyly or extra digits.)

Oral manifestations:

Frenulae and "clefts" are pathognomonic and characteristic. Clefts of the tongue associated with the strong bands of frenulae. Cleft palate in some cases. Pseudoclefts frequently due to the abnormal position of the frenulae (formed by thick bands over the jaw ridges).

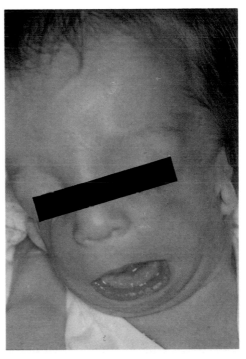

Fig. 4-9   Face of patient with mandibulofacial dysostosis (Courtesy of Dr. I. M. Rosenthal).

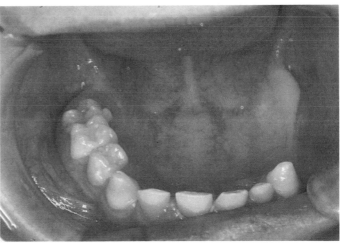

Fig. 4-10   Mandible of patient with incontinentia pigmenti. Note the congenital absence of several teeth on the left side (Courtesy of Dr. I.M. Rosenthal).

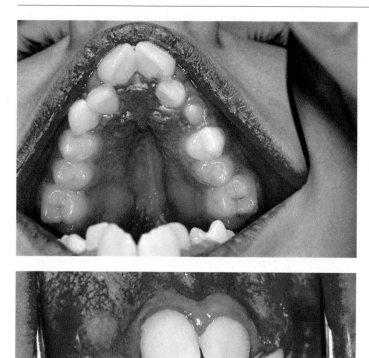

Fig. 4-11a and b   Maxilla of patient with Marfan syndrome.

Figure 4-11a

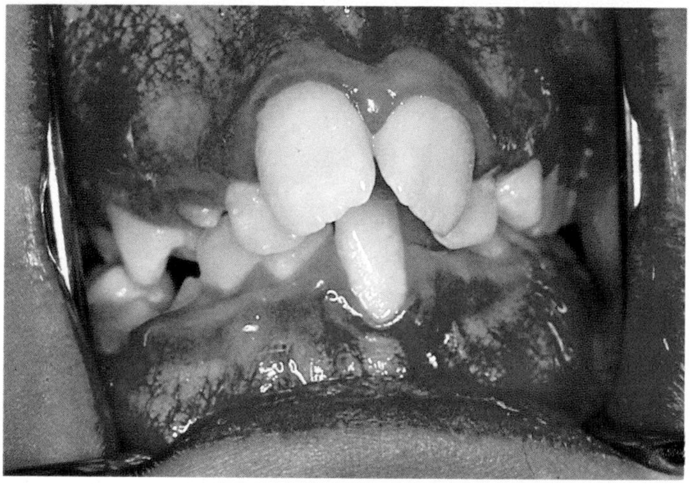

Figure 4-11b

Fig. 4-12 Face of patient with Hurler syndrome.

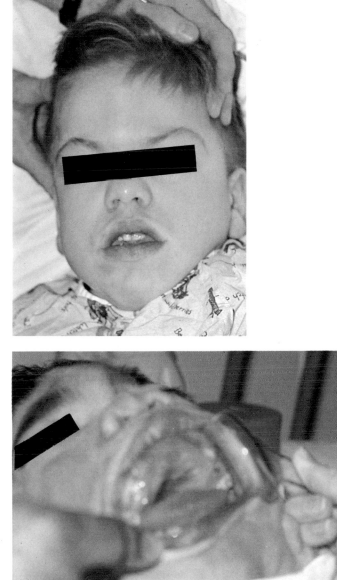

Fig. 4-13 Maxilla of patient with Hurler syndrome.

References

1. Benusis, K.P., S.M. Pueschel and C. Hum:
   Enamel hypoplasia in children with galactosemia associated with periods of poor control. J. Dent. Child. *45*: 73-75, 1978.

2. Boveri, T.:
   Über den Einfluß der Samenzelle auf die Larvencharaktere der Echiniden. Arch. Entwick. Organism. *16*: 340-363, 1903.

3. Cervenka, J., R.J. Gorlin and V.E. Anderson:
   The syndrome of pits of the lower lip and cleft lip and/or palate: genetic considerations. Am. J. Human Genet. *19*: 416-432, 1967.

4. Chai, C.K., H.R. Hunt, C.A. Hoppert and S. Rosen:
   Hereditary basis of caries resistance in rats. J. Dent. Res. *47*: 127-138, 1968.

5. Cohen, M.M. and R.A. Winer:
   Dental and facial characteristics in Down's syndrome (Mongolism). J. Dent. Res. *44*: 197-208, 1965.

6. Cohen, M.M., Jr.:
   Dysmorphic syndromes with craniofacial manifestations. In R. E. Stewart and G. H. Prescott (eds.), Oral facial genetics. St. Louis, Mosby, 1976.

7. Cudzinowski, L.:
   Von Gierke's disease: report of case. J. Dent. Child. *45*: 413-415, 1979.

8. Donaldson, V.H. and C.T. Kisker:
   Blood coagulation and hemostatis. In D.G. Nathan and F. A. Oski (eds.), Hematology of infancy and childhood. Philadelphia, Saunders, 1974.

9. Edwards, J.H., D.G. Harnden, A.H. Cameron, W.M. Crosse and O.H. Wolff:
   New trisomic syndrome. Lancet *1*: 787-790, 1960.

10. Fogh-Andersen, P.:
    Inheritance of harelip and cleft palate. (Thesis) Copenhagen, Nyt Nordisk Forlag, Arnold Busck, 1942.

11. Ford, C.E., P.W. Polani, J.C. de Almeida and J.H. Briggs:
    A sex chromosomal anomaly in a case of gonadal dysgenesis (Turner's syndrome). Lancet *1*: 711-713, 1959.

12. Garrod, A.E.:
    Inborn errors of metabolism. London, Henry Fowde, 1909.

13. Gorlin, R.J., J. Cervenka and S. Pruzansky:
    Facial clefting and its syndromes. Birth defects: *7(7)*: 3-49, 1971.

14. Gorlin, R.J., J.J. Pindborg and M.M. Cohen, Jr.:
    Syndromes of the head and neck (2nd ed.). New York, McGraw-Hill, 1976.

15. Hanson, J.W. and D.W. Smith:
    The fetal hydantoin syndrome. J. Pediat. *87*: 285-290, 1975.

16. Horowitz, S.L. and A. Morishima:
    Palatal abnormalities in the syndrome of gonadal dysgenesis and variants and in Noonan's syndrome. Oral Surg. *38*: 839-844, 1974.

17. Lejeune J., M. Gauthier and R. Turpin:
    Les chromosomes humaines en culture de tissus. C. R. Acad. Sci. *248*: 602-603, 1959.

18. Lewandowski, R.C., Jr. and J.J. Yunis:
    New chromosomal syndromes. Am. J. Dis. Child. *129*: 515-529, 1975.

19. Loevy, H.T.:
    Genetic influences on induced cleft palate in different strains of mice. Anat. Rec. *145*: 117-122, 1963.

20. Loevy, H.T.:
    In preparation.

21. Loevy, H.T., B.M. Jayaram, I.M. Rosenthal and R. Pildes:
    Partial trisomy 13 associated with cleft lip and cleft palate. Cleft Palate J. *14*: 239-243, 1977.

22. Loevy H. T., S. Pruzansky, E. Weiss, and I. M. Rosenthal:
Comparison of tooth development in a child with Turner's syndrome with her normal monozygotic twin. J. Dent. Res. *57*:187, 1978.

23. McKusick, V. A.:
Mendelian inheritance in man: catalogue of autosomal dominant, autosomal recessive and X-linked phenotypes (5th ed.). Baltimore, Johns Hopkins Press, 1978.

24. Myers, H. M., M. Dumas and H. B. Ballhorn:
Dental manifestations of phenylketonuria. J. Am. Dent. Assoc. *77*: 586-588, 1968.

25. Nora, J. J. and F. C. Fraser:
Medical genetics: principles and practice. Philadelphia, Lea and Febiger, 1974.

26. Patau, K., D. W. Smith, E. Therman, S. L. Inhorn and H. P. Wagner:
Multiple congenital anomalies caused by an extra autosome. Lancet *1*: 790-793, 1960.

27. Quick, A. J.:
Aspirin in hemophilia. In K. M. Brinkhous (ed.), Hemophilia and new hemorrhagic states. Chapel Hill, Univ. N. Carolina Press, 1970.

28. Steinle, C. J. and C. T. Kisker:
Pediatric dentistry for the child with hemophilia. New Eng. J. Med. *283*: 1325-1326, 1970.

29. Stewart, R. E.:
Taurodontism in X-chromosome aneuploid syndromes. Clin. Genet. *6*: 341-344, 1974.

30. Tjio, J. H. and A. Levan:
The chromosome number of man. Hereditas *42*: 1-6, 1956.

31. Turner, H. H.:
A syndrome of infantilism, congenital webbed neck cubitus valgus. Endocrinology *23*: 566-574, 1938.

Chapter 5

Tooth and Tongue Abnormalities

Developmental abnormalities of the dentition may cause serious problems for the patient, and are of major clinical relevance. The abnormalities may be hereditary or acquired. Included are variations in eruption and exfoliation pattern, number, position, shape, color, and texture of teeth. Early recognition and appropriate treatment of these problems is of great importance in pedodontics so that deleterious effects on the facial growth and development of the patient may be minimized or overcome.

Anomalies of tooth number

Numerical anomalies are characterized either by an excess or a deficiency in the normal complement of teeth.

Hypodontia

Hypodontia, the congenital absence of one or more teeth, is rarely found in the primary dentition but is not uncommon in the permanent dentition (Fig. 5-1). Egermark-Ericksson and Lund[17] studied approximately 3,500 Swedish children (ages 10 to 16) and found that hypodontia was more frequent in boys; several other reports provide similar data. Many cases of hypodontia, particularly those involving the lateral incisors, have genetic causes.

Certain syndromes of genetic origin are associated with hypodontia. In ectodermal dysplasia, there is a lack of development of all or almost all teeth (see Fig. 2-6). Management of this condition depends on its extent. In ectodermal dysplasia, an artificial prosthesis should be constructed initially when the child is about 3 or 4 years old. In less severe cases of hypodontia of one or more teeth, occlusion planning is necessary. Frequently placement of a space maintainer is indicated to keep teeth from moving into an abnormal position.

Supernumerary teeth

The presence of an excess number of teeth is reported as occurring in 0.2 to 4.5% of persons. This condition seldom involves the primary dentition[10]. The familial pattern of supernumerary teeth has been described frequently in the literature. Supernumerary teeth also may be found in association with certain disorders of genetic origin such as cleidocranial dysostosis, and in the region of the cleft in patients with cleft lip and palate. The most common site of supernumerary teeth is in the anterior region of the maxilla. Supernumerary teeth found in the midline are known as mesiodens (Fig. 5-2). Mesiodens may affect the development and eruption pattern of the maxillary permanent incisors either by erupting themselves or by interfering with the eruption pathway of these teeth (Fig. 5-4a and b, Fig. 5-5a and b).

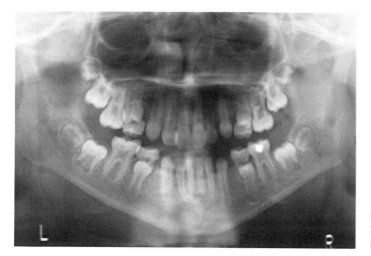

Fig. 5-1 Panoramic radiograph of an 11-year-old patient with all first pre-molars congenitally absent.

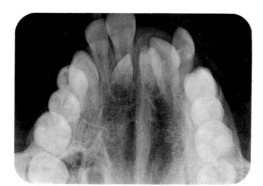

Fig. 5-2 Supernumerary tooth inter-fering with the eruption of tooth 8.

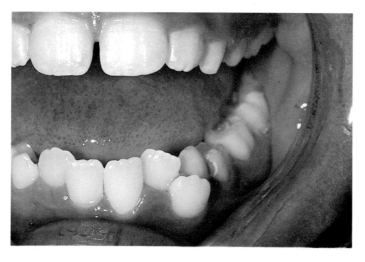

Fig. 5-3 Supernumerary mandibular lateral incisor.

Fig. 5-4a and b   Supernumerary tooth interfering with the eruption of tooth 9 in a 10-year-old boy.
2.5 months after surgical removal of the supernumerary.

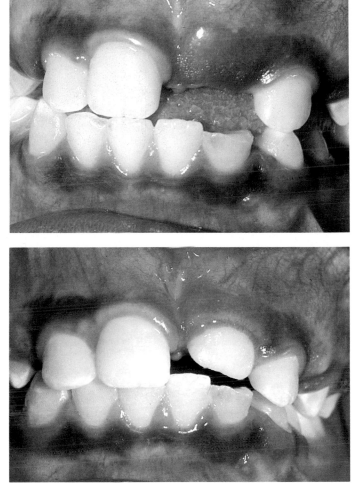

Figure 5-4a

Figure 5-4b

The molar and the premolar regions, in that order, are the next most frequent sites, but supernumerary teeth have been found in all locations in the arch (Figs. 5-3 and 5-6).

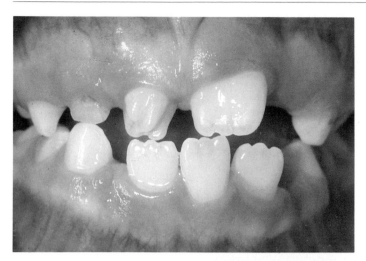

Fig. 5-5a and b   Supernumerary tooth erupted in the area of tooth 8.

Figure 5-5a

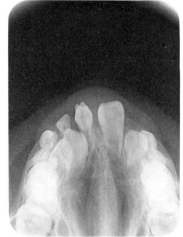

Figure 5-5b

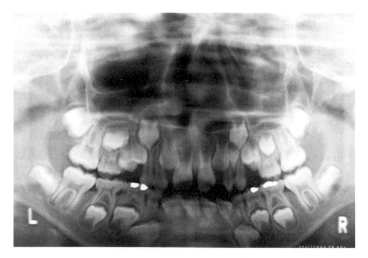

Fig. 5-6   Panoramic radiograph showing supernumerary canines on the maxillary right side.

Anomalies of form and size

Instances of macrodontia (teeth larger than the usual range) have been reported[19]. Microdontia, teeth which are smaller than the usual range, are also known. The teeth most frequently affected are the maxillary permanent lateral incisors and many such cases are familial[1].

Dens in dente

Dens in dente is an unusual developmental defect which results in enamel tissue within the tooth. The term *dens in dente* has been used since the 1850's but *dens invaginatus* is a more descriptive name. Because of enamel organ invagination during tooth development, an enamel-lined central cavity having a small external opening on the tooth surface but no communication with the dental pulp results. Maxillary permanent lateral incisors are the teeth most frequently involved.[39]

Dens evaginatus

This rare malformation has been reported under a variety of names, e.g., interstitial or supernumerary cusp. The affected tooth has a slender, enamel-covered projection rising from the buccal ridge to the central fissure of the occlusal surface. Depending on size, the tubercle may contain pulp tissue[37]. As these tubercles are high, they often fracture when the teeth occlude and the exposed pulp may necrotize. The anomaly is most frequent in patients of the Mongolian race[59].

Talon cusp

This is a cusp-like projection arising at the cingulum of an incisor (Fig. 5-7). It has been reported only in permanent teeth. Radiographically the projection is covered by enamel and dentin, and there is a deep developmental groove at the junction with the other part of the tooth. This developmental groove is highly susceptible to caries. Mellor and Ripa[33] describe 8 cases, 7 in the maxilla and 1 in the mandible (Fig. 5-7).

Taurodontism

According to Keith[28], taurodontism is a peculiar tooth form in which the body of the tooth and the pulp chamber are enlarged at the expense of the root. While this abnormality was considered at one time to be characteristic only of *Homo neanderthaliensis,* examples have been reported in modern man[24]. Molars with taurodontism have been found in several patients with triple X chromosomes and in patients with Klinefelter syndrome[57].

Fused and geminated teeth

Differential diagnosis of partially fused and geminated teeth is difficult. Fusion may occur between two normal teeth or between normal teeth and supernumerary teeth. (Figs. 5-8 and 5-9). Sometimes the pulp canals are united; fusion of tooth germs very early in embryonic development, leading to a single large tooth, have been reported[20]. Gemination is the development of two teeth from a single tooth germ with an incomplete separation. In fusion there is usually a reduction of the number of teeth in the arch while in gemination the number is usually normal (Fig. 5-10a to c).

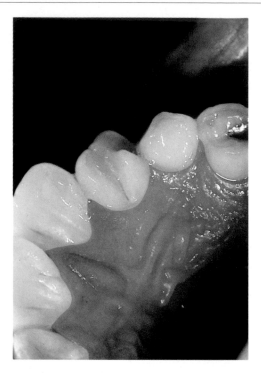

Fig. 5-7 Talon cusp in an 8-year-old boy.

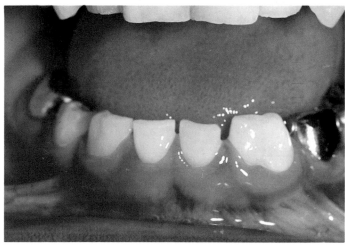

Fig. 5-8 Fused teeth in a 6-year-old girl.

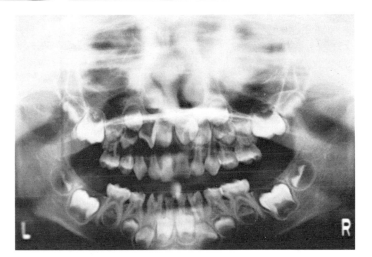

Fig. 5-9   Panoramic radiograph of the same patient as in Fig. 5-8.

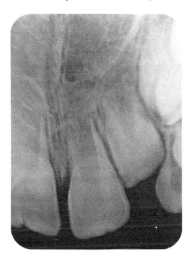

Figure 5-10a

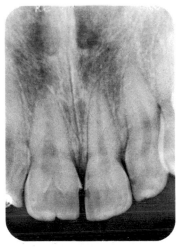

Figure 5-10b

Figure 5-10c

Fig. 5-10a to c   Very large central incisor possibly due to gemination (Courtesy of Dr. H. Freudenthal).

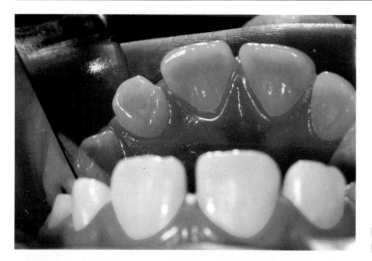

Fig. 5-11 Shovel-shaped teeth in a patient of Mexican origin.

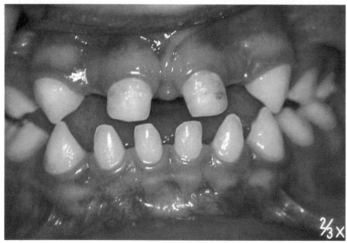

Fig. 5-12 Peg-shaped teeth in a patient with several congenitally missing teeth (Courtesy of Dr. B. Stone).

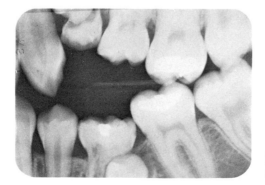

Fig. 5-13 Radiograph of a girl with several ankylosed primary molars.

Shovel-shaped teeth

Shovel-shaped teeth have a characteristic shape on the lingual side of the tooth. The lingual side is deeply concave, giving the tooth the more or less pronounced appearance of a shovel. The most common location is the anterior maxilla. Shovel-shaped teeth (Fig. 5-11) have been reported in Chinese, Japanese, Eskimos and several groups of North and South American Indians. The trait is rare among Blacks and apparently nonexistent in Whites[11, 16]. The distribution of this abnormality suggests genetic origin.

Peg-shaped incisors

Peg-shaped incisors have reduced mesiodistal width and proximal surfaces converging markedly toward the incisal margin, giving the tooth a conical shape. The teeth most commonly affected are maxillary lateral incisors. There seems to be a significant hereditary tendency for the trait, suggesting that missing and peg-shaped teeth are different expressions of the same gene or genes located in close proximity on the chromosome. Some investigators believe that it is an autosomal dominant inheritance with incomplete penetrance in some instances[1] (Fig. 5-12).

Anomalies in tooth position and eruption time

Transposition of teeth is not uncommon and the teeth most frequently involved are the permanent canines and the first premolars. This condition is usually unilateral and appears to be the result of an abnormal eruption pattern but bilateral examples have been reported[45].

Ankylosis

A localized union between the cementum of the tooth root and alveolar bone results in ankylosis. The most frequently affected teeth are the primary molars. The union of the tooth root with the alveolar bone causes a halt in the eruption pattern of the affected tooth and is usually diagnosed by the position of the tooth in the dental arch. This "submerged" condition may lead to various problems, including delayed exfoliation with consequent delayed eruption, impaction or dilaceration of the permanent tooth, difficulty of removal, or loss of arch length from the tipping of other teeth into the unoccupied occlusal space. Treatment varies, depending on the severity of the problem (see page 222). If there is any damage or space loss the tooth must be removed. In any event, ankylosed teeth must be evaluated frequently and be removed before they can damage the permanent dentition[5, 51]. If noted early, it is sometimes possible to luxate the ankylosed tooth by breaking the bony fusion and thereby permitting resumption of normal eruption. However, most occurrences are discovered too late for this treatment as the diagnosis is usually made from the "submerged" appearance of the tooth (Fig. 5-13). Tapping on the tooth will produce a dull sound. Once discovered, however, an assessment should be made of whether to leave the tooth undisturbed but under close observation for loss of arch length, to extract the tooth and place a space maintainer, or to build up the occlusal surface to establish mesiodistal width contacts and avoid supereruption of the antagonist tooth.

The teeth most frequently ankylosed are the mandibular primary second molars, and then in order, the mandibular primary first molars, maxillary primary second molars, and maxillary primary first molars[5].

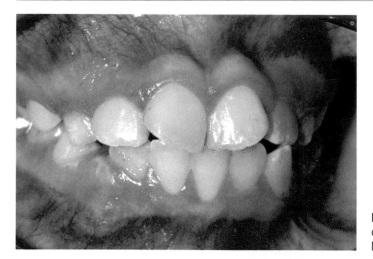

Fig. 5-14 Mesiopalatal torsion of central incisors (winging) in a girl of Mexican origin.

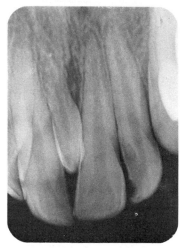

Fig. 5-15 Anterior crowding and rotation due to the presence of a mesiodens (Courtesy of Dr. H. Freudenthal).

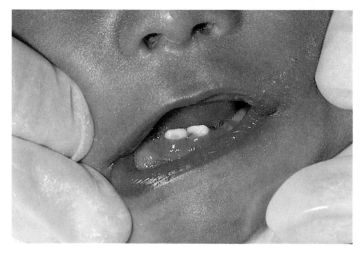

Fig. 5-16 Neonatal teeth in a 6-day-old boy.

Rotated central incisors

Mesio-palatal torsion of the maxillary central incisors, also described as "wing-like appearance" or "winging", is caused by rotation of these teeth in a manner such that the distal portion of the crown is turned labially and the mesial portion has a mesio-labial rotation (Fig. 5-14). "Winging" must be distinguished from crowding and malposition caused by a mesiodens (Fig. 5-15). "Winging" seems to be a trait characteristic of certain Oriental populations; it also has been described in several North and South American Indian populations[21].

Natal and neonatal teeth

Many reports of newborns with erupted (natal teeth) and of infants of less than one month with eruption teeth (neonatal teeth) have appeared in the literature. Usually the teeth affected are the mandibular incisors (Fig. 5-16). This rare eruption anomaly has for centuries been considered a good or bad omen depending on the culture. According to Bodenhoff and Gorlin[8], the incidence of natal and neonatal teeth is at least 1 in 3,000 births. About 15% of those affected have family members with a similar abnormality. It is not possible to have a more precise statistic as many observed cases go unreported. Usually, the pulp of the involved teeth is large and no root formation can be seen, accounting for the mobility. Natal and neonatal teeth have also been reported frequently in Ellis-van Creveld syndrome (chondroectodermal dysplasia), in Hallerman-Streiff syndrome (oculomandibular dyscephaly)[22], and in pachyonydria congenita[48].

Natal and neonatal teeth should not be confused with dental lamina or inclusion cysts which are found occasionally in newborns. Fromm[23] studied 1,367 newborns and found that 76% had inclusion cysts either along the midpalatine raphe (Epstein pearls) or on the buccal and lingual aspects of the dental ridges as well as other areas of the palate (Bohn's nodules), or dental lamina cysts found on the crest of the maxillary and mandibular dental ridges.

Teeth also may be present at birth in some patients with cleft lip and/or palate, but here they are usually not an anomaly of eruption but rather a position problem resulting from the cleft.

Structural defects of enamel

Many factors may cause defects in formation of the enamel of primary and permanent teeth. The appearance of the defect depends on the severity of the causal factor. Since the disturbance is usually localized, only one tooth or a very small number of teeth will be affected.

Enamel defects may manifest themselves either as a deficiency in the amount of enamel formed (hypoplasia) or in a deficiency of calcification of the enamel matrix (hypocalcification or hypomaturation). Hypoplastic defects of the enamel occur in association with many disturbances in development of the fetus, newborn, or young child[40]. Enamel hypoplasia of primary teeth has been reported in 50% of children who suffered neonatal tetany[40], in cerebral palsy[52], in patients with kernicterus following hemolytic disease[35], in association with phenylketonuria[36], in children of mothers who had rubella during pregnancy[25], and in 54% of children with neurological disorders[50]. Systemic disturbances apparently can affect ameloblastic activity and, depending on the severity, nature, and duration, can affect enamel formation. Enamel hypoplasia and hypomaturation result from altered metabolism of ameloblasts during tooth

111

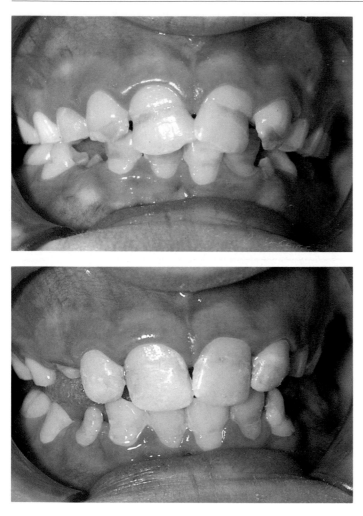

Fig. 5-17a and b   Enamel hypoplasia, (a) before and (b) after treatment with acid etch composite resin.

Figure 5-17a

Figure 5-17b

development and are manifested by irregularities and indentations on the enamel surface. As systemic factors may affect ameloblastic activity, all teeth in which enamel is developing at the time of disturbance will show the effects. Many of these disturbances occur during the first year of life and may manifest themselves by defective regions in the permanent incisors, canines, and first molars (Fig. 5-17a and b). Primary teeth may be affected if the systemic factor acted during prenatal or very early postnatal development.

Hereditary enamel defects, however, usually affect both the primary and permanent dentition and involve the entire crown of all or most teeth.
Localized hypoplasia of the enamel of some permanent teeth can also be associated with a periapical infection of a primary tooth. These teeth have also been called Turner teeth. This has been demonstrated by inducing periapical infection and enamel malformations in dogs[6], but experimentally induced infection of primary teeth did not always induce hypoplasia.

Amelogenesis imperfecta

The term amelogenesis imperfecta indicates defective enamel formation, but it is usually used to designate a particular hereditary defect of enamel formation. Rao and Witkop[41] indicate that the disease is rare (incidence of 1 in 14,000-16,000 children). Three major types of amelogenesis imperfecta: *hypoplastic, hypocalcified,* and *hypomaturation,* each with a number of subtypes based on clinical, genetic, and histological differences can be distinguished[56].

In general terms, the hypoplastic form of amelogenesis imperfecta results in enamel which is thinner than normal. The hypocalcified type is manifested by enamel which has developed to a thickness similar to normal teeth, but which is soft, friable, and easily detached from the tooth. In the hypomaturation type, enamel of normal thickness develops but it is abnormally hard and tends to chip away from the underlying dentin instead of wearing away as in the hypocalcified type. The most frequently encountered type of amelogenesis imperfecta seems to be hereditary hypocalcification.

Hypoplastic amelogenesis imperfecta

Five different sub-types have been described[41, 56]:

Type I Autosomal dominant; thin, smooth hypoplasia with eruption defect and resorption of teeth,

Type II Autosomal dominant; thin, rough hypoplasia,

Type III Autosomal dominant; randomly pitted hypoplasia,

Type IV Autosomal dominant; localized hypoplasia,

Type V X-linked dominant; rough hypoplasia.

Both dentitions are usually affected in all types; however, Type IV may be limited to the primary dentition. Type I is the most severe, with a greatly reduced amount of smooth enamel so that the teeth seem to be widely spaced. The enamel present is hard, shiny, and yellow-brown in color and intraoral radiographs usually fail to show it. In some patients the teeth fail to erupt and coronal resorption of the unerupted teeth may occur.

Type II is somewhat less severe than Type I, and some traces of enamel may be seen on radiographs. The enamel is thin and hard and may show roughness and pitting. The teeth are yellow-brown, but eruption problems have not usually been reported.

Type III is characterized by enamel of almost normal thickness with a large amount of pitting distributed over all the surfaces. As the thickness of the enamel is almost normal, there is no apparent increased spacing between teeth.

Type IV usually does not involve the permanent dentition, but if the permanent teeth are affected the changes are minimal, with some horizontal pitting and grooving.

Type V affects the sexes differently. In the male, the enamel is extremely thin, hard, and granular, while in the female, normal enamel and abnormal vertical banded enamel alternate.

Hypocalcified amelogenesis imperfecta

Only one type is known: autosomal dominant hypocalcification[41]; it is the most frequent type of amelogenesis imperfecta. This disease was formerly designated "hereditary brown teeth" because particularly the permanent teeth erupt with a dull surface varying in color from opaque white to light brown (Fig. 5-18). The condition is usually symmetrical but some teeth may be less affected than others in the same arch. The enamel is soft and can be peeled off. The tooth may be extremely sensitive as a result of enamel loss from abrasion and erosion.

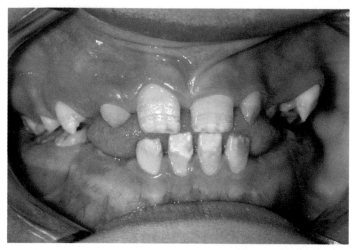

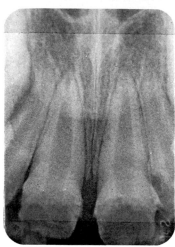

Fig. 5-18   Amelogenesis imperfecta.

Fig. 5-19a and b   Radiographs of a patient with amelogenesis imperfecta. Several other members of the family were also affected.

Figure 5-19a

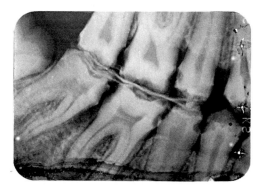

Figure 5-19b

Radiographic examination may show enamel indistinguishable from dentin because of lack of contrast (Fig. 5-19a and b). Chaudhry et al.[12] have estimated from histological studies that organic material concentration is considerably higher than normal. Large masses of calculus with complicating gingivitis are frequently associated with the defect.

Hypomaturation amelogenesis imperfecta

Two major groups and five subtypes have been described[56]:

Hypomaturation

Type I   X-linked recessive hypomaturation
Type II Autosomal recessive, pigmented hypomaturation
Type III Snow-capped teeth

Hypomaturation-hypoplasia with taurodontism

Type I   Autosomal dominant hypomaturation with occasional hypoplastic pits and taurodontism
Type II Autosomal dominant hypomaturation with thin hypoplasia and taurodontism

Of those cases of hypomaturation without taurodontism, Type I is characterized by enamel of normal thickness which can be easily penetrated by a dental explorer. Because of its softness, severe attrition of the enamel may occur. In female carriers, normal enamel bands alternate with bands of abnormal opaque-white enamel. In Type II, the enamel is of normal thickness but there is a lack of radiographic contrast. It is soft, with color varying from shiny milky-white to yellow-brown. In Type III only the incisal enamel of the anterior teeth or the occlusal enamel of posterior teeth (or both) is abnormal. The involved areas are either flecked or diffusely involved with opaque white patches, as the designation "snow capped" indicates. The inheritance pattern is not fully understood but some families have been reported in which the trait is autosomal dominant.

Two families with an amelogenesis imperfecta associated with taurodontism have been reported, one by Winter[55] and the other by Crawford[14]. Members of both families had a pattern of autosomal dominant inheritance. In the family described by Crawford, the teeth appeared widely spaced and the enamel thin and yellow-brown in color. In the family described by Winter, the hypoplastic enamel was of normal thickness with some of the subjects having local areas of random hypoplastic pitting.

Reports of more cases and family analysis will demonstrate whether some of the subtypes are actually variations of the same subtype instead of being unique entities.

The aim of the treatment of amelogenesis imperfecta is the improvement of facial esthetics and the establishment of an efficient masticatory apparatus while maintaining the health of the teeth and supporting structures and maintaining correct arch dimensions (Fig. 5-20). It is advantageous if the patient seeks treatment at an early age so that adequate evaluation and counseling can take place. Because the appearance of the teeth in these conditions does not improve with cleaning, there is frequently considerable apathy in the child and in the parent concerning oral hygiene. The teeth should be protected from attrition as soon as possible after eruption. Restorative dentistry should be provided and stainless steel crowns should be used to maintain or reestablish vertical dimension.

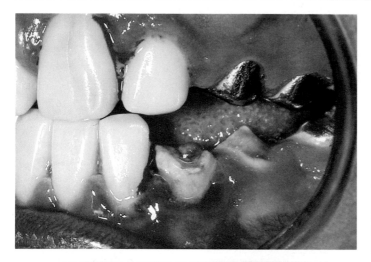

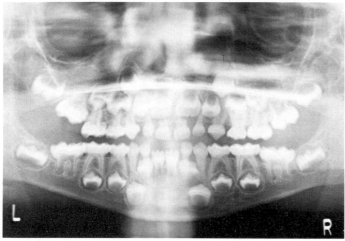

Fig. 5-20 Patient with amelogenesis imperfecta in treatment. Note pulp polyp of tooth 21.

Fig. 5-21 Panoramic radiograph of a 7-year-old boy with dentinogenesis imperfecta.

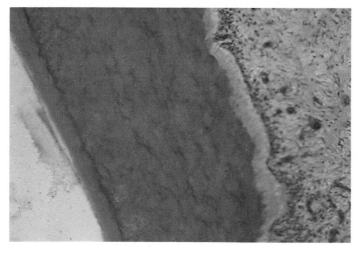

Fig. 5-22 Histological section of dentinogenesis imperfecta. Note the irregularities of the dentinal tubules.

Structural defects of dentin

Dentinogenesis Imperfecta

Dentinogenesis imperfecta is an hereditary anomaly transmitted as a Mendelian dominant trait. It may occur alone or in association with osteogenesis imperfecta. The condition also has been called hereditary opalescent dentin, hereditary dentin hypoplasia or dysplasia of Capdodont in honor of the person who first described the anomaly. It appears in both the primary and permanent dentition.

As dentinogenesis imperfecta is inherited as an autosomal dominant trait, there is usually a history of one affected parent. Sporadic occurrence is rare. Occasionally both parents of affected patients have normal teeth but there is evidence of the abnormality having occurred in previous generations. Usually all teeth are affected, but subjects in whom only some of the teeth are involved have been described[29, 44]. Variations of clinical expression of this defect among different family members have been reported[7], as have patients with normal coronal dentin with the defect present only in the roots.

Patients with dentinogenesis imperfecta have a gray-brown or pinkish opalescent discoloration of the teeth. The teeth have a particular shape with short roots and bell-shaped crowns (Fig. 5-21). The enamel may be normal or hypoplastic, easy to chip and fracture because of the poorly supported enamel. The teeth are subject to fast and excessive wear. The rapid attrition may cause exposure of the pulp chamber even though there is a reduction of pulp tissue. There is also a tendency to abscess formation.

While the outer part of the dentin appears histologically normal, the central portion of the tooth shows abnormal dentin characterized by a diminished number of tubules. These tubules are short and sometimes branched, and form an irregular wavy pattern[4]. The dentin is hypocalcified and irregular interglobular spaces are numerous (Fig. 5-22) Electron microscopic studies show irregularities in deposition of apatite crystals and in the configuration of the collagen fibrils[26]. Analysis of the extracted teeth has shown that both hardness of the dentin and radiographic absorption values are below those of normal dentin. Chemical analysis of the dentin has demonstrated high water and low inorganic content[4, 27].

Treatment of this condition is difficult, but if initiated early can be successful in preserving vertical dimension and improving appearance through placement of crowns on individually selected anterior and posterior teeth. As the disease is familial, proper counselling with the family will permit the evalution of patients soon after tooth eruption and before too much tooth structure has been lost through attrition. This also makes insertion of crowns easier.

Shell teeth

Other dentin defects with similarities to dentinogenesis imperfecta have been described as shell teeth or ghost teeth. In contrast to dentinogenesis imperfecta, shell teeth have abnormally large pulp chambers. Microscopic appearance of the dentin is abnormal[44] and the histologically normal enamel lies on irregularly calcified abnormal dentin. The dentin is thin, with large tubules in some areas and irregular matrix in others. The roots, if present, are short and very thin-walled.

Odontodysplasia

In 1922, Ballschmiede[3] described odontodysplasia, a condition of abnormal dentin with disarrangement of the dentinal tubules (particularly in the root) with large spherical bodies of calcified material embedded, giving the dentin a whorl-like appearance, and a calcification pattern completely obliterating the root canals. As a result of the early onset of the disturbance, most of the affected teeth have very short roots[31, 44].

Discoloration and stains of teeth

Tooth color is dependent on the translucency of the enamel with its blue, pink, and green tints, and on the color of the dentin, which varies from yellow to brown. Discolorations and stains may be caused by extrinsic or intrinsic factors. Extrinsic factors act through formation of a deposit on the surface of the enamel and usually can be removed by cleaning. Intrinsic factors act by affecting the calcified tissues internally.

Extrinsic stains

Extrinsic stains range in color from yellow to black depending on their etiology. Bacterial cell wall components such as muranic acid have been identified in some stains. Chromogenic bacteria producing green, brown, yellow, orange or black stains (Fig. 5-23) have been found in large numbers of children[30]. Brown or black stains are common and occur on the cervical third of the crown following the gingival line. Ultramicroscopy has demonstrated a large number of microorganisms associated with these discolorations[42, 49].

Very common green stains are more frequent in girls than in boys and often recur after removal. Usually the stained area appears as a green-yellow region on the cervical third of the labial surface of the maxillary teeth.

Black stains are usually found on the lingual and proximal surfaces of maxillary teeth. The primary teeth are most often affected, but permanent teeth occasionally have this type of stain. Such stains should not be confused with transient discoloration caused by food or medication. Reid and Beeley[42] collected gingival debris of children with black extrinsic stain and demonstrated that the material had higher calcium and phosphate concentration and lower protein content than the gingival debris of children without stained teeth. The stain apparently contains an insoluble iron compound formed by reaction between saliva chemicals and the compounds produced by bacterial action. This type of stain has also been found concurrent with a very low caries incidence[43].

Some foods, e.g., raspberries, also produce transient extrinsic stains on teeth. Defects in the enamel and poor oral hygiene increase such staining, which is related to the length of exposure and the number of times the teeth have been exposed to the agents. Certain medications, such as iron compounds administered orally for the treatment of anemia, also may produce dental extrinsic stains. Wellock et al.[53] have described extrinsic stains from the topical application of stannous fluoride in some patients.

Intrinsic stains

Many systemic conditions can alter the dental hard tissues during development and so alter the color of erupted teeth.

Patients with congenital erythropoetic porphyria, a disease caused by an inborn error of metabolism, show a pinkish-brown discoloration of the teeth (Fig. 5-24). The cause of the discoloration is the accumulation of porphyrin pigment in the teeth. Hemolytic anemia and the jaundice caused by Rh incompatibility may lead to localized yellow-green discoloration of primary dentition. The stain results from biliverdin deposition in enamel and dentin during the

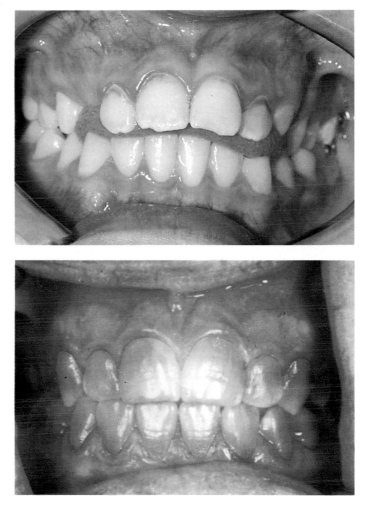

Fig. 5-23 Extrinsic green stain in a 9-year-old patient.

Fig. 5-24 Intrinsic tooth stain in patient with congenital erythropoietic porphyria (Courtesy of Dr. I. M. Rosenthal).

development of these tissues. The central incisors are discolored throughout but other teeth have the stain only in regions closer to the incisal and occlusal surfaces. Tissues developing after the hemolytic episode are not stained. Other hemolytic diseases may also alter tooth coloration.

Traumatic injuries followed by pulpal hemorrhage with extravasated blood components infiltrating into the dentin may cause discoloration.

Administration of tetracyclines to children during tooth development may result in yellow-brown tooth discoloration (Fig. 5-25). Although the use of tetracyclines has been curtailed in recent years, they were very useful antibiotics and were used occasionally in the treatment of the upper respiratory infections.

Incorporation of tetracyclines in dentin can be demonstrated by fluorescence. Enamel fluorescence, if present, is usually weak and is observed only after multiple or very high doses of tetracyclines. The incorporation and localization of tetracyclines into mineralized tissues is probably related to the

119

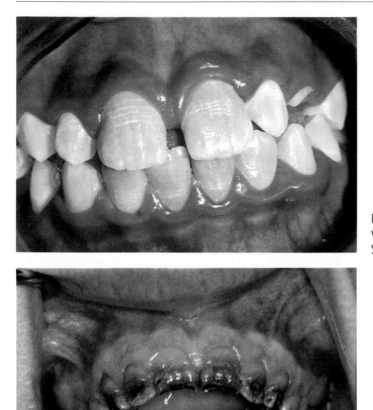

Fig. 5-25a Intrinsic stain in patient who received dietary fluoride at a young age.

Fig. 5-25b Intrinsic tooth stain in patient who received tetracycline therapy as a young child (Courtesy of Dr. Perry).

specific activity of the cell cycle at the time of administration[46]. The discoloration and fluorescence characteristics of the tetracyclines affect the appearance of the teeth, but do not appear to alter caries incidence. A study conducted in 100 3- to 12-year-old children with discoloration and fluorescence characteristics of tetracycline incorporation showed no hypoplastic enamel, and the number of decayed, missing, and filled surfaces was lower than in paired controls[9]. Dental fluorosis (mottled enamel) was recognized and described by McKay and Black at the beginning of the 20th century[32]. It was later demonstrated that excessive fluoride in drinking water was the substance responsible for this condition.

Other causes of non-endemic enamel opacities have been described, for instance, exanthematosis and fevers of various origins[47]. Trauma to the permanent teeth during development because of trauma to the primary teeth also can result in defects. A South African study[54] found that the maxillary permanent central incisors are most often affected by opacities.

Fig. 5-26a and b   Intrinsic tooth stain in patient who received tetracycline treatment (a) before and (b) after treatment with acid-etch composite veneer facing.

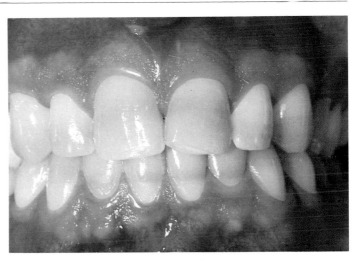

Figure 5-26a

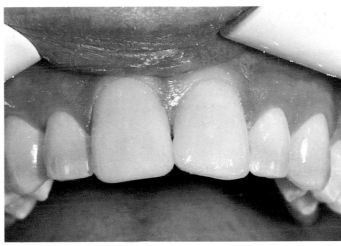

Figure 5-26b

Many attempts to treat stained enamel by selective removal and bleaching have been described as successful. The technique consists in the use of a bleaching solution containing 5 parts of 30% hydrogen peroxide, 5 parts of 36% hydrochloric acid, and one part of ether. Care must be used as the solution is highly flammable. A slight disking with wet fine disks is done during the 20 minute treatment. The bleaching solution is neutralized with a 5.25% solution of perchlorite followed by water rinse. If care is taken, the thickness of enamel removed will not affect the pulp tissue[2]. Care must be taken to avoid damage to the pulp. The treatment may have to be repeated.

Acid etching together with composite resin restoration is being used extensively for tooth discoloration affecting the enamel. This is a major contribution to esthetics. In cases of intrinsic enamel discolorations, the affected area is removed without removing any dentin. The enamel is etched with acid and manufacturer's instructions are followed for insertion of the composite resin material (Fig. 5-26).

Tongue abnormalities

Ankyloglossia

Ankyloglossia is an attachment of the tongue to the floor of the mouth or alveolar ridge. Complete ankyloglossia (Fig. 5-27) seems to be rare[38] but partial ankyloglossia (in which the abnormal lingual frenum extends nearly to the tip restricting tongue movement) is more frequent (Fig. 5-28). Witkop and Barros[58] give an incidence of 1 in 400 individuals in their Chilean study.

Fissured or furrowed tongue

Fissured or furrowed tongue is not uncommon. Grooves or furrows are present to some degree in most tongues, and deep furrows seem to be inherited according to genetic pattern. The condition has been described in many patients with Down syndrome[13].

Cleft tongue

Cleft tongue or lobulated tongue is a rare abnormality caused by the failure of fusion of the different *anlagen* that constitute the tongue. Lobulated tongue associated with the thick connective tissue bands and frenuli is a characteristic stigma of orofacial digital syndrome (OFD).

Macroglossia

Macroglossia refers to a condition which very rarely is due to a true muscular hypertrophy. Sometimes the enlargement is caused by a hemangiolymphangioma or lymphangioma or congenital neurofibromatosis. Partial enlargement of the tongue is seen in congenital hemifacial hypertrophy. Protruding tongue is frequently described in patients with Down syndrome and other congenital malformation syndromes. Whether this is a true macroglossia or simply a positional problem has not been determined.

Median rhomboid glossitis

Median rhomboid glossitis is a reddish area in the midline of the dorsum of the tongue, anterior to the circumvallate papillae. The reddish color is caused by the absence of filiform papillae. The abnormality is especially rare in children.

Microglossia

Microglossia and aglossia are rare abnormalities which are sometimes associated with other abnormalities as part of a syndrome. In some instances the tongue is not really absent but very reduced in size to give the impression of aglossia (Figs. 5-29 and 5-30).

Geographic tongue

Geographic tongue, also known as benign migratory glossitis, is a tongue anomaly frequently found in children. It is asymptomatic and often identified only during routine dental examination. The dorsum of the tongue shows smooth red areas, slightly raised and with a decreased number of filiform papillae. These raised areas may change location over time with increased keratinization in one area and increased desquamation in another. The etiology of the abnormality is not known but the condition is self limiting and does not require treatment. It is found primarily in children but has also been described in young adults[34] (Fig. 5-31).

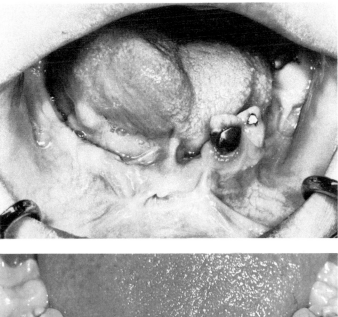

Fig. 5-27 Ankylogossia (Courtesy of Dr. M. Perko).

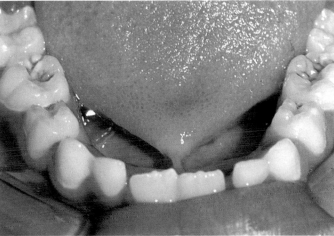

Fig. 5-28 Partial ankyloglossia.

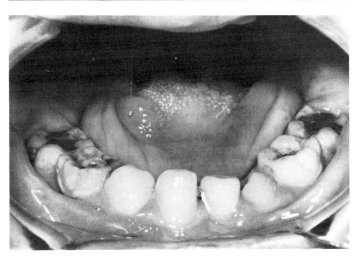

Figure 5-29 Microglossia (Courtesy of Dr. M. Perko[38]).

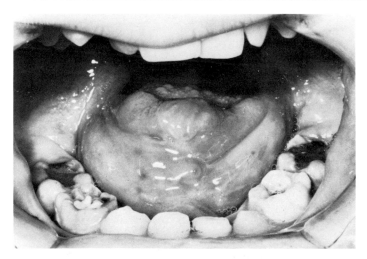

Figure 5-30   Microglossia (Courtesy of Dr. M. Perko[38]).

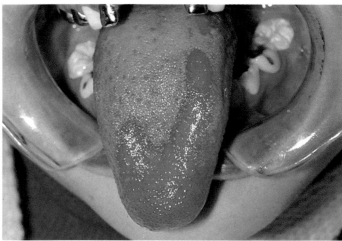

Fig. 5-31   Geographic tongue.

References

1. Alvesalo, L. and P. Portin:
   The inheritance pattern of missing peg-shaped and strongly mesio-distally reduced upper lateral incisors. Acta Odontol. Scand. *27*:563-575, 1969.

2. Bailey, R. W. and A. G. Christen:
   Effects of bleaching technic on the labial enamel of human teeth stained with endemic dental fluorosis. J. Dent. Res. *49*:168-170, 1970.

3. Ballschmiede, G.:
   Wurzellose Zähne. Beitrag für Kasuistik der Zahnanomalien in bezug auf Zahl und Größe. Inauguraldissertation, Greifswald, 1921. Zahnarzt. Rundschau (50):751, 1922.

4. Bergman, G., B. Engfeldt and I. Sundvall-Hagland:
   Studies on mineralized dental tissues. VIII. Histologic and microradiographic investigation of hereditary opalescent dentine. Acta Odontol. Scand. *14*:103-117, 1956.

5. Biederman, W.:
   Etiology and treatment of tooth ankylosis. Am. J. Orthod. *48*:670-684, 1962.

6. Binns, W. H. and A. Escobar:
   Defects in permanent teeth following pulp exposure of primary teeth. J. Dent. Child. *34*:4-14, 1967.

7. Bixler, D., P. M. Conneally and A. G. Christen:
   Dentinogenesis imperfecta: genetic variations in a six-generation family. J. Dent. Res. *48*:1196-1199, 1969.

8. Bodenhoff, J. and R. J. Gorlin:
   Natal and neonatal teeth. Folklore and fact. Pediatrics *32*:1078-1093, 1963.

9. Brearley, L. J. and J. R. Porteous:
   Characteristics and caries experience of tetracycline affected dentitions. J. Dent. Res. *52*:503-516, 1973.

10. Brook, A. H.:
    Dental anomalies of number, form and size: their prevalence in British schoolchildren. J. Int. Assoc. Dent. Child. *5*:37-53, 1974.

11. Carbonell, V. M.:
    Variation in the frequency of shovel-shaped incisors in different populations. In D. R. Brothwell (ed.), Dental anatomy. London, Pergamon, 1965.

12. Chaudhry, A. P., O. N. Johnson, D. F. Mitchell, R. J. Gorlin and W. L. Bartholdi:
    Hereditary enamel dysplasia. J. Pediat. *54*:776-785, 1959.

13. Cohen, M. M. and R. A. Winer:
    Dental and facial characteristics in Down's syndrome. J. Dent. Res. *44*:197-208, 1965.

14. Crawford, J. L.:
    Concomittant taurodontism and amelogenesis imperfecta in the American Caucasian. J. Dent. Child. *37*:171-175, 1970.

15. Dahlberg, A. A.:
    Rotated maxillary central incisors. J. Japan Orthod. Soc. *17*:157-169, 1958.

16. Devoto, F. C. H., N. H. Arias, S. Ringulet and N. H. Palma:
    Shovel-shaped incisors in a Northeastern Argentine population. J. Dent. Res. *47*:820-823, 1968.

17. Egermark-Eriksson, I. and V. Lind:
    Congenital numerical variations in the permanent dentition. Odontol. Revy *22*:309-315, 1971.

18. Eidelman, E. and K. A. Rosenzweig:
    Ellis-Van Creveld syndrome. Oral Surg. *20*:174-179, 1965.

19. Ekman-Westborg, B. and P. Julin:
    Multiple anomalies in dental morphology: macrodontia, multipuberculism, central cusps and pulp invaginations. Oral Surg. *38*:217-222, 1974.

20. Ellisdon, P. S. and K. F. Marchall:
    Connation of maxillary incisors. Brit. Dent. J. *129*:16-21, 1970.

21. Escobar, V., M. Melnick and P. M. Conneally:
    The importance of bilateral rotation of maxillary central incisors. Am. J. Phys. Anthropol. *45*:109-115, 1976.

22. Falls, H.F. and W.J. Schull:
Hallermann-Streiff syndrome: a dyscephaly with congenital cataracts and hypotrichosis. Arch. Ophthalmol. *63*:403-420, 1960.

23. Fromm, A.:
Epstein's pearls, Bohn's nodules and inclusion cysts of the oral cavity. J. Dent. Child. *39*:275-287, 1967.

24. Goldstein, E. and M.A. Gottlieb:
Taurodontism: familial tendencies demonstrated in eleven of fourteen case reports. Oral Surg. *36*:131-144, 1973.

25. Gullikson, J.S.:
Tooth morphology in rubella syndrome children. J. Dent. Child. *42*:479-482, 1975.

26. Herold, R.C.:
Fine structure of tooth dentine in human dentinogenesis imperfecta. Arch. Oral Biol. *17*:1009-1013, 1972.

27. Hodge, H.C., S.B. Finn, H.B.G. Robinson, R.S. Manly, M.L. Manly, G.V. Huysen and W.F. Bale:
Hereditary opalescent dentine. III. Histological chemical and physical studies. J. Dent. Res. *19*:521-536, 1940.

28. Keith, A.:
Problems relating to the teeth of the earlier forms of prehistorical man. Proc. Roy. Soc. Med. (Odont. Sect.) *6*:103-119, 1913.

29. Kustaloglu, O.A.:
Hereditary dentinogenesis imperfecta. Dent. Radiogr. Photogr. *35*:7-10, 1962.

30. Leung, S.W.:
Naturally occurring stains on the teeth of children. J. Am. Dent. Assoc. *41*:191-197, 1950.

31. Logan, J., H. Becks, and S. Silverman, Jr.:
Dentinal dysplasia. Oral Surg. *15*:317-333, 1962.

32. McKay, F.S. and Black, G.V.:
An investigation of mottled teeth: an endemic development imperfection of the enamel of the teeth heretofore unknown in the literature of dentistry. Dent. Cosmos *58*:477-484, 627-644, 781-792, 894-904, 1916.

33. Mellor, J.K. and L.W. Ripa:
Talon cusp: a clinically significant anomaly. Oral Surg. *29*:225-228, 1970.

34. Meskin, L.H., R.S. Redman and R.J. Gorlin:
Incidence of geographic tongue among 3,668 students at the University of Minnesota. J. Dent. Res. *42*:895, 1963.

35. Miller, J. and R.M. Forrester:
Neonatal enamel hypoplasia associated with haemolytic disease and with prematurity. Brit. Dent. J. *106*:93-104, 1959.

36. Myers, H.M., M. Dumas and H.B. Ballhorn:
Dental manifestations of phenylketonuria. J. Am. Dent. Assoc. *77*:586-588, 1968.

37. Oehlers, F.A.C.:
The tuberculated premolar. Dent. Pract. *6*:144-148, 1956.

38. Perko, M.:
Tongue malformations. Quintessence Int. *3*(3):9-16, 1972.

39. Poyton, H.G. and G.A. Morgan:
Dens in dente. Dent. Radiogr. Photogr. *39*:27-33, 1966.

40. Purvis, R.J., G.S. MacKay, F. Cockburn, W.J. McK. Barrie, E.M. Wilkinson and N.R. Belton:
Enamel hypoplasia of the teeth associated with neonatal tetany: a manifestation of maternal vitamin D. deficiency. Lancet *2*:811-814, 1973.

41. Rao, S. and C.J. Witkop, Jr.:
Inherited defects in tooth structure. Birth Def. Orig. Art. *7*(7):153-184, June 1971.

42. Reid, J.S. and J.A. Beeley:
Biochemical studies on the composition of gingival debris from children with black extrinsic tooth stain. Caries Res. *10*:363-369, 1976.

43. Reid, J.S., J.A. Beeley and D.G. MacDonald:
Investigation into black extrinsic tooth stain. J. Dent. Res. *56*:895-899, 1977.

44. Rushton, M.A.:
Anomalies of human dentine. Ann. Roy. Coll. Surg. Eng. *16*:94-117, 1955.

45. Sist, T.C. and A.J. Drinnan:
Transposition – an unusual dental anomaly. N.Y. State Dent. J. *37*:158-161, 1971.

46. Skinner, H.C.W. and J. Nalbandian:
Tetracyclines and mineralized tissues: review and perspectives. Yale J. Biol. Med. *48*:377-397, 1975.

47. Small, B.W. and J.J. Murray:
Enamel opacities: prevalence, classifications and etiological considerations. J. Dent. *6*:33-42, 1978.

48. Soderquist, N.A. and W.B. Reed:
Pachyonychia congenita with epidermal cysts and other congenital dyskeratoses. Arch. Dermatol. *97*:31-33, 1968.

49. Theilade, J., J. Slots and O. Fejerskov:
The ultrastructure of black stain on human primary teeth. Scand. J. Dent. Res. *81*:528-532, 1973.

50. Via, W. F., Jr. and J. A. Churchill:
Relationship of enamel hypoplasia to abnormal events of gestation and birth. J. Am. Dent. Assoc. *59*: 702-707, 1959.

51. Vorheis, J. M., T. Gregory and R. E. McDonald:
Ankylosed deciduous molars. J. Amer. Dent. Assoc. *44*: 68-72, 1952.

52. Watson, A. O., M. Massler, and M. A. Perlstein:
Tooth ring analysis in cerebral palsy. Am. J. Dis. Child. *107*: 370-378, 1964.

53. Wellock, W. D., A. Maitland and F. Brudevold:
Caries increments, tooth discoloration and state of oral hygiene in children given single annual application of acid phosphatase – fluoride and stannous fluoride. Arch. Oral Biol. *10*: 452-460, 1965.

54. Wilson, R. M. and P. Cleaton-Jones:
Enamel mottling and infectious exanthemata in a rural community. J. Dent. *6*: 161-165, 1978.

55. Winter, G. B., K. W. Lee and N. W. Johnson:
Hereditary amelogenesis imperfecta: a rare autosomal dominant type. Brit. Dent. J. *17*: 157-164, 1969.

56. Winter, G. B. and A. H. Brook:
Enamel hypoplasia and anomalies of the enamel. Dent. Clin. North Am. *19*: 3-24, 1975.

57. Witkop, C. J., Jr.:
Clinical aspects of dental anomalies. Int. Dent. J. *26*: 378-390, 1976.

58. Witkop. C. J., Jr. and L. Barros:
Oral and genetic studies of Chilean 1960, Part I. Oral anomalies. Am. J. Phys. Anthropol. *21*: 15-24, 1963.

59. Yip, W. K.:
The prevalance of dens evaginatus. Oral Surg. *38*: 80-87, 1974.

Chapter 6

Preventive Aspects of Pedodontics

Plaque control, oral hygiene instruction, nutritional and dietary counselling, and fluoride administration are fundamental aspects of good preventive dentistry and should be part of every pedodontic practice. Pit and fissure sealants have been introduced successfully in the last decade as additional means of preventing dental caries.

Preventive dentistry also consists of encouraging the patient to assume responsibility for his oral health. The idea of the dentist as the person who cures, and the patient only as a passive recipient of treatment is no longer acceptable, but concepts and rationale underlying prevention must be understood by the patient if he is to cooperate, and this problem, like others in pedodontics, requires explanation to the patient at a level appropriate to his age.

The development of good hygiene habits should take place early in life. Preschool children should be encouraged to develop these habits and continue them throughout life. It is difficult, however, to motivate young children as their manual dexterity is usually not well developed nor are they able to follow complex instructions. Starkey[66] points out that before age 7 it is unrealistic to expect adequate manual dexterity in a child, and a successful preventive program requires parental participation. Tsamtsouris[71] suggests that parents should clean their children's teeth and then let the child practice without forcing the issue. Since adoles-

cents are usually interested in personal appearance and peer acceptance, these aspects can be used to motivate teenagers to acquire habits of good dental hygiene.

Changing habits is a time-consuming process and cannot be accomplished in a short-term program. Prolonged interaction and supervision are required until the practice of concerned care becomes a new habit. Kaplan[26] outlines the positive and negative conditions that influence motivation in preventive measures in dentistry. The negative conditions which have to be overcome include: lack of understanding of dental health and disease, good dentition with little or no experience of dental problems, or, conversely, previous bad experience with dentistry and exposure to non-motivated or skeptical health professionals.

Dental plaque

Several investigators have demonstrated the influence of dental plaque on the etiology of dental caries. Its elimination is an important step in preventive dentistry. Dental plaque can be defined as a soft, adherent tooth deposit made up of bacteria and a matrix of bacterial products and salivary polymers. It is thought that dental plaque is formed through a process involving the attachment or entrapment of bacteria in mucinous salivary material deposited as a pellicle on the tooth surface. This deposition is followed by bacterial growth and multiplication. The formation of the acquired tooth pellicle results from selective adsorption of salivary glycoproteins to the tooth surface, and is a process that is renewed soon after tooth brushing. It seems that some proteinaceous components of saliva, not as yet entirely identified, are adsorbed on tooth surfaces, simultaneously promoting bacterial clumping. Oral bacteria further contribute a matrix of dextrans, levans, and extracellular polysaccharides which may contribute to the adhesiveness and nutrition of the plaque colonies. The longer the plaque remains on the tooth, the more bacterial flora will adhere and multiply. Several different microorganisms have been found in dental plaque, and it is thought that these are involved in the production of acid that dissolves tooth structure and causes caries. As the plaque becomes older, the fall in pH after sugar is applied becomes greater and it is more difficult to neutralize the acid produced. The patient and his family must learn that dental plaque increases susceptibility to dental caries and enhances the development of decay. Once this is understood, cooperation can often be obtained.

Dental plaque scoring

Epidemiologists have devised several plaque scoring tests. The most widely used are those described by Greene and Vermillion[23], Podshadley and Haley[54] and Martens and Maskin[35]. The last authors modified Greene and Vermillion's test by increasing the accuracy of recording, thus making it a good method for detailed plaque scoring. With the aid of erythrocin tablets or any other suitable disclosing solution, the presence of plaque is demonstrated and the amount and location recorded. The tooth is divided into 5 areas

for scoring (Fig. 6-1A). A score is given for each tooth recorded. Usually the buccal surfaces of three maxillary teeth and lingual surfaces of three mandibular teeth are evaluated. The surfaces evaluated in the primary dentition are the buccal surfaces of A, C, and I and the lingual surfaces of K, M, and S. In the permanent dentition the buccal surfaces of 3, 6, and 12 and the lingual surfaces of 19, 22, and 28 are usually chosen. If these teeth are not present, the antemeres may be used. Scores are assigned as follows:

0 – no debris present
1 – one tooth subdivision with debris
2-4 – the number of tooth surfaces on which debris is demonstrated (Fig. 6-1).

The sum of the individual scores of the 6 tooth surfaces examined constitutes the score for the mouth at a given time (PHP-M). This test is repeated at intervals to evaluate improvement of oral hygiene habits.

After bacterial plaque present has been quantified, its presence must be demonstrated to the patient, his parents, or both depending on the age of the patient (Fig. 6-2a and b). The patient is then shown how to remove the microbial mass and the area is stained again with a disclosing dye to check the thoroughness of cleaning. The patient is instructed to repeat this process each day at a regular convenient time and the presence of plaque and the gingival health conditions are reevaluated a week later.

Toothbrushing methodology

The removal of dental plaque is accomplished by toothbrushing and dental flossing. Dental floss is not indicated for use by small children. A study of the use of dental floss at the second grade level did not show beneficial results, but rather demonstrated its

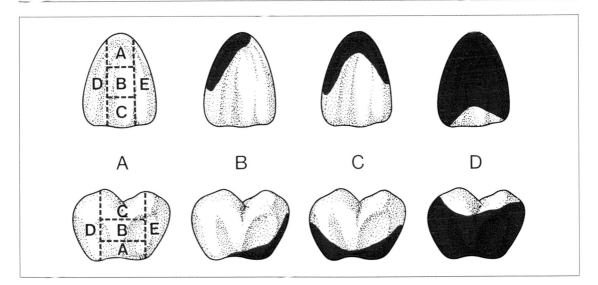

Fig. 6-1 Scoring method; (A) teeth marked in sections to allow proper scoring of plaque deposits; (B) score of 1; (C) score of 3; (D) score of 4.

misuse[9]. Terhune[69] demonstrated, however, that some 8 and 9-year-old children were able to learn how to use floss, but were much slower in learning then 10 and 11-year-old subjects.

Several different methods of toothbrushing have been advocated. The four methods most frequently used are:

ROLL METHOD: The toothbrush is placed with the bristle ends apically and the sides of the bristles touching the gingival tissue of the teeth. Lateral pressure is applied and the brush is moved towards the occlusal surface of the teeth. This rolling motion is repeated with segments of two teeth being brushed at one time. The lingual surfaces are brushed in the same manner.

HORIZONTAL SCRUBBING METHOD: The toothbrush is used horizontally with back and forth brushing strokes on both buccal and lingual surfaces.

CHARTERS' METHOD: The ends of the toothbrush bristles are placed in contact with the teeth and gingiva with the bristles at a 45° angle to the plane of occlusion. A lateral and downward pressure is then placed upon the brush, and the brush is vibrated gently back and forth.

MODIFIED FONES METHOD: The teeth are closed and the brush is placed in the buccal sulcus. The bristles are placed facing the teeth and the brush is rotated lightly and quickly in circles moving from the posterior to the anterior region. After repeating these motions on the other side of the mouth, the lingual surface of the teeth is cleaned by a flicking movement from the gingival tissues to surface. The occlusal surfaces of the posterior teeth are cleaned by a scrubbing motion.

Each of the methods has disadvantages. The roll method, frequently advocated for adults, and the Charters' method require

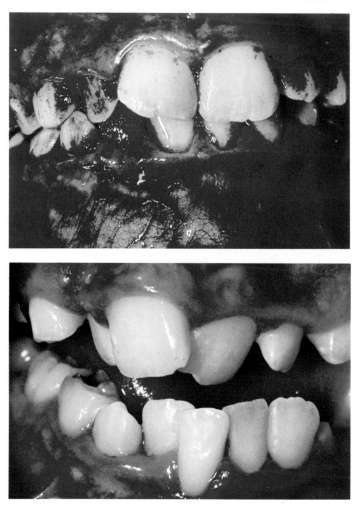

Fig. 6-2a and b   Disclosing solution in use to demonstrate dental plaque. Note plaque accumulation on tooth.

Figure 6-2a

Figure 6-2b

considerable manual dexterity. The same can be said for the Fones method, for which two different types of motion must be mastered. Prolonged use of the horizontal scrubbing method may lead to abrasion of the teeth and damage to the gingiva.

Several investigators have attempted to compare the effectiveness of plaque removal of these techniques. Studies have shown that the horizontal scrub technique is more effective than other brushing techniques in adults[18, 61] as well as in children[2, 38, 63]. Anaise[2] instructed 4 different groups of chil-

dren 11 to 14 years of age in the different techniques and compared the mean plaque score after 23 days. The horizontal scrubbing method was most effective in these groups and Charters' method was the least effective. Sangnes[63] compared the roll method to the horizontal scrub method in 6-year-old children brushing alone or having their teeth brushed by parents. Results indicate that the horizontal scrub technique performed by the parents was the most effective, and the roll method performed by the children the least effective in reducing plaque.

McClure[38] evaluated a group of children 3 to 5 years of age and concluded that some of these children were completely unable to master toothbrushing technique and that parental assistance was indispensable. The horizontal scrub method proved more effective than the roll technique when either the parent or the child brushed, although parental brushing was always more effective in this age group. The horizontal scrub method is indicated because of its speed and reduced dexterity requirements.

None of the methods appear to be effective on the proximal surfaces even in volunteer adult college students[18]. This seems to indicate the need for interproximal flossing at least in older patients. Berenie et al.[4] studied the relationship between the frequency of toothbrushing and oral hygiene and concluded that brushing once a day was insufficient for good oral hygiene, and that good oral hygiene requires at least two brushings a day, with a soft bristle toothbrush.

The effectiveness of electric toothbrushing has been studied by various investigators in handicapped and normal children. Some children who had difficulty in brushing because of their handicaps showed an improvement in oral hygiene when an electric toothbrush was used[29]. In normal children no major difference was found between electric and manual toothbrushes[51].

Several dentifrices containing a variety of agents have been developed in the hope of formulating a dentifrice with cariostatic activity. Of the different formulations, those dentifrices containing fluoride have shown some anticaries action, but even in this group dentifrices containing sodium fluoride have not shown positive clinical results. Dentifrices containing stannous fluoride and calcium pyrophosphate were recognized in 1960[1] by the American Dental Association as "effective anticaries" dentifrices and are available commercially under different brand names. Other fluoride compounds in dentifrices also have shown promising results. These include sodium monofluorophosphate[16, 21] and acidulated fluoride phosphate[8]. A small increase in fluoride concentration on the enamel surfaces of teeth treated by four different dentifrices containing fluoride in vitro was demonstrated by Kirkegaard in 1977[30].

Dietary counselling

Standards and tables for adequate diets have been in existence since the mid nineteen-forties and are revised as new knowledge is acquired. The tables are known as Recommended Dietary Allowance tables (RDA). Tables of the Minimum Daily Requirements (MDR) are prepared by the U.S. Food and Drug Administration, and are used primarily for labeling purposes. RDA values are useful for patient nutritional advice, the main aim of this advice being the establishment of a balanced diet that supplies the many requirements for healthy life. Individual adjustments must be made when counselling different ethnic and cultural groups because habits and customs have an influence on dietary patterns.

The objectives of dietary counselling in pedodontics are:

1. to explain to parents and children the nutritional values of different foods so that a nutritionally balanced diet may be achieved;
2. to identify the frequency of eating of foods containing sucrose and to quantify their damaging effects on dental health;
3. to offer a choice of acceptable substitutes that are non-cariogenic or of lesser cariogenicity, taking into consideration the personal needs and the motivations of the child and his family.

Since the first experiments of Lavoisier at the end of the 18th century and his famous statement "La vie est une fonction chimique" (life is a chemical function), great progress has been made in the basic understanding of food metabolism and in the science of nutrition. Awareness of adequate nutrition in the maintenance of good health and in prevention of disease has increased considerably in recent years. Much research is still needed in the study of the composition of foods and how their composition affects and alters human life.

In considering the role of various nutrients as a source of energy, two groups have been differentiated. The body requires certain nutrients in large quantities as primary sources of main chemical building blocks. These compounds are oxidized and yield the energy necessary for metabolic reactions, for thermal equilibrium, physical activity, and for other processes of life. This group consists of carbohydrates, proteins, and fats. A second group of required nutrients, necessary only in small amounts, are the vitamins and minerals. In addition, water is an important component of the diet, not as an energy furnishing element *per se,* but because it is indispensable in body chemistry. Some nutritionists also include fiber among nutrients. While not directly related to the chemistry of nutrition, its mechanical role is important to normal digestion. The nutritional requirements for other substances, particularly some trace elements, are not fully understood and further investigation probably will demonstrate still other minerals or trace elements to be essential in human nutrition.

The aim of nutrition is the production of energy. The energy produced through ingestion of food is measured in calories. The "calories" to which nutritional texts refer are kilocalories (in terms of physics). While food is usually described as containing calories, in reality it contains energy potential measured in calorie units. The caloric needs of an individual depend on the energy needs for maintenance of the individual, the energy requirements for specific dynamic actions, and the energy requirements for growth and maintenance of health. All of these needs vary with age and type of physical activity. Tables of nutritional requirements assembled by various investigators are available in specialized nutrition texts[49].

Carbohydrates

Carbohydrates (sugars and starches) are a major dietary source of energy. They are also important chemical components of body constituents such as glycoproteins, nucleic acids, and heparin. The amount of carbohydrates consumed in the diet is dependent on the economic and cultural development status of the individual, as carbohydrates are usually easily available and low in cost.

Proteins

The importance of proteins lies in the fact that they are composed of amino acids. Amino acids, once absorbed through the intestine, are utilized as building blocks of the cell. Some amino acids are called essential because they are not synthesized in the human body and must be obtained from food. These include: histidine, isoleucine, leucine, lysine, methionine, phenylalanine, threonine, tryptophan, and valine. Growing children also require arginine. The evaluation of the quality of a protein depends on body needs for growth maintenance, repair and reproduction. Nutritionists often qualify protein sources as "high quality" and "low quality" depending on the quantities of the different amino acids available in the source. "High quality" protein sources include meat and cheese, and "low quality" sources include vegetables such as beans (low in methionine), peanuts, and wheat products (low in lysine). When a protein is low in an important amino acid, it is considered unbalanced and this lack must be compensated through other proteins which contain larger amounts of that amino acid. This is critical because amino acid imbalances can be damaging to the growth and health of the individual.

Protein requirements are dependent on several conditions, and are relatively high in children because of growth and development. Through consumption of proteins, the body acquires nitrogen. If the nitrogen intake of foods is equal to the nitrogen elimination via the urine, the skin, and feces, the patient is in nitrogen balance. If the nitrogen intake is larger than that eliminated, the patient is in anabolism, or positive balance. Negative balance is termed catabolism or tissue destruction. These metabolic conditions are dependent on nutrition and endocrine balance. Acute bacterial, viral, or other infections, as well as accidental or surgical trauma can lead to negative nitrogen balance. Diets deficient in protein during tooth development can alter tooth morphology and tooth eruption patterns in laboratory animals[42, 52].

Fats

While an extensive literature relates fats to various diseases, they are nevertheless an important and essential part of the diet. Fatty acids are components of the cells and include phospholipids, a component of the cell membranes. Further, certain vitamins (A, D, E, and K) are fat soluble and are ingested as part of the fat that is eaten.

Vitamins and minerals

The need for small amounts of certain substances for maintenance of health in addition to carbohydrates, fats, and proteins was recognized already at the beginning of the 20th century. The word vitamin (vitamine) was coined in 1913 by Casimir Funk who discovered the cure for beriberi by using extracts of grain hulls. Vitamins are compounds that are needed as catalysts for adequate cellular metabolism. In man, most of them must be supplied in the diet. There are fat soluble vitamins such as A, D, E, and K, and water soluble vitamins such as vitamin C and those of the B complex.

Certain inorganic substances also have been found to be essential for life processes. These can be divided into two groups:

Group 1 includes calcium, phosphorus, magnesium, sodium, potassium, sulfur, iron, and chlorine which are necessary in relatively large quantities.

Group 2 includes trace minerals such as copper, manganese, zinc, iodine, cobalt, molybdenum, seleninum and fluorine.

In addition to their metabolic functions, calcium and phosphorus are important components of bones and teeth and are especially required during bone and tooth formation. Some of these inorganic substances are recirculated by the human body, but when heavy losses take place the ingested supply must be increased to replace them. An example is iron which is lost in severe bleeding. During growth periods there is also need for a large dietary supply of these inorganic substances. Detailed studies of nutritional requirements for minerals and electrolytes are available[49].

Foods are usually classified in 4 major groups and a system of exchange is established to allow inclusion of foods of each group in amounts suitable to the preparation of a varied diet.

The four major groups are:

A. Milk group: this group includes milk, different types of cheese, ice cream, and other dairy products. Three servings from this group are needed daily by children, 4 servings by adolescents, and 2 servings by adults.
B. Meat group: this group includes meats, eggs, fish, poultry, beans, peas, nuts, etc. Two servings a day are recommended for all age groups.
C. Vegetable and fruit group: two subgroups are recognized; yellow (such as carrots and turnips) and green (such as beans and spinach). Four or more servings per day are recommended for all age groups.
D. Cereals group: this group includes a wide variety of grains such as wheat, rice, corn, rye, barley, etc. Four or more daily servings are recommended for all ages.

The nutritional needs of the child change greatly with growth and development. These changes are dependent on sex, physiological conditions, and the physical activities of the youngster.

Diet and dental caries

The importance of dietary carbohydrates in the development of dental caries has been demonstrated in laboratory animals[64]. The severity of the condition varies with the type of carbohydrate. It is significantly increased by sucrose and increased slightly by raw wheat starch. It is thought that starches are less cariogenic than sugars because the molecules are hydrolyzed in the gastrointestinal tract. Thus, their sugar components are not easily available for cariogenic activity on the tooth surface.

Since the beginning of this century, several investigators have demonstrated that a carbohydrate substrate is necessary for acid formation through bacterial action. A low pH caused by rapid acid formation in the presence of sugars, particularly sucrose, seems to be a favorable condition for the development of oral bacteria associated with dental decay[17, 24, 44]. The cariogenic effects of refined sugar have been demonstrated in several studies[34]. One of the major early investigations was done by Gustaffson et al.[24] in Vipeholm, Sweden in 1954. Patients in a mental institution were given a basic diet which was supplemented with foods containing sugar for some groups. The results indicated that although the incidence of dental decay did not parallel the total amount of sugar ingested, a correlation existed between caries and the nature of the sweetened food and the frequency with which it was eaten. Recent investigations in laboratory animals apparently demonstrate that various carbohydrates have different effects on cariogenic microorganisms, sucrose being more cariogenic than glucose[32]. Patients on a diet with no sugar because of hereditary fructose intolerance have a very low incidence of dental caries[36]. Many laboratories currently are investigating this question but the evidence points to the cariogenic effects of diets rich in refined sugar.

The mouth, with its optimal temperature and moisture, is an excellent environment for bacterial growth. The large number of indigenous flora which have been described include microorganisms involved with production of dental decay. Bacteria derive their nutritional requirements directly from ingested food and indirectly from saliva and tissue fluids. Foods that remain in the oral cavity for long periods of time can be excellent nutrients for bacteria.

In order to counsel properly about a healthier and less caries-inducing diet, the nutritional pattern of the patient must be analyzed to establish quantitative and qualitative nutritional content. Nizel[49] has established a simplified technique for diet analysis which is widely used and is based on the four different food groups.

Initially the patient or parent is instructed to keep a food diary for a specified period of time, usually 5 days, and preferably including one weekend or a holiday, as diets frequently change on special occasions. It is important not only that food eaten at meal times, but also food and beverages taken between meals be recorded, and that the diet be the usual one without major changes during the trial period. The parent should not only record the type of food or beverage, but also the amount consumed, the manner of preparation, and types and quantities of additives (such as fats or sugars) used. Special forms can be furnished to the patient for record keeping. These have the psychological value of calling the attention of the patient to the importance of this aspect of preventive dentistry. It is essential that the record be detailed, accurate, and specific.

Certain problems should be remembered in evaluating this dietary history. Usually a 3 to 5-day survey is a more representative sample of diet than a 24-hour survey which can be uncharacteristic and incomplete (especially if done by recall). Even a 3 to 5 day recall diet may have been of a non-representative period, but this is less likely. A parent anxious to please the professional may provide incomplete or erroneous information about quantity and quality with the best of intentions. Further, the food provided for consumption and the food actually consumed can be different, depending on place and type of supervision during meal times. In evaluating the dietary history, notice should be taken that ethnic and cultural aspects can play an important role in types of food supplied.

A demonstration of the manner in which the diary should be kept is usually helpful. The best way is to record the diet of the last 24 hours in detail with the parent or patient. This can be considered as day 1 of the diary and will demonstrate to the parent how specific and detailed the record should be.

Once the diet diary is obtained, the next step is the evaluation of the number of sugar exposures in a day. All foods and beverages containing sugar, as well as dried fruits such as prunes, raisins, apricots, etc., should be underlined.

A table similar to Table 6-1 is useful in tallying the total and the average daily sugar exposures. Table 6-2 shows a tally table for the evaluation of food ingested, by food groups. This table also includes the recommended daily serving for each group. After evaluating and recording each day's food ingestion in the appropriate column, the calculated average is compared to the column of recommended amounts and the difference between the two columns recorded. Evaluation of these two tables will provide the practitioner with adequate information about type and quantity to enable him to provide adequate advice for a balanced and non-cariogenic diet. Demonstration of that group which is inadequately consumed is also easy with this type of tally table. The patient should also be questioned about food allergies, as elimination of certain foods from the diet may produce imbalanced nutritional habits. Careful examination of a child, combined with the information obtained from a dietary history, may raise questions about the adequacy of the child's nutrition and the patient may be referred to a pediatrician for further evaluation and treatment of the general condition. Because the number of daily sugar exposures is very important in caries prevention, as are the retentive properties of the sweets ingested, snack substitutes in the form of fresh fruit, vegetables, or cheese should be recommended. Nuts are not indicated as a snack for young children because of the danger of aspiration. A follow-up evaluation of the diet after a few months is essential for best results.

Table 6-1

Sweets consumption*

When eaten Meal	Sugar in Solution			Retentive Sweets			Solid Sweets		
	Between	During	End	Between	During	End	Between	During	End
1st day									
2nd day									
3rd day									
4th day									
5th day									
Total									
Grand total									

*Modified after Nizel[49]

Fluorides

Fluorides in drinking water in the optimum amount of 1 part per million will reduce dental caries significantly if ingested during the first 10 to 12 years of life[40]. This beneficial effect seems to be mostly post-natal; prenatal exposure does not seem to be cariostatic in later life[28].

Epidemiologic studies have demonstrated the unequivocal advantage of optimum water fluoridation for dental caries prevention. Studies of this question have been conducted since the mid-nineteen thirties and a large amount of data has been accumulated. In 1939, Dean et al.[12] evaluated the relationship between mottled enamel and dental caries by evaluating the incidence of dental decay in four midwestern cities of the United States with different natural fluoride contents in the drinking water. The four cities studied were located in close proximity and only children 12, 13, and 14 years old were evaluated. A more detailed study evaluating the same problem was conducted in eight Chicago suburban communities by Dean et al.[11]

Elmhurst, Maywood, Aurora and Joliet, with more than 1 ppm of fluoride in the water, were compared with Evanston, Oak Park, Waukegan, and Elgin with much less fluoride in the drinking water. Several other studies have also demonstrated the beneficial effect of fluoride in drinking water in reducing

Table 6-2

Dietary tabulation*

Groups	Milk Group	Meat Group	Vegetable/Fruit Group	Bread/Cereal Group
Recommended Servings	3-4	2 or more	4 or more	4 or more
1st day				
2nd day				
3rd day				
4th day				
5th day				
Average/day				
Deviation				

*Modified after Nizel[49]

dental decay. Since the mid-nineteen forties fluorides have been added to water supplies in many parts of the world, chiefly in metropolitan centers and noticeable reduction of dental decay has ensued.

Fluorides are a normal component of all food and are invariably present in the diet, especially in diets containing much seafood. Fluoride is rapidly absorbed by the gastrointestinal tract, apparently as an ion, and is absorbed faster in solution than in solid forms. Once absorbed, fluoride is either deposited in the hard tissues of the skeleton and teeth or is excreted in the urine[53]. There is a direct relation between fluoride in drinking water and fluoride content of the urine[39]. In developing bone and bone under-

going remodeling[73], fluoride is incorporated in the form of fluorohydroxyapatite[47].

Higher than optimum content of fluoride, however, adversely affects dental enamel and produces a condition of endemic fluorosis called mottled enamel[41]. Mottling is a dystrophic condition which appears as an opaque white color mottled with brown spots or yellow, brown, or black bands. This problem was described first in Italy at the turn of the century. It has been found in parts of the Rocky Mountain region of the United States and in other parts of the world where the fluoride content of the water is several parts per million.

Exposure of domestic animals and man to excessive quantities of fluoride can also produce serious problems of fluoride toxicosis. These may arise from high concentrations of naturally occurring fluoride in the drinking water or through contamination from industrial wastes. The effects of fluoride toxicosis have been studied extensively, particularly in domestic animals as these animals develop characteristic lameness and skeletal deformities[50]. Long bones, metacarpals, metatarsals and phalanges showed exostoses and increased diameter, while the animals were usually emaciated and failed to thrive. Bone defects in humans also have been demonstrated from fluoride toxicosis[33, 45].

The beneficial effect of optimal amounts of fluoride arise from systemic and topical tooth alterations. During tooth development, fluoride is incorporated into enamel and dentin. After eruption, fluoride has a topical effect, altering enamel structure and increasing its resistance to environmental factors. Recent studies have indicated that fluoride may interfere with bacterial growth and metabolism[27].

While communal water fluoridation remains the first choice for partial control of dental caries, in areas where communal water is not fluoridated other means of providing fluorides systematically have been studied and demonstrated to be effective. These alternatives include professionally applied topical fluorides, individual diet supplements, self-applied topical fluorides, and mouth rinses.

Use of fluoride tablets either in the drinking water or given directly to the patients has been studied in various countries[14, 20]. The effectiveness of tablets used by children in the home has been studied by Arnold et al.[3] Children ingested 1.0 mg fluoride (as NaF) daily under parental supervision, and proved it effective in both deciduous and permanent dentitions. According to Nikiforuk[48] the dosage schedule for fluoride in such a program was: age 0-2 years: 0.25 mg/day;

2-4 years: 0.50 mg; 4-6 years, 0.75 mg/day and over 6 years, 1 mg/day. Such a regimen obviously requires major cooperation, interest, and motivation of the parents. As fluoride in very high quantities (300-700 mg for a 20-pound child) can be toxic or even lethal, the number of tablets prescribed at any one time must be kept below the lethal dose, and the tablets should be kept out of the reach of children (Table 6-3). In addition to tablets, fluorides have been added to milk (1.0 mg fluoride)[62] with great cariostatic success. Fluoridated table salt is available in some communities, and has been shown to be effective when used regularly[37]. Care must be taken that such programs are used only in regions where the natural fluoride content of the drinking water is known, to avoid excessive fluoride intake.

With the rising cost of health care, several attempts have been made to develop effective caries reduction programs using self-applied topical methods. Fluoride suitable for use in public health programs for large groups of patients, in school settings, and in individual programs in the home include toothbrushing with fluoride solution, paste, or gel, rinsing with a mouth rinse containing fluoride, and use of trays containing fluoride gel.

Individual brushing of teeth by children using fluoride solution, gels or pastes can be effective for caries reduction. Daily rinsing with 0.05% NaF solution is also an effective means of reducing caries development[70]. Good results were demonstrated when fitted trays containing sodium fluoride gel (pH7) were used each school day for 6 minutes over a 21-month period[15]. These methods are suitable for use in regions without fluoride, and have been reviewed by Ripa[57] who recommends use of one of the following programs, depending on the individual condition of the patient:

Brushing: once a month with a prophylactic

Table 6-3

Recommended daily dosages of fluoride supplements*

Natural fluoride in existing water	Age of child (years)	
	0-2.0	3-12
0 -0.25 ppm	0.50 ml. 1 tab.	1.0 ml. 2 tab.
0.25-0.45 ppm	0.25 ml. 0.5 tab.	0.75 ml. 1.5 tab.
0.50-0.75 ppm	0 0	0.5 ml. 1 tab.

* Adapted from Nikitoruk[48]

paste or gel is the preferred method for the preschool child who is not yet able to "swish" properly. Parents are instructed to brush the patient's teeth first with the usual dentifrice.

Mouth rinsing: older children able to rinse properly are instructed to use a solution containing 5ml (one teaspoon) of either an APF solution or a neutral NaF solution for 30 seconds, once daily, after regular toothbrushing.
The solution can be prepared from a concentrated solution. A tablet containing 2.2mg of NaF in 4.4ml water will provide a solution containing 0.05% of NaF.

Custom trays: individual mouth trays are prepared for the child (age 12 years and over) who is instructed to place 5 to 10 drops of an acidulated phosphate fluoride gel in each tray and to keep this tray in contact with the teeth for 5 minutes five times a week.
The combined use of biannual self-applications of 2.2% phosphate fluoride prophylactic paste and weekly 0.2% NaF mouth rinses resulted in a significantly lower caries incidence in a school population of students aged 8-10, tested over a 2-year period[56].

Daily use during the school week of a rinse containing 1.0mgF-/5ml in phosphate solution at pH 4 by high school students reduced caries by 25%[19].
Topical application of several different compounds by dental professionals has been used with positive results for several years. Initially sodium fluoride topical solutions were applied with a caries reduction of up to 33%. Studies using stannous fluoride show slightly better results (36% caries reduction)[6]. More recently, acidulated sodium fluoride phosphate has been tested with 61% caries reduction[7]. Evidence accumulated since 1942[5] indicates that partial control of dental caries can be obtained by the use of professionally applied fluorides. Since that time, there has been continuing research to develop compounds and techniques which will have a higher cariostatic effect; many fluoride compounds have been tested and proven to be effective. In areas of optimal public water fluoridation, the dentist still must evaluate possible benefits of individualized use of fluorides as dental caries develop, even in zones of fluoridation. Any inhibition in caries development is beneficial to the patient, especially when "high-

risk" patients can be identified. Originally, 4 applications of 2% aqueous solution of sodium fluoride, 2 to 7 days apart, were made at ages 3, 7, 11 and 13 to protect newly erupted teeth[31]. A thorough prophylaxis was performed before the first fluoride application. The 2% fluoride solution is relatively stable and can be stored in plastic containers for 2-3 weeks. More recently Mercer and Muhler[43] have shown that 8% stannous fluoride solution applied only once every 6 months during routine dental recall visits is highly effective. Difficulties in routine use caused by chemical instability and unpleasant taste and odor made it desirable to continue the search for other means of fluoride application.

Of the various fluoride compounds tested, acidulated phosphate fluoride was developed with the aim of obtaining maximum fluoride uptake[13]. This is a mixture of sodium fluoride and orthophosphoric acid and, while it produces high immediate fluoride uptake and great depth of penetration, the fluoride concentration subsequently falls[67]. Acidulated phosphate fluoride must be kept in plastic bottles because it etches glass and porcelain, but it can be flavored and colored without reducing effectiveness. The gel is placed in trays that fit over the patient's dental arches, care being taken to have the teeth as free as possible of saliva before insertion of the tray which is kept in place for 4 minutes. Depending on the type of tray used, efforts are made to cause the gel to flow into the interproximal spaces of the teeth. The patient is instructed not to rinse, eat, or drink for 30 minutes. Recent laboratory tests have suggested that use of stannous fluoride with acidulated phosphate fluoride is a more effective cariostatic treatment than sodium fluoride, but more laboratory testing is necessary. The high uptake of ammonium fluoride by enamel also has been demonstrated, but further clinical tests are necessary[72].

Pit and fissure sealants

The protective effect of fluorides is considerably less in the fissure areas than on smooth surfaces. It is thought that this is due to the thinness of the enamel at the base of the fissure and the morphology at the base which allows food debris to remain over long periods of time so that acid attack subsequently takes place. The recent development of commercially available pit and fissure sealants has been an important addition to preventive dentistry. The technique of acid etching with phosphoric acid was initially described by Buonocore in 1955[6]. Since then, several chemicals have been tested in vitro. At present the agents generally used for clinical etching are 50% citric acid or orthophosphoric acid of varying concentrations. Chelating agents such as EFTA have been rejected for this procedure as the necessary changes are not produced within suitable clinical time[65]. The effect of etching has been described as the removal of the outer thin layer of aprismatic enamel, permitting the interlocking of the resin which can flow into the spaces and polymerize there. There is a mechanical interlocking of the resin, 10 to 25 μm deep, with the etched surface rather than true adhesion[25].

The majority of commercially available fissure sealants consist of a resin that polymerizes, either under the effect of an ultraviolet light source or by chemical means following the mixing of the components. It is likely that materials with longer shelf life and less temperature sensitivity will be developed.

The ideal material to be used as a sealant should have the following properties:

1. The material should be non-toxic and not irritating to the tissues
2. It must be able to adhere to the tooth as a thin layer

3. The consistency and viscosity before polymerization must permit flow and penetration easily into small areas during clinical use
4. The mechanical, compressive and tensile properties of the material once polymerized should be sufficient to withstand mastication and to resist wear
5. Shrinkage or expansion of the material after polymerization should be as low as possible, to avoid marginal leakage
6. Water absorption and solubility after polymerization should be as low as possible to assure resistance to displacement and discoloration
7. The material should have optical properties that allow it to be seen but be harmonious with tooth structure.

Resins of cyanoacrylate[10, 58, 68], polyurethane[60], and dimethacrylate types[59] have been tested clinically. The dimethacrylate types such as bisphenol A and glycidylmethacrylate (also referred to as Bis-GMA) have shown greatest durability. Results after two years of clinical trials of 4 different commercially available fissure sealants demonstrated that at least two, Nuva Seal (80%) and Epoxylite (51.5%), remained on the tooth surface and were intact with demonstrable caries reduction when compared to controls[60].

Comparative studies on the retention of the sealants on permanent and primary teeth demonstrate that permanent teeth retain the material better than the primary[55, 58], but even primary teeth retain the material in a number of cases. Indications are that sealants are occasionally useful in mentally retarded children[55].

The pits and fissures to be sealed should be deep and narrow but not decayed. Tissues that show regions of decalcification on radiographs should not be sealed but treated by removal of the decayed tissue. Tooth eruption should be sufficiently advanced so that no overlapping mucosal tag remains on the occlusal surface. Sealants should be applied soon after the eruption of the first permanent molars and again when the second permanent molars and premolars have erupted (12-13 years). The sealant should be reevaluated at each 6 month follow-up visit and replaced as necessary.

Application procedure

Absolute moisture control is of major importance in adequate sealant application. The enamel should be cleaned properly with a rubber prophylactic cup and suitable paste before application and debris should be removed carefully with thorough rinsing. The acid is then applied with a brush or cotton pellet and allowed to remain on the area to be etched for the correct time. Depending on the particular product, this is normally 30 seconds to one minute. Longer conditioning (up to 90 seconds) apparently improves sealant retention on the occlusal surfaces of primary teeth[22]. The acid is then flushed off the tooth surface, and the tooth dried. Correctly etched enamel has a dull white appearance. The sealant is applied and allowed to polymerize in the manner appropriate to the particular material. By scrupulous attention to technique and control of moisture, preferably with the use of a rubber dam, good results can be obtained.

In areas of low fluoride concentration in the public water supplies, the application of sealants also should be accompanied by some type of topical fluoride schedule as the sealants do not reduce the incidence of interproximal caries.

References

1. American Dental Assoc. Council on Dental Therapeutics:
Evaluation of Crest toothpaste. J. Am. Dent. Assoc. *61*:272-274, 1960.

2. Anaise, J.Z.:
The toothbrush in plaque removal. J. Dent. Child. *42*:186-189, 1975.

3. Arnold, F.A., Jr., F.J. McClure and C.L. White:
Sodium fluoride tablets for children. Dent. Progr. *1*:8-12, 1960.

4. Berenie, J., L.W. Ripa and G. Leske:
The relationship of frequency of toothbrushing, oral hygiene, gingival health and caries-experience in school children. J. Public Health Dent. *33*:160-171, 1973.

5. Bibby, B.G.:
A new approach to caries prophylaxis: a preliminary report on the use of fluoride applications. Tufts Dent. Outlook *15*(4):4-8, 1942.

6. Buonocore, M.G.:
Simple method of increasing the adhesion of acrylic filling materials to enamel surfaces. J. Dent. Res. *34*:849-853, 1955.

7. Buonocore, M.G. and B.G. Bibby:
Fluoride dentifrices, topical fluorides and fluoridation. *In* Pharmacotherapeutics of oral disease. Kutscher, A.H., E.V. Zegarelli and G.A. Hyman (eds.). New York, McGraw-Hill, 1966.

8. Bullen, D.C.T., F. McCombie and L.W. Hole:
Two year effect of supervised toothbrushing with an acidulated fluoride-phosphate solution. J. Canad. Dent. Assoc. *32*:89-93, 1966.

9. Bryn, K.J.:
A report on the feasibility of a plaque control program with the use of dental floss at a second grade level in a school setting. J. Indiana Dent. Assoc. *52*:437-441, 1973.

10. Cueto, E.I. and M.G. Buonocore:
Sealing of pits and fissures with an adhesive resin: its use in caries prevention. J. Am. Dent. Assoc. *75*:121-128, 1967.

11. Dean, H.T., P. Jay, F.A. Arnold Jr. and E. Elvove:
Domestic water and dental caries. II. A study of 2,832 white children aged 12-14 years of 8 suburban Chicago communities including Lactobacillus acidophilus studies of 1,761 children. Public Health Rep. *56*:761-792, 1941.

12. Dean, H.T., P. Jay, F.A. Arnold Jr., F.J. McClure and E. Elvove:
Domestic water and dental caries including certain epidemiological aspects of L. acidophilus. Public Health Rep. *54*:862-888, 1939.

13. DePaola, P.F. and J.R. Mellberg:
Caries experience and fluoride uptake in children receiving semiannual prophylaxis with an acidulated phosphate fluoride paste. J. Am. Dent. Assoc. *87*:155-159, 1973.

14. Driscoll, W.S., S.B. Heifetz and D.C. Korts:
Effect of chewable fluoride tablets on dental caries in school children: results after six years use. J. Am. Dent. Assoc. *97*:820-824, 1978.

15. Englander, H.R., P.H. Keyes, M. Gestwicki and H.A. Sultz:
Clinical anticaries effect of repeated topical sodium fluoride applications by mouthpieces. J. Am. Dent. Assoc. *75*:638-644, 1967.

16. Finns, S.F. and H.C. Jamison:
A comparative clinical study of three dentifrices. J. Dent. Child. *30*:17-25, 1963.

17. Fosdick, L.S. and D.Y. Burrill:
The effect of pure sugar solutions on the hydrogen in concentration of carious lesion. Fortnightly Rev. *6*:7-10, 1943.

18. Frandsen, A.M., J.P. Barbano, J.D. Suomi, J.J. Chang and R. Houston:
A comparison of the effectiveness of the Charters', scrub, and roll methods of toothbrushing in removing plaque. Scand. J. Dent. Res. *80*:267-271, 1972.

19. Frankl, S.N., S. Fleisch and R.R. Diodati:
The topical anticariogenic effect of daily rinsing with an acidulated phosphate fluoride solution. J. Am. Dent. Assoc. *85*:882-886, 1972.

20. Gedalia, I.:
Fluoride tablets. Int. Dent. J. *17*:18-30, 1967.

21. Goaz, P.W., L.P. McElwaine, H.A. Biswell and W.E. White:
Effect of daily applications of sodium monofluorophosphate solution on caries rate in children. J. Dent. Res. *42*:965-972, 1963.

22. Gourley, J.M.:
A one year study of a fissure sealant in two Nova Scotia communities. J. Canad. Dent. Assoc. *40*:549-552, 1974.

23. Greene, J.C. and J.R. Vermillion:
Simplified oral hygiene index. J. Am. Dent. Assoc. *68*:7-13, 1964.

24. Gustaffson, B.E., C.E. Quensel, L.S. Lanke, C. Lundqvist, H. Grahnen, B.E. Bonow and B. Krasse:
The Vipeholm dental caries study: the effect of different levels of carbohydrate intake on caries activity in 436 individuals observed for five years. (Sweden). Acta Odontol. Scand. *11*:232-364, 1954.

25. Gwinnett, A.J.:
Morphology of the interface between adhesive resins and treated human enamel fissures as seen by scanning electron microscopy. Arch. Oral Biol. *16*:237-238, 1971.

26. Kaplan, R.I.:
Preventive dentistry – fact or fad. J. Am. Coll. Dent. *40*:217-224, 248, 1973.

27. Kashket, S., V.M. Rodriguez and F.J. Bunick:
Inhibition of glucose utilization on oral streptococci by low concentrations of fluoride. Caries Res. *11*:301-307, 1977.

28. Katz, S. and J.C. Muhler:
Prenatal and postnatal fluoride and dental caries experience in deciduous teeth. J. Am. Dent. Assoc. *76*:305-311, 1968.

29. Kelner, M.:
Comparative analysis of the effects of automatic and conventional toothbrushing in mental retardates. Penn. Dent. J. *30*:102-108, 1963.

30. Kirkegaard, E.:
In vitro fluoride uptake in human dental enamel from four different dentifrices. Caries Res. *11*:24-29, 1977.

31. Knutson, J.W. and W.D.:
The effect of topically applied sodium fluoride on dental caries experience. Public Health Rep. *58*:1701-1715, 1943.

32. Krasse, B.:
The effect of caries-inducing streptococci in hamsters fed diets with sucrose or glucose. Arch. Oral Biol. *10*:223-226, 1965.

33. Latham, M.C.:
The effects of excessive fluoride intake. Am. J. Public Health *57*:651-660, 1967.

34. Losee, F.L.:
Enamel caries research: 1962-1964. J. Am. Dent. Assoc. *70*:1428-1432, 1965.

35. Martens, L.V. and L.H. Meskin:
An innovative technique for assessing oral hygiene. J. Dent. Child. *39*:12-14, 1972.

36. Marthaler, T.M. and E.R. Froesch:
Hereditary fructose intolerance: dental status of 8 patients. Brit. Dent. J. *123*:57-99, 1967.

37. Marthaler, T.M. and C. Schenardi:
Inhibition of caries in children after 5-1/2 years of fluoridated table salt. Helv. Odontol. Acta. *6*:1-6, 1962.

38. McClure, D.B.:
A comparison of toothbrushing technics for the preschool child. J. Dent. Child. *33*:205-210, 1966.

39. McClure, F.J. and C.A. Kinser:
Fluoride domestic waters and systemic effects. II. Fluorine content of urine in relation to fluorine in drinking water. Public Health Rep. *59*:1575-1591, 1944.

40. McClure, F.J.:
Water fluoridation. The search and the victory. Bethesda, Md., U.S. Dept. Health. Ed. Welfare, 1970.

41. McKay, F.S.:
Mottled enamel: the prevention of its further production through a change of the water supply at Oakley, Ida. J. Am. Dent. Assoc. *20*:1137-1149, 1933.

42. Menaker, L. and J.M. Navia:
Effect of undernutrition during prenatal period on caries development in the rat. IV. Effects of differential tooth eruption and exposure to a cariogenic diet on subsequent dental caries incidence. J. Dent. Res. *52*:692-697, 1973.

43. Mercer, V.H. and J.C. Muhler:
Comparison of single topical applications of sodium fluoride and stannous fluoride. J. Dent. Res. *51*:1325-1330, 1972.

44. Miller, W.D.:
The microorganisms of the human mouth. Philadelphia, S.S. White, 1890.

45. Moller, P.F. and S.V. Gudjonsson:
Massive fluorosis of bone and ligaments. Acta Radiol. *13*:269-294, 1932.

46. Murray, J.J.:
Fluorides in caries prevention. Bristol, Wright, 1976.

47. Neumann, W.F., M.W. Neuman, E.R. Main, J. O'Leary and F.A. Smith:
The surface chemistry of bone. II. Fluoride deposition. J. Biol. Chem. *187*:655-661, 1950.

48. Nikiforuk, G.:
Fluoride supplements for prophylaxis of caries. Can. Dent. Hyg. *10*:43-46, 1976.

49. Nizel, A.E.:
Nutrition in preventive dentistry: science and practice. 2nd Ed. Philadelphia, Saunders, 1980.

50. Obel, A.L.:
A literary review on bovine fluorosis. Acta Vet. Scand. *12*:151-163, 1971.

51. Owen, T.L.
A clinical evaluation of electric and manual toothbrushing by children with primary dentitions. J. Dent. Child. *39*:15-21, 1972.

52. Paynter, K.J. and Grainger, R.M.:
The relation of nutrition to the morphology and size of rat molar teeth. J. Canad. Dent. Assoc. *22*:519-531, 1956.

53. Perkinson, J.D. Jr., I.B. Whitney, R.A. Monroe, W.E. Lotz and C.L. Comar:
Metabolism of fluoride in domestic animals. Am. J. Physiol. *55*:383-389, 1955.

54. Podshadley, A.G. and J.V. Haley:
A method for evaluation of oral hygiene performance. Pub. Health Rep. *83*:259-264, 1968.

55. Richardson, B.A., D.C. Smith and J.A. Hargreaves:
Study of a fissure sealant in metally retarded Canadian children. Community Dent. Oral Epidemiol. *5*:220-226, 1977.

56. Ringleberg, M.I., A.J. Conti and D.B. Webster:
An evaluation of single and combined self-applied fluoride programs in schools. J. Public Health Dent. *36*:229-236, 1976.

57. Ripa, L.W.:
Self-application of topical fluoride: review and recommendations for use in a private office program. Quintessence Int. *7*(11):51-58, 1976.

58. Ripa, L.W. and W.W. Cole:
Occlusal sealing and caries prevention: results 12 months after a single application of adhesive resins. J. Dent. Res. *49*:171-173, 1970.

59. Rock, W.P.:
Fissure sealants: results obtained with two different sealants after one year. Brit. Dent. J. *133*:146-151, 1972.

60. Rock. W.P.:
Fissure sealants. Further results of clinical trials. Brit. Dent. J. *136*:317-321, 1974.

61. Rodda, J.C.:
A comparison of four methods of toothbrushing. N.Z. Dent. J. *64*:162-167, 1968.

62. Russoff, L.L., B.S. Kanikoff, J.B. Frye, J.E. Johnston and W.W. Frye:
Fluoride addition to milk and its effect on dental caries in school children. Am. J. Clin. Nutr. *11*:94-101, 1962.

63. Sangnes, C.:
Effectiveness of vertical and horizontal toothbrushing techniques in the removal of plaque. II. Comparison of brushing by six year old children and their parents. J. Dent. Child. *41*:119-123, 1974.

64. Shaw, J.H.:
The effect of carbohydrate-free and carbohydrate-low diets on the incidence of dental caries in white rats. J. Nutr. *53*:151-162, 1954.

65. Silverstone, L.M.:
Fissure sealants. Laboratory studies. Caries Res. *8*:2-26, 1974.

66. Starkey, P.:
Instructions to parents for brushing the child's teeth. J. Dent. Child. *28*:42-47, 1961.

67. Stearns, R.I.:
Incorporation of fluoride by human enamel. III. In vivo effects of nonfluoride and fluoride prophylactic pastes and APF gels. J. Dent. Res. *52*:30-35, 1973.

68. Takeuchi, M., T. Shimizu, T. Kizu, M. Eto, M. Nakagawa, T. Ohsawa and T. Oishi:
Sealing of the pit and fissure with resin adhesive: IV. Results of five-year field work and a method of evaluation of field work for caries prevention. Bull. Tokyo Dent. Coll. *12*:295-316, 1971.

69. Terhune, J.A.:
Predicting the readiness of elementary school children to learning an effective dental flossing technique. J. Am. Dent. Assoc. *88*:1332-1336, 1973.

70. Torell, P.:
Two-year clinical tests with different methods of local caries preventive fluoride application in Swedish school children. Acta Odontol. Scand. 23:287-322, 1965.

71. Tsamtsouris, A.:
Preventive measures for the preschool child. J. Pedod. 2:30-38, 1977.

72. Wei, S.H.Y. and E.M. Schulz, Jr.:
In vivo microsampling of enamel fluoride concentrations after topical treatments. Caries Res. 9:50-58, 1975.

73. Zipkin, I., F.J. McClure, N.C. Leone and W.A. Lee:
Fluoride deposition in human bones after prolonged ingestion of fluoride in drinking water. Pub. Health Rep. 73:732-740, 1958.

Chapter 7

Dental Caries, Pulp, and Periodontal Diseases

Dental caries

Dental caries is one of the most prevalent diseases of mankind and is ubiquitous in civilized populations. Unlike many other diseases, its incidence tends to increase with improved socio-economic conditions. There are wide variations in caries incidence, depending on cultural and socio-economic differences; these are related in part to eating habits, including increased consumption of refined sugars. Since the work of W. D. Miller in 1889[25], the etiology of dental caries has been associated with acid dissolution of the mineral tooth components, the acid being produced by oral bacteria using dietary carbohydrates as a substrate.

Extensive evidence has been presented that bacteria are necessary for the progress of caries attack. The role of microorganisms in the etiology of dental caries was demonstrated unequivocally by Orland and his co-workers[28, 29]. In these experiments, a high intake of cariogenic diet alone was insufficient to produce dental caries in germfree animals. When a bacterial population isolated from conventional rat mouth was introduced with the same diet, dental caries developed. Various mechanisms of pathogenesis have been proposed and are being studied in several research laboratories. Progress in microbiological research may make it possible to specify which organisms are primarily involved. Fitzgerald and Keyes[11] demonstrated that hamster caries could be transmitted from animal to animal. Dental caries can be considered a transmissible infection with colonization of tooth surface by a group of bacteria capable of fermenting dietary carbohydrate *in situ*. The acid produced, acting at susceptible sites, can initiate the carious process by demineralization of the enamel surface. Like any other infectious disease, treatment is through the eradication of the etiological agent, removal of the affected tissue, and increased host resistance. Host immunity can be obtained by the acquisition of specific immunological defenses, and much research is devoted to this goal at present.

Caries prevention can be achieved only by adequately modifying dietary habits and the environment in which bacteria act, and in reducing tooth permeability. The bacteria found in the carious lesion metabolize sucrose, producing dextran (an adhesive polysaccharide) from the glucose moiety and lactic acid from the fructose moiety. As caries development is dependent on the relationship of tooth surface, oral microorganisms, and dietary foodstuff, control of decay depends on the effective modification of these factors and their interactions. Adequate prevention methods (Chapter 6) should be given priority in the effort to reduce decay.

Enhancing the resistance of the tooth to carious attack is another approach to reducing caries. Sealants and fluorides are used extensively at present in this approach.

Trace elements also may be effective in decay prevention and further research will determine their role in the process.

Several saliva factors seem to play a role in the etiology of tooth decay[35]. Saliva has a sugar buffering capacity and salivary viscosity also is an important factor.

Classification of dental caries

According to the anatomical position, dental caries can be either pit and fissure caries or smooth surface caries. In both types, the breakdown of enamel follows the direction of the enamel rods. In pit and fissure caries the initial spread is narrow, but when the dentin is reached there is a lateral spread of the lesion following a conical shape in the dentin, with the apex of the cone towards the pulp and the base of the cone at the dentinoenamel junction (Fig. 7-1).

In smooth surface caries the external surface of the lesion is broader but the spread follows a similar pattern at the level of the dentinoenamel junction. Thus it is possible to distinguish lesions which affect only the enamel and others which affect both the enamel and dentin, the severity depending on the depth of penetration of the lesion.

Clinically the caries attack may range from a very rapid, deeply penetrating destruction to a slowly progressing lesion. The two types usually can be differentiated by the color and consistency of the carious dentin. An arrested lesion is usually dark, with color varying from dark yellow to brown-black (Fig. 7-2), leathery surface, and usually is not sensitive to mild stimulation. Clinically, the active, rapidly progressing lesion has a soft, lightly stained, friable surface (Fig. 7-3). Some carious lesions have both characteristics indicating either a reactivation or retardation of the process[21].

Structural aspects of dental caries

Early enamel caries are characterized by partial dissolution of calcified tissue with the lesion progressing towards the dentino-enamel junction. The greatest zone of demineralization in early caries is located more centrally in the affected enamel, suggesting some remineralization on the surface. The various zones have different refractive indices, indicating variations in density and mineralization.

Small carious lesions usually have a "cone shape". Larger lesions have a truncated cone because of proximity to the pulp and a apparent slowing of the lesion in the dentinal-pulpal region.

After the carious process has reached the dentin, phases of activity followed by phases of arrest and possible reactivation are noticeable. The dentin reacts to these attacks by forming calcific barriers with occlusion of dentinal tubules by secondary mineralization or development of sclerotic tracts[38]. A calcitraumatic line (basophilic line) usually can be demonstrated histologically as a limit of permeability of the dentin. (Fig. 7-4) The regularity or irregularity of the secondary dentin formed may depend on the severity and incremental progress of the lesion[21]. Not all dentinal tracts become sclerotic; some lose their odontoblastic processes and are filled by cell debris and organic matter. These are called "dead tracts" and are permeable.

Histopathologic studies of demineralized and ground tooth sections demonstrate that the carious lesion is made up of several zones of carious activity. These layers are not neatly limited but are dependent on the progress of the process. The layers usually observed are:

External layer of destruction: in this layer the dentin is necrotic and decalcified with large cavities containing organic remnants and microorganisms (Fig. 7-5).

Fig. 7-1   Fissure caries spread at the level of the dentinoenamel junction.

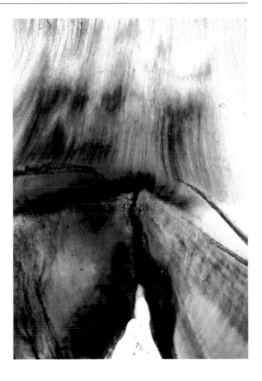

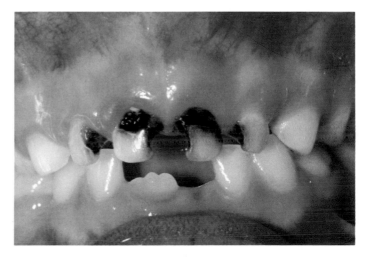

Fig. 7-2   Dental caries, arrested. Note the dark color of the lesion.

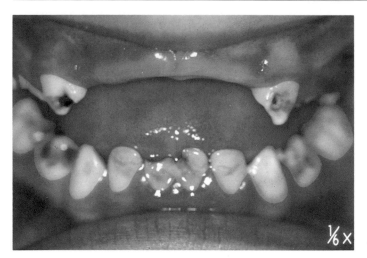

Fig. 7-3   Dental caries, active. Note the light color of the lesion.

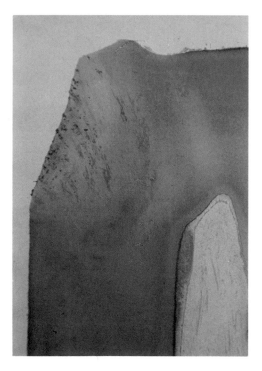

Fig. 7-4   Histologic section through a tooth with dental caries. Note the dark stained limiting layer around the carious process and the development of reparative dentin.

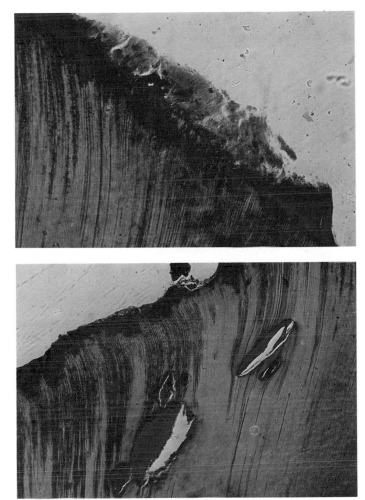

Fig. 7-5 Outer caries layer of dentin showing necrotic and decalcified tissue.

Fig. 7-6 Histological section through dental caries showing the infected layer.

The infected layer: in this layer the dentin is decalcified but still recognizable. The distended tubular structure is invaded with microorganisms (Fig 7-6).

The layer of decalcification: in this layer the dentin has lost much mineral content but the tubules do not contain microorganisms.

The translucent layer: this layer is occluded with highly mineralized sclerotic occluded dentinal tubules. The closure of the tubules may constitute a barrier against fast penetration of bacteria and toxic material into the pulp.

Reparative dentin layer: formation of reparative dentin under the lesion is also a block against further damage to the pulp by the bacteria and toxic material which infect the carious tissues. There is a good correlation between the amount of reparative dentin laid down, superficial destruction, and the speed of destruction by the carious process (Fig. 7-7).

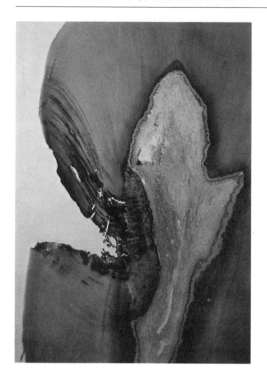

Fig. 7-7 Histological section showing the formation of secondary dentin.

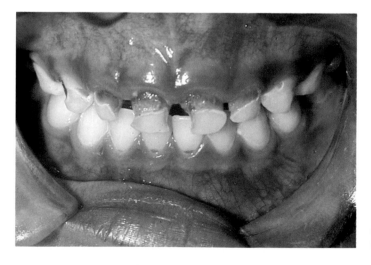

Fig. 7-8 Extensive dental caries in a 3-year-old boy due to extended nursing time.

Fig. 7-9 a to c Anterior caries in a 3-year-old boy (a) intraoral photograph; (b) radiograph of wire to stabilize the crown; (c) polycarbonate crowns in place.

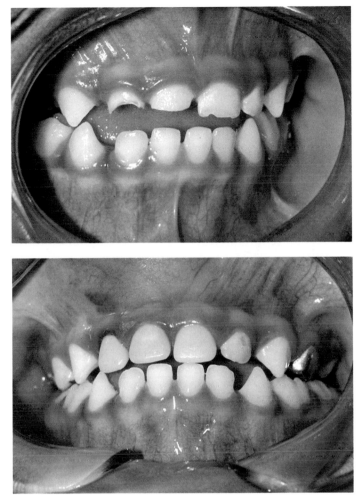

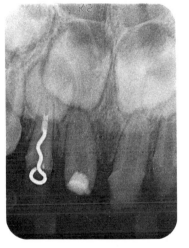

Nursing bottle caries

The term nursing bottle caries was originally used by Fass[10] who described the problem of extensive dental caries in very young children who had been bottle fed for a long time or often had been given a pacifier dipped in sweetened fluid.

The problem of increased incidence of caries with bottle feeding seems to be related not only to the number of times the bottle is provided but also to its content[6]. Studies also demonstrate that frequent "on demand" breast feeding of small children can lead to a pattern of extensive tooth destruction of the primary teeth[15]. In either case, the caries process can be demonstrated on the labial and incisal areas of the maxillary anterior teeth and in more advanced examples on the molar regions too (Fig. 7-8) In very advanced cases the mandibular anterior teeth are also affected. Treatment of the condition often involves complete oral rehabilitation with crowns (Fig. 7-9a to e). Many times this treatment must be rendered under general anesthesia because of the young age of the patient.

Clinical assessment and treatment of the carious lesion

Optimal treatment of carious lesions depends on:

1. Complete removal of carious tissues
2. Preservation of pulp able to react to stimuli without irreversible pathological changes
3. Establishment of a hermetically sealed and lasting restoration

Complete removal of the carious tissues

Treatment of a carious lesion should result in the total arrest of the process and preservation of pulp vitality if possible. This can be attained best with total removal of all infected tissue. After all the infected dentin is removed, the exact cavity outline is established. The type of restoration to be placed depends on the amount of healthy tooth structure available and the type of support this structure can give. If the carious process is too extensive silver amalgam restorations cannot be placed because inadequate cavity walls will result in cusp fractures. In these cases prefabricated stainless steel crowns are better than silver amalgam restorations.

Primary teeth present special problems in restoration because of their unique morphology. In many cases the causes of failure of restorations are faulty design and inadequate manipulation of the restorative material.

When primary teeth are prepared the usual sound principles of cavity preparation must be observed. That is, all carious tissue must be removed, the remaining enamel be well supported, and the pulp not endangered.

The major differences between cavity preparations in primary and permanent teeth is the shape of the teeth and contact areas, the morphology of the pulp, and the general configuration of the enamel rods (Figs. 7-10 to 7-12).

The shape of the primary molars must be emphasized. The crowns of these teeth have such a barrel shape that a definite enamel bulge can be noticed with a marked constriction at the gingival margin. The floor of the proximal box of a class II cavity preparation should break contact, but not be placed too far apically of this bulge. If the floor of the proximal wall is placed too far apically a new axial wall must be established by moving it pulpally. This endangers the pulp tissue, possibly even causing pulp exposure.

The width and depth of the cavity preparation should be designed to avoid the pulp tissue, in particular the horns which normally can be found rather close to the dentino-enamel junction, and especially the mesiobuccal pulp horn of the primary first molars[37].

The narrow occlusal surface of the primary molars makes the preparation of a class II cavity rather difficult. The extension into the proximal surface must be done carefully to avoid widening the area and endangering pulp support.

The contact area between primary teeth is broader and flatter than in permanent teeth, making bitewing evaluation indispensable for detection of interproximal caries. Unlike permanent teeth, the direction of the enamel rods in primary teeth is inclined towards the occlusal surface in the interproximal area. This is an important consideration in cavity preparation of primary teeth as the gingival floor of the proximal box should follow the inclination of the rods and no bevel should be prepared.

The dental age, the extent of the decay, the general condition of oral hygiene, and the shape of the tooth will decide whether the tooth can be restored with a silver amalgam restoration or a stainless steel crown is needed. Usually MOD preparations are not indicated in small children but sometimes they can be placed in selected cases (usually in second primary molars).

Figs. 7-10 to 7-12　Dental cavity preparations for primary teeth.

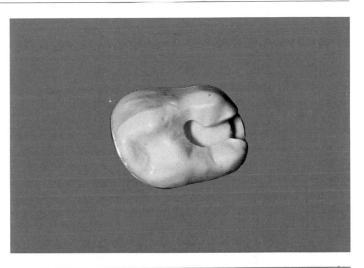

Figure 7-10

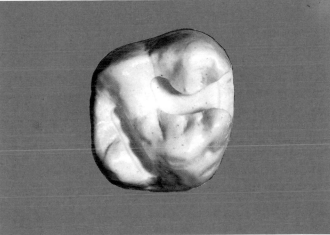

Figure 7-11

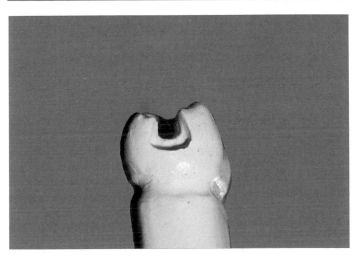

Figure 7-12

Pulp preservation

Accurate diagnosis of the condition of the pulp must be obtained before any restoration may be considered. Restoration of a deep carious lesion can be successful only if the pulp is sound and vital.

In general, for the diagnosis of the type of dental caries and the possible involvement of the pulp in the pathologic process, the clinician evaluates the following:

1. Age, color, texture, and size of the lesion
2. Presence or absence of pain
3. Radiographic appearance
4. Pulp vitality

The diagnosis of the pulp status in the treatment of the tooth with a deep lesion is difficult because the methods of evaluation are not very precise. The color of the lesion often may indicate its speed of progress. A consequence of slow progress is a distinct darkening of the carious dentin. This may suggest that reparative secondary dentin has walled off the dental pulp from the process. This, in combination with absence of pain, may permit somewhat optimistic prognosis of pulp vitality. While excellent detailed descriptions of pulp pathology are found in many textbooks, intraoral diagnosis depends on the skill and care of the examiner and his clinical judgment. The major question is the assessment of pulp vitality. When pulpal damage is present, one must ascertain whether it is reversible or will lead to pulp degeneration.

Pain is not a reliable indicator of the condition of the pulp, but may serve as an indicator of the presence of an inflammatory process. It may also indicate changes transmitted to the pulp through the dentin. Note should be taken, however, that total lack of pain cannot be considered an indication of pulp health. In many carious lesions pulp inflammation may have caused pulpal necrosis. Hasler and

Mitchell[18] demonstrated histological pulpitis in 58% of asymptomatic carious teeth. Pulp testing either by hot or cold stimuli or with an electric pulp tester is of relative value only, as the response is also dependent on the depth of the carious lesion and the reliability of the child.

Unfortunately, radiographic evidence also has its limitations. Radiographs can show the proximity of the carious process to the pulp tissue, and periapical radiolucencies may suggest pathologic changes of the pulp and periapical tissue. The contour of the pulp chamber may indicate pulp response and secondary dentin formation but the two-dimensional nature of the technique interferes with an accurate localization of the secondary dentin.

By considering all the information available, guidelines can be developed for the extent of tissue removal needed to assure adequate treatment. Undoubtedly, success or failure of the treatment of pulp exposures depends on whether bacterial infection of the pulp has occurred.

Pulp tissue diseases

Treatment of any tooth, with or without pulpal involvement, demands an understanding of pulp physiology and pathology. Pulp diseases often are the result of earlier treatment and are an important consideration in treatment planning.

Normal dental pulp is composed of connective tissue rich in ground substance and fibroblasts and contains blood vessels and nerve fibers (Figs. 7-13 and 7-14). At the dentinal borders of the pulp there is a continuous layer of odontoblastic cell bodies. Like other connective tissue in the body, pulp tissue has repair mechanisms; however, limiting factors may greatly interfere with

Fig. 7-13   Normal human pulp tissue.

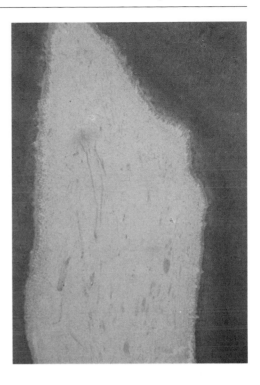

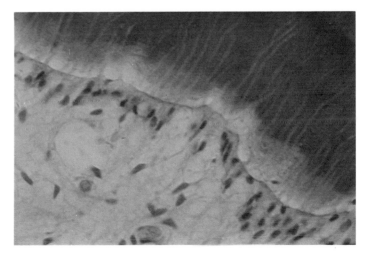

Fig. 7-14   High magnification of the odontoblastic area and normal pulp tissue.

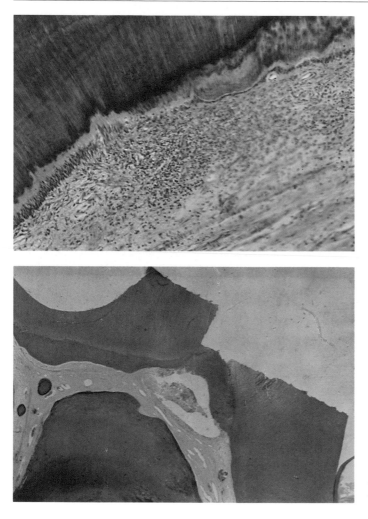

Fig. 7-15 Inflammatory reaction of the pulp from dental caries.

Fig. 7-16 Pulp necrosis associated with recurrent dental caries under filling. Note zone of abscess.

repair potential. Therefore even early stages of pulpitis (inflammation of the pulp) may be irreversible if not treated properly and promptly.

The etiology of pulpitis is irritation to the pulp tissue. This may be physical, chemical, or more frequently bacterial. Pulpitis may be partial or total, depending on the amount of pulp tissue involved in the inflammatory process (Fig. 7-15). An acute pulpitis may become chronic if not treated or, if severe enough, may result in tissue destruction and abscess formation.

A pulp with a total acute pulpitis may become completely abscessed, with invasion of the periapical tissues. In such cases, extreme pain and tenderness accompanies tissue degeneration. In chronic pulpitis, the pulp degenerates and ultimately necrotizes (Figs. 7-16 and 7-17). A granuloma with chronic inflammatory cells may develop, if the degeneration invades the periapical region. In general, pulpal pathology is characterized by a slowly progressing degeneration of pulpal tissue with accompanying inflammation and degeneration of the regions

Fig. 7-17 Complete necrosis associated with pulp exposure.

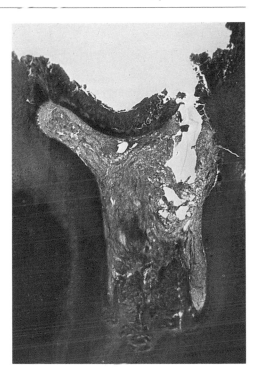

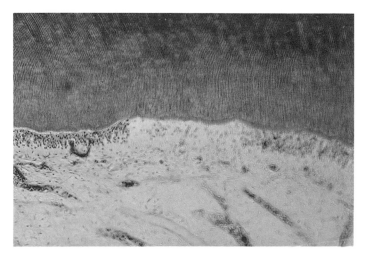

Fig. 7-18 Zone beneath cavity preparation with aspirated odontoblasts in dentinal tubules.

161

involved. Occasionally, sudden and massive degeneration can follow traumatic injury. As the dental pulp is a continuation of the dentin, it can be damaged not only by dental caries but also by dental procedures in the dentin and by chemicals placed on the dentin.

Intrapulpal effects of deep cavity preparations are usually significant. Immediately following cavity preparation a degeneration zone with absence of odontoblasts can be demonstrated (Fig. 7-18). Depending on the age of the pulp and its health, the unharmed cells may initiate cell division and repopulate the pulp space beneath the damaged dentinal tubules and reparative dentin will be formed. Injuries to the dental pulp during operative dentistry are usually the result of thermal, chemical, or mechanical insult. Thermal damage occurs when the heat generated by the rotating instruments is not moderated by properly applied cooling. Obviously the damage to the pulp is related to the distance between the cavity floor and the pulp tissue (the smaller the distance, the greater the possibility of damage) and the age and condition of the pulp tissue before the operative procedures. Chemical damage is usually caused by agents applied as sterilizers or disinfectants or to acids in restorative materials. Zinc phosphate cements and silicate cements seep through the open dentin tubules and are highly irritating to pulp tissue. Irritation by other restorative materials such as composites has been demonstrated. Suitable cavity liners should be used if at all possible[5]. Mechanical damage can occur when the pulp is accidentally exposed and not treated.

Microleakage also may affect the pulp. Leakage usually occurs at the interface between the restoration and the cavity wall. Microleakage and pulp damage may be reduced greatly by the use of cavity varnishes and liners. The more nearly hermetic the closure of the restoration, the better the chance of pulp recovery from injury.

Histologic studies have shown the morphology and distribution of nerve fiber in pulp tissue in health and in disease conditions[9]. Some degeneration is seen in nerve fibers of specimens with irreversible pulpitis, but the degeneration seems less severe than that in surrounding tissue. As these nerve fibers seem to be intact longer than the surrounding tissue, they probably would be able to conduct sensory impulses while the rest of the pulp tissue was degenerating. At some point, with progress of the pulpitis and necrosis of the tissue, degeneration and dissolution of the nerve fibers takes place. With severe degeneration of these fibers, they probably are no longer able to conduct sensory stimuli.

Hyperemia

Hyperemia is the first state of pulpal response to irritation. It frequently results from operative procedures, traumatic occlusion, or irritating chemicals present in restorative materials. The symptoms of hyperemia are sharp pain of short duration, elicited by cold or sweets. Hyperemia is completely reversible if treated promptly by elimination of the etiological factor.

Acute pulpitis

The clinical symptoms of acute pulpitis are characterized by thermal sensitivity, particularly to cold. If all the pulp is involved in the inflammatory process, the patient may complain of intermittent pain which may start spontaneously or through thermal stimulation. Like any other type of acute inflammation, pulpitis is accompanied by increased blood flow, more cell elements in the region,

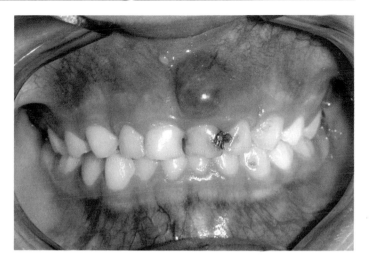

Fig. 7-19   Tooth discoloration with pulp necrosis. Note also the presence of a dentoalveolar abscess.

and some edema. Because the pulp chamber is constricted, these changes compress the nerve fibers and pain develops. If the activity is confined to the pulp chamber, no major radiographic changes can be detected. Percussion tests do not provide significant results, but electric vitality tests often produce a response at levels lower than normal. If the etiological factor is removed, acute pulpitis may be reversible.

Acute suppurative pulpitis

Severe acute pulpitis may be accompanied by abscess formation with attendant leukocyte infiltrates, liquefaction, and pus formation. The size of the abscess may vary from a very small area at a pulp horn to all of the pulp tissue of the tooth. The pain is usually severe and it is not always possible for the patient to identify the specific tooth. If periapical tissue is not involved, no major radiographic changes will be seen. Radiographs are of great value because they may demonstrate the etiological factor, such as a deep restoration close to the pulp tissue. Depending on the amount of leukocyte infiltration, the electrical pulp test response may be erratic,

but heat usually increases and cold relieves the pain. Treatment consists of relieving pressure by opening the pulp chamber and removing the injured tissue.

Chronic pulpitis

The symptoms of a chronic pulpitis are less severe than those of the acute condition. The patient may occasionally experience pain stimulated by thermal changes. Electrical stimuli usually have to be greater than normal to elicit a response and pressure tests will be inconclusive unless periapical tissue is involved. If the cause of irritation is removed early in the inflammatory process, the inflammation may be reversible.

Dentoalveolar abscess

Acute pulpitis may lead to a complete liquefaction of all the pulp tissue in the pulp chamber and canal with the development of a dentoalveolar abscess (Fig. 7-19). In this condition the symptoms are severe pain, swelling and redness, the classical picture of dental emergency. The tooth may be mobile, very tender to touch, and sensitive to heat. The patient may have elevated temperature and be toxic and irritable. Radiographs are useful if the etiology is associated with a pre-existing granuloma or cyst, and may help in showing a deep restoration or cavity. Treatment consists of immediately providing good drainage through the pulp chamber if at all possible. Sometimes extreme fluctuant swelling is present, indicating bone destruction by pus. In this case an incision should be made into the abscess. Antibiotic therapy also may be necessary.

Necrotic pulp with or without periapical involvement

As a necrotic pulp is not sensitive, its presence is usually detected through a dental examination. The extent of the tooth change, its restorability, and the condition of the periodontal tissue will determine whether endodontic treatment or extraction is indicated.

Internal root resorption

This is a pathological process starting at the borders of the pulp chamber, involving destruction of dentin, and progressing outward. It may occur following pulp disease, but can also occur following trauma. If diagnosed very early, endodontic treatment with removal of the dentinoblasts may arrest the process. If the process is too far advanced, the tooth must be extracted (Figs. 7-20 and 7-21).

Pulp therapy

Pulp therapy can be indirect or direct, pulpotomy or pulpectomy.

Indirect pulp capping

The objective of indirect pulp therapy is the preservation of pulp under deep lesions by improvement of the defense mechanism where there is danger of pulp exposure. This treatment tries to promote healing of the pulp by the sclerosis of the dentinal tubules and formation of reparative dentin. Under ideal conditions the pulp will show signs of only mild inflammation and will respond to the carious injury by production of reparative dentin of the regular tubular type. The technique consists of eliminating the infected dentin but leaving that dentin which, although altered and possibly demineralized, is not infected with microorganisms. The type of medication used is not critical but sterilizing solutions or solutions irritating to the odontoblasts must be avoided. It is essential that the medication and the cavity be sealed against contamination from the oral environment and for that purpose zinc oxide-eugenol paste remains the agent of choice. Healing time is 6 to 8 weeks, and care must be taken to assure proper closure of the cavity during this period. If symptoms develop, pulpotomy or pulpectomy is indicated.

Direct pulp capping

Direct pulp capping is the treatment of a dental pulp exposed accidentally or during excavation of caries. This technique is used in permanent teeth. The prognosis is guarded in cases of carious exposure as the condition of the pulp may not be favorable. Nyborn[27] and Seltzer and Bender[34] have demonstrated that calcium hydroxide used in direct pulp capping can be effective by forming a calcific barrier but much controversy exists concerning the effectiveness of the direct pulp capping procedure. It is contraindicated in primary teeth.

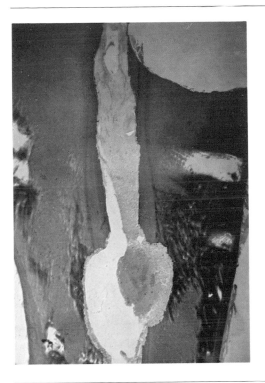

Fig. 7-20 Histological section of internal root resorption.

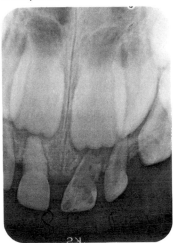

Fig. 7-21 Radiograph of tooth F of a 6-year-old boy showing internal resorption while tooth E shows obliterated calcified root canal (Courtesy of Dr. H. Freudenthal).

When the treatment is successful, the dental pulp capped with medication containing calcium hydroxide has the ability to bridge the exposure with reparative dentin. The tooth remains free of symptoms, reacts adequately to vitality testing, and has a normal radiographic appearance. When a minute pulp exposure has occurred and direct pulp capping is attempted, it is advisable to close the cavity with an appropriate restoration. Reevaluation of the tooth should occur after a period of 30 to 60 days.

Pulpotomy

Pulpotomy is the surgical removal of the coronal portion of the pulp. The healthy radicular pulp tissue is then treated to promote healing of the surgical site. Since the initial work of Teuscher and Zander[39] using calcium hydroxide, numerous investigators have used that material with varying degrees of success. Phanuef et al.[30] demonstrated that different forms of calcium hydroxide will affect pulp differently, creating dentinal bridges in some cases but not in others.

Doyle et al.[8] investigated pulpotomies in primary teeth and concluded that formocresol is superior to calcium hydroxide as a therapeutic agent. There is, however, a difference in the treatment of those permanent teeth in which an attempt at root closure is considered. (See page 168). After proper analgesia, with a rubber dam in place, the roof of the pulp chamber is removed with a large round bur at slow speed. The coronal pulp is amputated with a sharp sterile spoon excavator. After the bleeding is controlled, the radicular pulp tissue is examined and an almost dry cotton pellet containing formocresol is placed in the chamber for a shorter (5 minutes) or a longer (7 days) period to

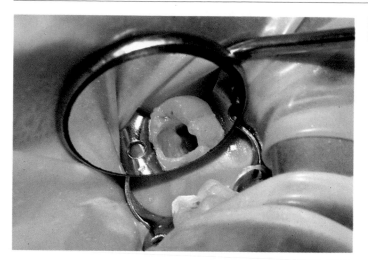

Fig. 7-22   Pulpotomy of tooth T in a 6-year-old boy.

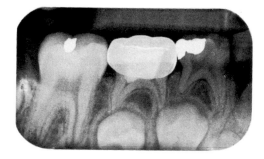

Fig. 7-23   Radiograph of a pulpotomy one year after treatment.

sterilize the area. If only a 5-minute application is used the pellet should be moist.

The formocresol dressing then is removed and the cavity is filled with zinc oxide-eugenol paste and a permanent restoration is placed. The 5-minute application of formocresol has been used successfully in cases of minimal pulp exposure (Figs. 7-22 and 7-23).

Failure of pulpotomy frequently will result in internal resorption. For this reason careful follow-up radiographs are essential.

Pulpectomy

While endodontic treatment of non-vital permanent teeth is common practice, root canal treatment of primary teeth with non-vital infected pulp has been discouraged because the anatomy of the root canals and pulpal connections between different canals makes this procedure difficult. There is also the problem of possible damage to the succedaneous tooth[4]. During physiologic root resorption, secondary dentin formation may create major aberrations in the morphology of the root canals. These variations may create extremely fine and torturous canals, making tissue removal, shaping, and obturation extremely difficult. Furthermore, the normal anatomy of primary molars differs from that of permanent molars. The roots of primary molars are curved, making manual manipulation very

Fig. 7-24a and b   Eruption of tooth 8 with E still in place without root resorption. Tooth had root canal therapy.

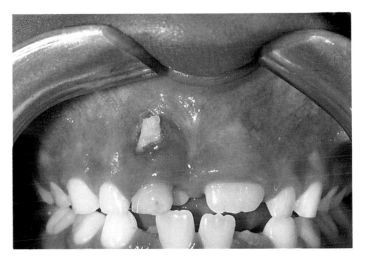

Figure 7-24 a

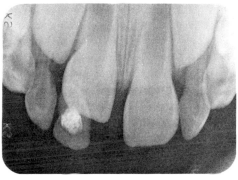

Figure 7-24 b

difficult, while those of permanent molars are straighter and easier to control in endodontic instrumentation.

Indications for pulpectomy of primary teeth include:

A. The absence of a permanent tooth, requiring retention of the primary tooth until a favorable occlusion has developed.
B. A second primary molar present when the first permanent molar has not yet erupted. (The tooth, if restorable, remains a better space maintainer than an appliance.)
C. The condition of the radicular pulp after pulpotomy indicates advanced hyper-

emia and poor prognosis for the pulpotomy.
D. Systemic condition of the patient precludes extraction.

Contraindications for pulpectomy are:

A. Advanced root resorption indicating that the tooth will not remain in the arch much longer.
B. Damaged clinical crown, making proper isolation of the field and restoration impossible.
C. Inadequate periodontal support.
D. Evidence of internal resorption or carious damage to the bifurcation.

In 1953, Rabinowitch[31] published a report of very successful endodontic procedures in primary teeth, but his technique involved an average of 7.7 visits for a treatment of a tooth with a non-vital pulp. This requires major parental and patient cooperation.

According to Bennett[2], in teeth with vital pulp the canals are instrumented 0.5mm short of the radiographic root tip, irrigated, dried, cultured, and sealed with eugenol for 3-7 days. On the second visit, the canals are mechanically enlarged, and camphorated P-chlorophenol is inserted as a medication. The canals are filled with a resorbable paste, usually of zinc oxide-eugenol. In treating teeth with non-vital pulp, two-thirds of the root canal content is removed after establishing drainage for the abscess, and camphorated P-chlorophenol is sealed in as a medicating agent. Following this treatment, the tooth is treated in the same manner as those with vital pulp.

The filling material must be resorbable concurrently with the roots. Therefore gutta percha and silver points are contraindicated. Even though resorption does not always take place in a tooth treated in this way (Fig. 7-24), the endodontically treated tooth must be checked carefully to assure correct time of exfoliation and correct placement of the permanent tooth in the arch.

In cases of permanent teeth with an open apex it is often possible to attain the development of a calcified apical seal by the use of careful endodontic technique, proper cleaning of the canal, and good closure while the calcified material is forming. This provides the barrier necessary for condensation of gutta percha or other permanent closure material. Once the pulp chamber has been opened, the canal(s) is properly cleaned and a paste containing calcium hydroxide is placed close to the apical third[12]. Care should be taken not to exceed the apex. The root canal(s) is sealed and the progress of the treatment is reevaluated after a few months. Induction of calcified material deposition takes place after a period of 6 month to two years. (Good seal has been reported in even shorter periods of time[13]). The canal then is permanently filled following routine endodontic procedures.

Periodontal disease

Periodontal disease occasionally is encountered in pedodontics. Moreover, epidemiologic studies demonstrate that periodontal disease of adults may have its inception in early childhood. In many cases the destructive phase of the disease can be demonstrated in patients in their teens[22].

Many times, however, the initial stages of periodontal involvement are neglected or not recognized because of other problems such as dental caries and malocclusion. Still, early recognition, treatment, and prevention of periodontal pathology in the child and adolescent can prevent later tooth loss.

Periodontal disease is a slowly progressing destructive disease. However in the mixed dentition the physiologic changes that are occurring make diagnosis difficult. The presence of inflammation resulting from processes such as exfoliation and eruption accompanied by inadequate oral hygiene complicate the clinical picture and make evaluation and determination of deviations from normal problematic. Probing in the primary dentition is also difficult because the anatomy of the roots of the primary teeth make placement of a probe parallel to the root surface difficult without striking the root. Erupting teeth also are problematic because crown morphology may interfere with the probing and the greater sulcular depth may give a false reading. During eruption of permanent teeth, measurement may vary even more.

According to Rubin[33], the gingiva of children is more reddish than that of adults because

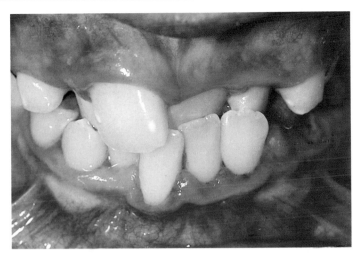

Fig. 7-25 Gingivitis in patient with severe tooth crowding.

of thinner epithelium and higher vascularity. The connective tissue is also less rich in collagen fibers giving the gingiva a more flaccid texture. Normal gingiva of children is more flaccid marginally, and less firmly attached to the tooth which is still erupting, with a hyperplastic tendency and rounding of the gingival margin. The periodontal membrane is wider in children, with less dense fibers, has an extensive blood and lymph vessel supply with increased amount of ground substance. The alveolar bone is less calcified than in adults, and there are larger marrow spaces.

In general, the young child with primary dentition may have gingivitis, herpetic gingivitis, gingivitis due to phenytoin or to self-mutilating habits, or periodontal problems associated with the abnormal pull of an enlarged frenum. In addition to these pathological conditions the child may show periodontal abnormalities associated with tooth movement resulting in root blunting and loss of periodontal support during the mixed dentition or early permanent dentition. Gingivitis also can be exaggerated as a result of hormonal changes of puberty.

Gingivitis

Gingivitis is the most common periodontal problem found in children. It may be the result of poor oral hygiene, food impaction, or trauma. Eruption of teeth may be accompanied by gingivitis, particularly if poor oral hygiene or other factors create a *locus minoris resistentia* (Fig. 7-25). Therapy must be directed toward the elimination of all irritants.

Acute herpetic gingivostomatitis is a common infectious disease in childhood. The condition is caused by the herpes simplex virus and is accompanied by fever, irritability, vesiculation of the oral mucosa, inflamed gingiva, and regional lymphadenopathy. The vesicles rupture 24 hours after formation, and result in small painful ulcerations having a yellow-gray depressed center and a raised red marginal halo. As these ulcerations are very painful, the patient has difficulty in eating and drinking. The lesions usually heal within 10 to 14 days unless a secondary infection occurs. It is important to force fluids to avoid dehydration. Occasionally intravenous fluids must be used for a few days.

Acute necrotising ulcerative gingivitis is most frequent in older children and young adults.

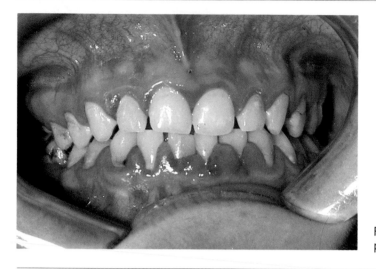

Fig. 7-26   Gingivitis in patient taking phenytoin therapy.

The patient usually shows signs of systemic illness, malaise, and loss of appetite. There is an acute local marginal inflammation of the gingiva with erythema and punched out, crater-like depressions covered by a gray pseudomembranous membrane. Several different microorganisms are usually found in these lesions including *B. vincentii* and *F. dentium.* The onset of the disease is usually sudden with pain, tenderness, profuse salivation, and often gingival bleeding. The treatment of uncomplicated cases of ANUG is debridement with irrigation and periodontal curettage where possible. As the area is very sensitive, this treatment may require several sessions. Antibiotics are not usually required in uncomplicated cases.

Gingivitis associated with endocrine changes such as those occurring during puberty may influence and aggravate gingival inflammation. During the pubertal period, pre-existing gingival inflammation may become very severe in relation to the magnitude of the irritants.

Gingivitis associated with drug therapy. Certain drugs such as phenytoin may influence the body response to poor oral hygiene. Patients taking phenytoin should be checked frequently to remove irritants that could cause gingivitis, because this drug will exacerbate the response to any gingival irritation (e.g. plaque). The incidence of phenytoin gingivitis varies with the duration and dosage of the therapy. Thorough oral hygiene will decrease the hyperplasia, and it may disappear with change to another anticonvulsant. Sometimes, however, phenytoin cannot be substituted. Surgery may be necessary for some patients if the hyperplasia is of long duration and many collagen fibers are present in the gingival tissue (Fig. 7-26).

Gingivitis associated with mouth breathing has been described by many investigators who have found it to be an aggravating factor in marginal gingivitis[19]. Studies comparing children with histories of medical complications caused by enlarged adenoids to healthy normal nosebreathing children demonstrate that mouthbreathers have more severe gingivitis than non-mouthbreathers. Dehydration is a possible associated factor but no statistical difference in plaque scores has been demonstrated between the two groups[19].

Congenital fibromatosis is a genetic disease of autosomal dominant inheritance. The gingiva is fibrous and pink in color, with increased fibers but no large increase in blood vessels. Both dentitions may be affected, and the tissue may completely cover the crowns of the teeth. Surgical treatment is the best therapy, even though the gingival fibromatosis will usually recur.

Gingival recession and recession of the periodontal tissue with increased length of the anatomical crown is usually caused by a mutilating finger traumatizing the gingival tissue. Recession may be seen around permanent teeth in patients with malocclusion, traumatizing habits, abnormal frenum attachment and anterior crossbite.

Periodontosis

There is much disagreement about the exact nature of the condition variously called periodontosis, juvenile periodontosis, or precocious periodontosis.

Whether periodontosis is a specific non-inflammatory degenerative condition starting in the periodontal tissues or a particularly severe periodontitis of several regions of the oral cavity is still controversial. Some investigators believe that periodontosis is a variant of periodontitis with a degenerative phase overshadowing the inflammation[1].

Clinically, periodontosis can be identified by early tooth mobility, diastema formation, migration of teeth, and advanced deep alveolar bone loss with little inflammation. The development of gingival inflammation and deep periodontal pockets is a later stage of the disease.

In periodontosis, the alveolar bone is destroyed with a widening of the periodontal space before the gingiva is actively involved. When the process is complicated by marginal periodontitis, the alveolar bone at the crest is also affected. The disease affects more girls than boys, and some data indicate that periodontosis may be familial and inherited as an X-linked dominant trait with varied penetrance[23]. It does not usually affect primary teeth, as do systemic diseases such as cyclic neutropenia, hypophosphatasia, and Papillon-LeFèvre syndrome. However, it has been reported in a 4.5-year-old girl[26].

Periodontitis

Advanced adolescent periodontitis, especially when involving the permanent incisors and first molars, may be a sequela to preexisting gingivitis and usually results from poor oral hygiene and neglect. It is not associated with anomalies and no distinctive laboratory findings have been reported. It should therefore be distinguished from periodontal disease associated with certain systemic diseases.

Periodontal disease as oral manifestation of systemic conditions

Several systemic disturbances can cause periodontal destruction in children resulting in loss of teeth. The loss may be in the primary dentition, the permanent dentition, or both.

Diabetes mellitus has been associated with early onset of periodontal disease in children. An increased gingival response to plaque has been found in diabetic children[32] but the alveolar bone remains unaffected in most cases. Bernick[3] reported 6 cases of some bone loss among 50 diabetic children.

Hypophosphatasia is characterized by diminished serum and tissue alkaline phosphatase levels. The serum phosphate concentration is normal but calcium may be elevated. The defect interferes with bone mineralization through a defect of synthesis of bone matrix. The genetic pattern of inheritance is autosomal recessive. A characteristic oral manifestation, and often one of the

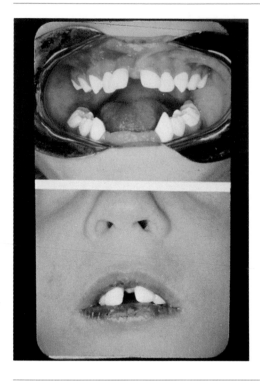

Fig. 7-27   Hypophosphatasia in 6-year-old girl (Courtesy of Dr. I. M. Rosenthal).

first signs of the disease, is the increased mobility and loss of the primary anterior teeth in the first years of life (Fig 7-27) but with little attendant gingival inflammation. The affected primary teeth have reduced cementum and enlarged pulps[20].

Papillon-LeFèvre syndrome is a rare disease characterized by hyperkeratosis of the wrists, ankles, palms of the hand, and soles of the feet, and is also characterized by premature loss of primary and permanent teeth. Several cases associated with parental consanguinity suggest a possible autosomal recessive pattern of inheritance[13].

Histiocytosis X is a condition which manifests itself with various clinical signs such as granulomatous lesions with histiocytic proliferation. Many patients have bone lesions. More severely affected children also have visceral involvement. Radiographs of the bones usually show bone lesions of a "punched out" type. Oral manifestations are frequently present[36] and include ulcerative necrotizing gingivitis and alveolar bone loss around both the primary and permanent teeth. Cyst-like lesions in the angle of the mandible or even in the body of the mandible may be seen on radiographs. Abnormal eruption patterns may occur in the areas of bone loss.

Neutropenia is a reduction of the number of circulating neutrophils from reduced production or excessive peripheral destruction. When the neutrophil count drops below 1500 per mm^3 the patient's susceptibility to infection increases significantly. Oral manifestations of the disease are persistent ulcerative gingivitis with alveolar bone loss in either or both dentitions, and occasionally ulcerations of the lip, tongue, or palate[17].

Leukemia is the most common childhood malignancy. Acute lymphocytic leukemia (ALL) accounts for about two-thirds of the cases and acute non-lymphocytic leukemia

(ANLL) acounts for about one-fifth. The several types of acute non-lymphocytic leukemia include acute myelocytic leukemia, erythroleukemia, eosinophilic leukemia, promyelocytic leukemia, and monoblastic leukemia. Chronic myelocytic leukemia (CML) accounts for about 3% of the cases in childhood.

Children with ALL may have fever, pallor and gingival bleeding. Lymphadenopathy and splenomegaly are usually present and thrombocytopenia is often found. Diagnosis is established by bone marrow examination. With modern therapy many of these patients can be treated successfully and permanent remission can be achieved. During remission these patients should receive appropriate dental care with special emphasis on oral hygiene and prevention of dental caries.

Children with ANLL have a poor prognosis. Remission can be obtained in about two-thirds of the patients but is of short duration. Measures should be taken to assure the dental comfort of the patient.

Dental treatment should be postponed in ALL patents If possible until remission is achieved. Once remission is established preventive dentistry measures similar to those instituted for patients with hemophilia are of great importance to avoid emergencies secondary to dental neglect. On rare occasions it may be necessary to proceed with dental treatment and clear infection before remission. In these cases appropriate antibiotic therapy is essential.

Oral ulcers can be a complication of some of the chemotherapeutic agents utilized in the treatment of leukemia. If the drug responsible is discontinued, the ulcers will heal. Palliative measures include topical anesthetic spray and protection of the ulcers with oral adhesive with or without addition of powdered thrombin[24]. Occasionally xerostomia may develop secondary to chemotherapy or radiation. Prophylactic measures against dental caries, including nutrition control and scrupulous oral hygiene, are essential. Topical application of fluorides may be indicated[26].

Hemorrhage and infection can occur in patients with leukemia. Hemorrhage after dental surgery is related to the degree of thrombocytopenia although other defects in the clotting mechanism may also be present. Radiographically detectable jawbone changes have been described in children[7].

Increased susceptibility to infection is also frequently found in children with leukemia and is often related to the granulocytopenia.

Establishing and maintaining a good oral hygiene program can greatly decrease the oral manifestations of the disease by reducing local irritants to the gingival tissues. Care must be taken to remove all oral irritants such as dental caries and sharp surfaces on teeth and appliances. Meticulous follow-up is necessary in these patients to avoid dental emergencies. Because salicylates interfere with platelet function, they should be avoided.

References

1. Anderson, D.C. and R. Farbman:
   Periodontosis: real or imagined? J. D. C. Dent. Soc. 53:27-30, 1978.

2. Bennett, C.G.:
   Pulpal management of deciduous teeth. P.D.M. 22:1-38, 1965.

3. Bernick, S.M., D.W. Cohen, L. Baker and L. Laster:
   Dental disease in children with diabetes mellitus. J. Periodontol. 46:241-245, 1975.

4. Binns, W.H., Jr. and A. Escobar:
   Defects in permanent teeth following pulp exposure of primary teeth. J. Dent. Child. 34:4-14, 1967.

5. Brannstrom, M. and H. Nyborg:
   Pulpal reaction to composite resin restorations. J. Prosthet. Dent. 27:181-189, 1972.

6. Crawford, J.G., R.G. Testa and B.C. Stone:
   Breast feeding vs. bottle feeding as related to dental caries incidence: a review of the literature. Israel J. Dent. Med. 23:19-26, 1974.

7. Curtis, A.B.:
   Childhood leukemias. Osseous changes in jaws on panoramic dental radiographs. J. Am. Dent. Assoc. 83:844-847, 1971.

8. Doyle, W.A., R.E. McDonald and D.F. Mitchell:
   Formocresol versus calcium hydroxide in pulpotomy. J. Dent. Child. 29:86-97, 1962.

9. England, M.C., E.G. Pellis and A.E. Michanowicz:
   Histopathologic study of the effect of pulpal disease upon nerve fibers of the human dental pulp. Oral Surg. 38:783-790, 1974.

10. Fass, E.N.:
    Is bottle feeding of milk a factor in dental caries? J. Dent. Child. 29:245-251, 1962.

11. Fitzgerald, R.J. and P.H. Keyes:
    Demonstration of the etiologic role of streptococci in experimental caries in the hamster. J. Am. Dent. Assoc. 61:9-19, 1960.

12. Frank, A.L.:
    Therapy for the divergent pulpless tooth by continued apical formation. J. Am. Dent. Assoc. 72:87-93, 1966.

13. Galanter, D.R. and S. Bradford:
    Hyperkeratosis palmoplantaris and periodontosis: the Papillon-LeFèvre syndrome. J. Periodontol. 40:40-47, 1969.

14. Gallagher, C.S. and A.P. Mourino:
    Root-end induction. J. Am. Dent. Assoc. 98:578-580, 1979.

15. Gardner, D.E., J.R. Nordwood and J.E. Eisenson:
    At-will breast feeding and dental caries: four case reports. J. Dent. Child. 44:186-191, 1977.

16. Goepferd, S.J.:
    Leukemia and its dental implications. J. Dent. Handicapped 4:44-49, 1979.

17. Gorlin, R.J. and A.P. Chaudhry:
    The oral manifestations of cyclic neutropenia. Arch. Dermatol. 82:344-348, 1960.

18. Hasler, J.E. and D.F. Mitchell:
    Painless pulpitis. J. Am. Dent. Assoc. 81:671-677, 1970.

19. Jacobson, L.:
    Mouthbreathing and gingivitis. I. Gingival conditions in children with epipharyngeal adenoids. J. Periodont. Res. 8:269-277, 1973.

20. Kjellman, M., V. Oldfelt, A. Nordenram and M.O. Nordenram:
    Five cases of hypophosphatasia with dental findings. Int. J. Dent. Surg. 2:152-158, 1973.

21. Loevy, H.:
    Pulpal reactions to dental caries. M.S. thesis, University of Illinois, Chicago, 1959.

22. Marshall-Day, C.D., R.G. Stephens and L.F. Quigley Jr.:
    Periodontal disease: prevalence and incidence. J. Periodontol. 26:185-203, 1955.

23. Melnick, M., E.D. Shields and D. Bixler:
Periodontosis: a phenotypic and genetic analysis.
Oral Surg. *42*:32-41, 1976.

24. Michaud, M., R.L. Baehner, D. Bixler and A.H. Kafrawy:
Oral manifestations of acute leukemia in children.
J. Am. Dent. Assoc. 1145-1150, 1977.

25. Miller, W.D.:
Microorganisms of the human teeth. Philadelphia,
S.S. White, 1890.

26. Moffitt, J.H.:
Juvenile periodontosis: report of a case. J. Dent.
Child. *41*:452-455, 1974.

27. Nyborg, H.:
Healing processes in the pulp on capping. Acta
Odontol. Scand. *13*:Suppl. 9-130, 1955.

28. Orland, F.J., J.R. Blayney, R.W. Harrison, J.A.
Reyniers, P.C. Trexler, F. Ervin, H.A. Gordon and
M. Wagner:
Experimental caries in germ-free rats innoculated
with enterococci. J. Am. Dent. Assoc. *50*:259-272,
1955.

29. Orland, F.J., R. Blayney, R.W. Harrison, J.A. Reyniers, P.C. Trexler, M. Wagner, H.A. Gordon and
T.D. Luckey:
Use of the germ-free animal technic in the study
of experimental dental caries. I. Basic observa-
tions on rats reared free of all microorganisms.
J. Dent. Res. *33*:147-174, 1954.

30. Phaneuf, R.A., S.N. Frankl and M.P. Ruben:
A comparative histological evaluation of three calcium hydroxide preparations on the human primary
dental pulp. J. Dent. Child. *35*:61-75, 1968.

31. Rabinowitch, B.Z.:
Pulp management in primary teeth. Oral Surg.
6:671-676, 1953.

32. Ringelberg, M.L., D.O. Dixon, A.O. Francis and R.
W. Plummer:
Comparison of gingival health and gingival crevic-
ular fluid flow in children with and without diabetes. J. Dent. Res. *56*:108-111, 1977.

33. Ruben, M.P., S.N. Frankl and S. Wallace:
The histopathology of periodontal disease in children. J. Periodontol. *42*:473-484, 1971.

34. Seltzer, S. and I.B. Bender:
Some influences affecting repair of the exposed
pulps of dogs' teeth. J. Dent. Res. *37*:678-687,
1958.

35. Shannon, I.L. and R.P. Feller:
Parotid saliva flow rate, calcium, phosphorus and
magnesium concentrations in relation to dental
caries experience in children. Pediatr. Dent.
1:16-20, 1979.

36. Sigala, J.L., S. Silverman Jr., H.A. Brody and J.H.
Kushner:
Dental involvement in histiocytosis. Oral Surg.
33:42-48, 1972.

37. Stoner, J.E.:
Dental caries in deciduous molars. Brit. Dent. J.
123:130-134, 1967.

38. Takuma, S., H. Sunohara, H. Watanabe and K. Yama:
Some structural aspects of carious lesions in
human dentin. Bull Tokyo Dent. Coll. *10*:173-181,
1969.

39. Teuscher, G.W. and H.A. Zander:
A preliminary report on pulpotomy. Northwestern
Univ. Grad. Bull. *39*:4-8, 1938.

Chapter 8

Cephalometrics

Efforts in the past 50 years to eliminate empiricism have allowed the development of scientific approaches to the study of facial growth and enhanced establishment of a descriptive pattern useful in therapy. One of the pioneers in this field was B. H. Broadbent who was involved in the development of standardized radiographic techniques through which the growth of a subject could be studied over a period of years.

Cephalometric radiography was first described by Broadbent[2] and Hofrath[10]. To study the growing child over time Broadbent developed a craniostat that permits a constant target-film distance of 60 inches and a fixed orientation of the head in the Frankfort horizontal position. Hofrath's method was slightly different in orienting the head of the patient. These techniques have been used over many years and permit better understanding of changes of head and face from birth to adulthood.

The aim of cephalometric analysis is the evaluation of jaw to jaw and tooth to jaw relationships. Comparison of serial cephalograms helps in observation and analysis of growth patterns and in prediction of possible growth patterns.

The difference between lateral skull and cephalometric radiographs must be understood. The craniostat is used for serial studies or of relations between structures which require a fixed target firm distance and a fixed head position. A lateral skull radiograph is an invaluable diagnostic aid but does not involve a craniostat. It is used for diagnosis of bone anomalies such as fractures, impactions, supernumerary teeth, pathologic bone changes, etc.

Cephalometry is the study of anatomical landmarks. For comparison of several skull radiographs, it is necessary to adopt certain landmark points and planes that are not subject to much variation and are easy to locate.

In cephalometric analysis these different landmarks are identified and the points connected to form lines, planes, and angles. The search for such planes and landmarks has been a major concern and several different types of analysis have been advocated. Among them are the systems of Downs, Steiner, Reidel, Tweed, Bjork, and others[8]. However, common sense in the evaluation of cephalometric data is of primary importance and excessive rigidity and concern with numbers can lead to diagnostic errors and therapeutic mismanagement.

Cephalometric analysis permits evaluation of the following questions:

A. Are both jaws harmoniously related to one another and to the cranial base?
B. In case of disharmony is the problem mild, moderate, or severe?
C. Is either jaw orthognathic, prognathic, or retrognathic?

Many cephalometric machines are marketed. It is imperative that the positioner permit a precise repositioning of the head at successive examinations. Tilting of the head may affect the X-ray beam direction and can create an apparent size reduction of one section of the head and elongation of sections on the other side. In considering the head holder, the following characteristics are important. The head holder should not allow the patient to move, thereby altering the relation to the source. The ear rods should fit comfortably, without distorting the external ear area; they should be easy to manipulate so that alignment can be made quickly and without discomfort to the patient. Ear rods and their holders should be of a material and shape that will not produce a shadow which will interfere with the radiographic image of the head.

Over the years the 5 foot anode-objective distance has become standard. It has the advantage of providing interchangeability of records among operators for both research and clinical use.

Different investigators prefer different film size. An 8" x 10" film is used in many laboratories interested in clinical diagnosis while 10" x 12" or 12" x 14" are used by many researchers in the field to show the entire skull.

High definition films require increased X-ray exposures, but use of intensifying screens reduces exposure time. Exposure time therefore depends upon the machine, the type of film, and the screen used[14].

The greater the distance between the X-ray source and the head, the smaller the degree of enlargement, but the power of the X-ray beam must be increased proportionally by the square of the distance from the film.

There are many sources of errors in cephalometrics. Some are caused by the tracing; some by the conversion of the three-dimensional body into a two dimensional radiograph; some by the relative position of the head; and others by the X-ray source and film.

Other errors may arise from the lack of perceptiveness of the eye, the thickness of the tracing pencil, the film contrast, and the type of film emulsion. The identification of landmarks should be as consistent as possible and depends on the experience and training of the examiner. That small errors may easily occur during the mechanical tracing or replication, duplication, and superimposition must be kept in mind even if many of the currently popular landmarks have been selected because they could be visualized fairly easily on conventional cephalometric radiographs. Even with very good radiographs there may be lack of clarity of some landmarks because of superimposed structures. Digital computer techniques currently are being introduced to reduce human error and to improve the accuracy of caphalometry[15].

Many factors must be controlled to obtain satisfactory cephalometric films:

A. distortion is controlled by selecting an anode-target to avoid overenlargements;
B. angulation of the X-rays must be at true right angles to the film surface;
C. axis of the central X-ray beam must be at true right angle to the reference plane (usually the midsagittal plane);
D. position of the head usually is controlled by positioning the ear post; it must conform to 2 planes of reference to assure correct alignment (Frankfort horizontal and left and right Porion points).

Anatomical landmarks used in examining and evaluating the films and most frequently used in head plate tracing are:

Point *A* (subspinale):
deepest midline point on the maxilla between anterior nasal spine and the alveolar crest of the maxillary incisor
Anterior Nasal Spine (ANS):
most anterior tip on norma lateralis of nasospinal projection of the maxilla

Articulare (Ar):
intersection point on the dorsal contour of the mandibular ramus and the anterior part of the temporal bone

Point *B* (supramentale):
deepest midline point in the concavity between the lower incisor alveolar crest and pogonion (Po)

Basion (Ba):
midline point at the inferior margin of the anterior border of the foramen magnum

Gnathion (Gn):
midpoint between pogonion (Po) and menton (M) (anatomical point) *or* point on the chin determined by the angle formed by the facial line and mandibular plane (constructed point)

Gonion (Go):
midpoint on the curvature of the mandible between the mandibular ramus plane and mandibular plane

Menton (M):
lowest point on the symphyseal area as seen on norma lateralis

Nasion (N):
most anterior point of the nasofrontal suture

Orbitale (O):
most inferior point on the lower margin of the orbit

Posterior Nasal Spine (PNS):
most posterior tip on the palatal shelf on norma lateralis

Porion (P):
most superior point of the skeletal external auditory meatus (anatomical point) *or* most superior point of the earpost of the cephalostat as seen on the lateral cephalometric radiograph (mechanical point)

Pogonion (Po):
most anterior prominent point on the midline of mandibular symphysis

Pterygomaxillary fissure (Ptm):
junction point of the anterior surface of the pterygoid process of the sphenoid bone and the posterior margin of the maxilla

Sella (S):
point representing the geometric center of the pituitary fossa (sella turcica)

Planes most frequently used as basis of evaluation include:

Frankfurt Horizontal (FH):
plane determined by a line connecting P and O. (This reference plane passes through the center of the face)

SN Plane (SN):
plane determined by a line connecting S and N. (This plane separates the anterior cranial base from the face, and is usually considered a stable reference for superimposure in longitudinal studies)

Palatal Plane (Pal. P1):
plane determined by a line connecting ANS and PNS

Occlusal Plane (Occ. P1):
plane determined by a line passing through half the incisal overbite or open bite and half the height of the molars

Esthetic Plane (E line):
line determined by a tangent to the soft tissues of the chin passing at the level of the tip of the nose.

Cephalometric evaluation

The demarcation between the brain case and the face is the *cranial base.* There is an *anterior cranial base* associated with the upper face and a *posterior cranial base* associated with the mandible with the spheno-occipital junction dividing these 2 parts of the cranial base. A line drawn from the center of sella turcica (in the sphenoid bone) to the fronto-nasal junction at Nasion easily separates the brain case from the face. This line is commonly referred to as the SN line or plane (Figs. 8-1 and 8-2). It was described initially by Broadbent[37] and later used by Brodie, and still serves as one of the

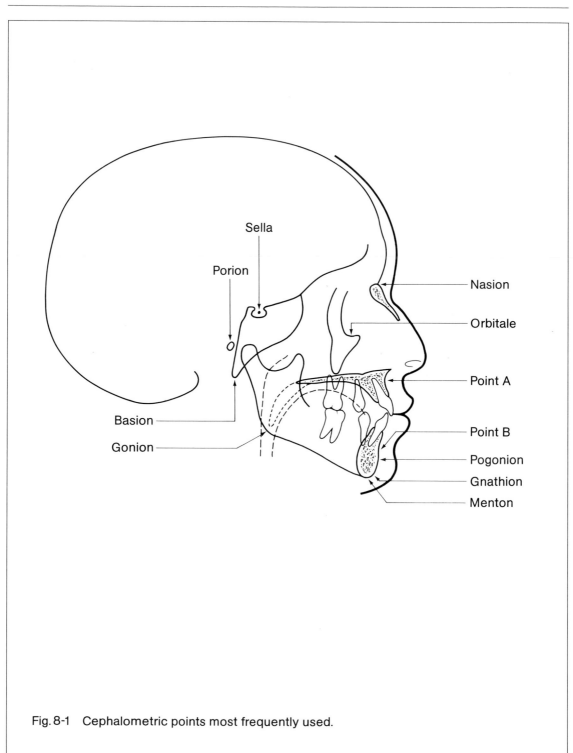

Fig. 8-1   Cephalometric points most frequently used.

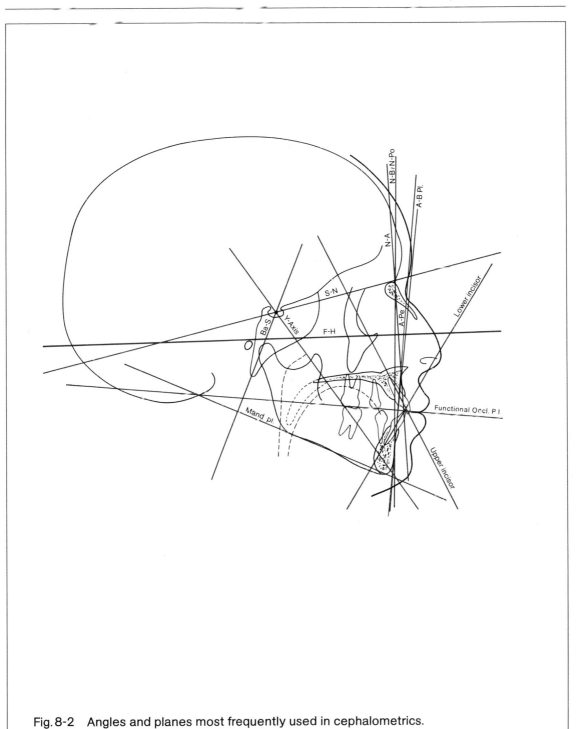

Fig. 8-2   Angles and planes most frequently used in cephalometrics.

baselines from which growth of the face as related to the cranium may be assessed[4].

Sella turcica was considered as a fixed point in the cranium by Brodie[4]. While this is probably not completely true, it is an easy point to locate and can be established reproducibly with a good degree of accuracy. Nasion as a point is dependent on growth and development of the skeletal orbits and eye position. Unequal growth of the two bones bordering the frontonasal suture as well as the appositional growth in the area may cause some migration of this suture affecting N. For practical purposes however, SN is a very useful landmark and is relatively stable after 8 years of age when the sphenoethmoidal suture has apparently completed its growth.

When Broadbent[3] started to evaluate the variation in growth he selected a point on the curvature between the occipital condyle and the squama of the occipital base and called it Bolton. He drew a line from Bolton to N and referred to the plane described by this line as the Bolton plane. By connecting Bolton point, S and N, he constructed the Bolton triangle. A perpendicular line may be constructed from S to the Bolton plane; the bisection of this line is referred to as point R (registration point) and has been used extensively as a point of registration. However, as growth of the mastoid process takes place, the location of Bolton point is more difficult to determine and therefore construction of the Bolton triangle is unreliable. Values have been attributed to the measurements in "normal" individuals, but it must be remembered that normal individuals do not always have these ideal values. Walker and Kowalsky[18] studied the ANB angle in 800 normal individuals and found that while the ideal angle is usually given as 2°, the sample showed the overall mean to be 4.5°, depending on sexual dimorphism and age variation. Variations in measurements related to age, sex or racial characteristics are evident in many measurements and must be taken into consideration for diagnostic purposes.

In 1948 Downs published a series of values derived from linear angular measurement of normal facial and dental patterns[7]. He used as his sample 20 individuals ranging in age from 12 to 20 years with excellent occlusion.

His Downs' analysis has been accepted as a standard and has been modified over the years. It is used as a method of evaluation of skeletal and dental patterns for classification of facial types. Downs described facial angle, angle of convexity, the Y axis, mandibular plane angle, and anterior posterior relation to the denture base (A-B plane to facial plane). After these initial studies of Downs several other investigators defined and evaluated new angles. The cephalometric analysis used in most laboratories is the one first proposed by Downs plus additional information.

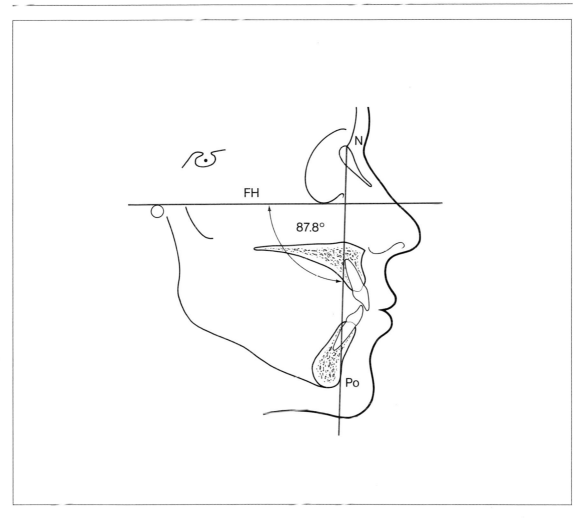

Facial form assessment

Facial plane and facial angle

These are used as a guide for the profile inclination. The *facial plane* is established by N and Po. The *facial angle* is the angle formed by the facial plane and FH. The established normal value for Caucasians is about 87°. Since this angle describes the relative antero-posterior position of the mandible, a small angle indicates a retrusion and a large angle an anterior position of the chin with a range of 82° (recessive chin) to 95° (protrusive chin). In young children this angle is acute and becomes more obtuse with increasing age. It is an important factor in growth prediction because it facilitates the prediction of the amount and direction of mandibular development.

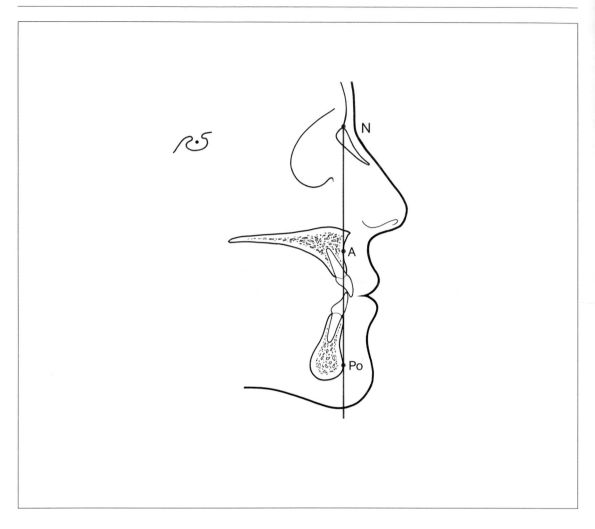

Angle of convexity

This angle is formed by a line drawn from nasion (N) to point A and from point A to pogonion (Po). The angle of convexity is a means of evaluation of the relationship of the maxillary part of the face to the total profile and measures the convexity or concavity of the facial profile. In Downs' Caucasian sample, this angle was a straight line (180°): if the facial plane coincides with the angle of convexity the value of the angle is 0° with a range of +10° (convex) to −8.5° (concave). Reidel's[16] value for this angle is +4.2° in children 8-11 years old and +1.6° for adults (age 18-36). This angle is normally flatter in other groups such as Japanese and Chinese. A flat angle indicates that the upper face, middle face, and lower face are on the same plane. An increase in convexity may be caused either by protrusion of the maxilla or a retrusion of the mandible.

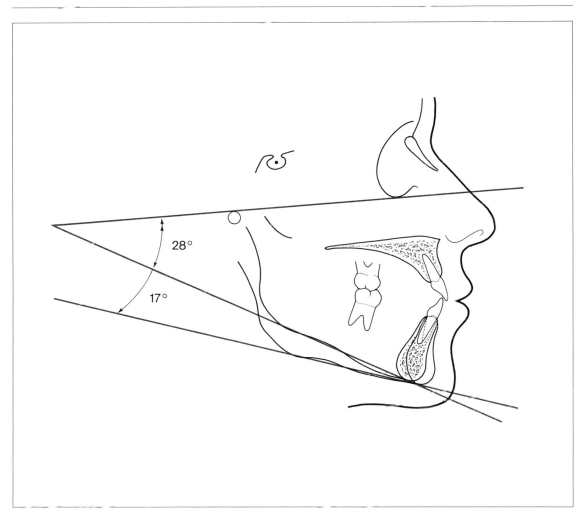

Mandibular plane and angle

The mandibular plane passes at the level of the lower border of the mandible. The angle formed by this plane and FH is usually referred to as the mandibular angle or the Frankfurt mandibular angle (FMP). The normal value for this angle is from 17° to 28° with a mean of 21.9°. The size of the angle is dependent in part on the relation between the body and the ramus of the mandible. A large angle may be associated with a short ramus and a small angle with a more horizontal mandibular plane. In some laboratories the angle between the mandibular plane and SN is measured. In this case the value is larger, 32.2°[6].

185

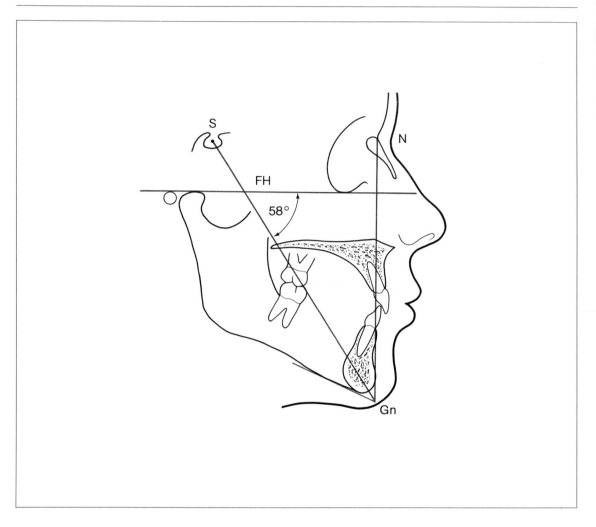

Y axis and Y axis-FH angle

The line drawn from sella (S) to gnathion (Gn) is called the Y axis. The angle formed by FH and Y axis indicates the direction of growth of the lower part of the face. Usually the value is about 58°. A very small angle indicates a forward growth of the mandible. A large angle indicates downward or even a posterior growth. According to Downs' analysis, the mean value for his sample was 59.4° with a range of 53° (class III) to 66° (class II).

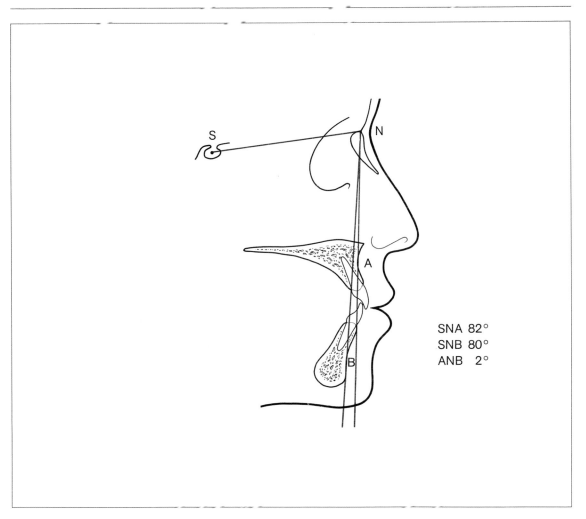

SNA 82°
SNB 80°
ANB 2°

SNA and SNB angles

Reidel studied the anteroposterior position of the maxilla and mandible as related to cranial base (SN) and evaluated the SNA and SNB angles. The value for young children (age 8 to 11) for SNA was 80.7° compared to 82.1° for adults. For SNB the mean value for children was 78.02° and adults 79.9°, indicating that both maxilla and mandible tend to become more prognathic with growth.

Dental pattern assessment

The aim of the study of the relation between incisors is to determine whether this relationship is in balance and harmonious. The norms used are primarily based on the values established by Downs[7] and Steiner[17]. While not too much importance should be attached to individual values and variations, it is desirable to have the total data before treatment is initiated. Several different reference angles and planes can be traced and used to evaluate the position of the central incisors and their relationship to each other and to the face.

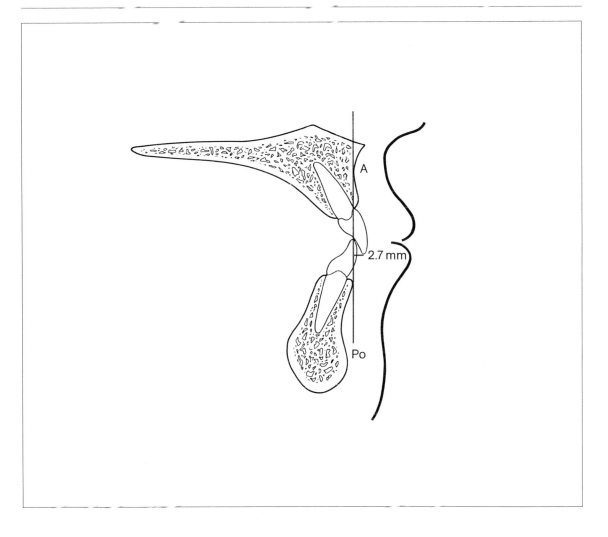

1 to A-Po and N-Po

Downs proposed that the amount of protrusion of the maxillary central incisors can be evaluated by measuring the distance in mm of the incisal edge of that tooth to a line connecting A to Po. The mean value for this distance is +2.7 mm with a variation from +5 to −1mm in a group of patients age 12 to 17. Reidel[16] used the facial plane (N-Po) instead of A-Po for this evaluation and found a mean value of +6.35mm in his sample of children 8 to 13 years with excellent occlusion and +5.3mm in a group of older patients. This difference can be explained by the decrease in convexity as age increases.

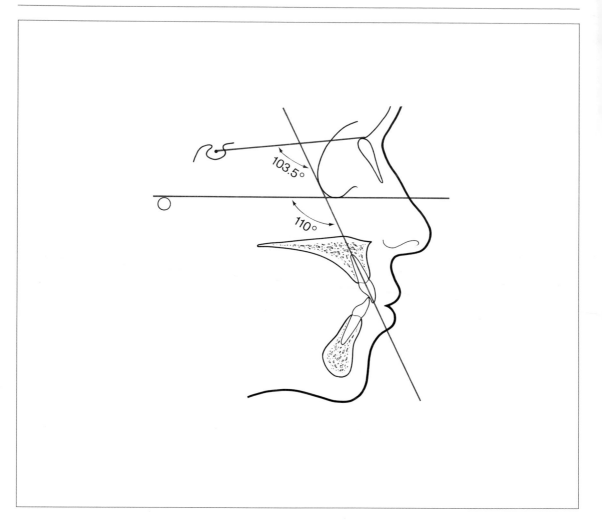

1 to SN and FH

The position of 1 can also be analyzed in relation to SN and FH. Reidel[16] compared the angle measurements of the junction of the long axis of the central incisor and SN. Very little variation was seen with increasing age and the angle was measured as 103.5°. If the angle of the long axis of 1 to FH is measured instead, the mean value is 110° since FH and SN are not parallel. There is a slight sex difference in these measurements, males being more protrusive.

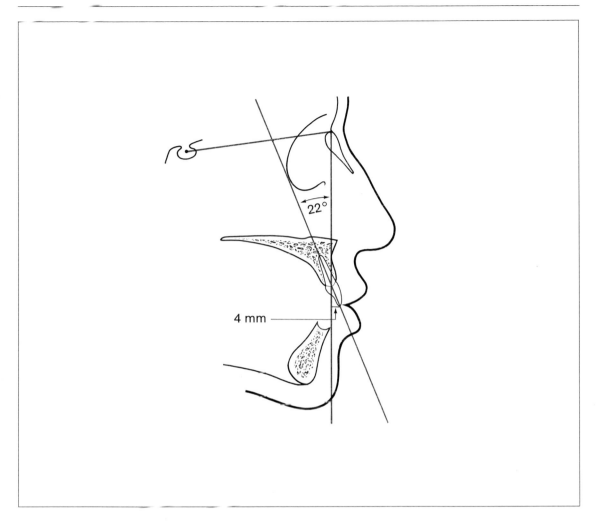

1 to NA

In 1953 Steiner published a paper[17] in which he studied the relationship of the maxillary central incisor to A both linearly and as an angle measurement using the angle formed by 1 and the long axis of NA. This angle was found to be 22°. According to Steiner the maxillary central incisor should lie on the NA line in such a manner that the most anterior point of its crown is 4 mm in front of this line.

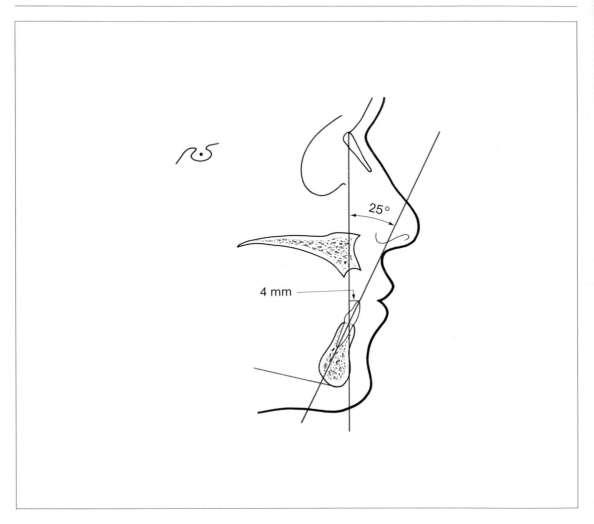

1 to NB

In the same manner as the maxillary incisor is related to NA the mandibular central incisor may be related to NB angularly and linearly. Steiner considered the angular measurement to be 25° and the most anterior point of the incisor to be 4 mm in front of this line.

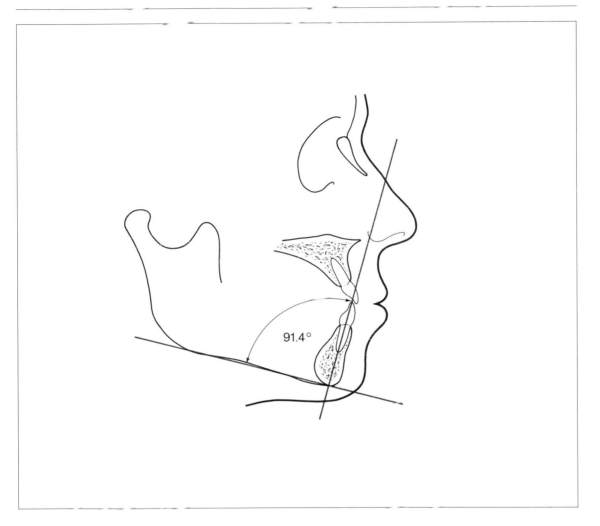

1 to Mandibular plane

Many investigators have studied the angle of the long axis of the mandibular incisor to the mandibular plane (IMPA). The value varies slightly depending on how MP is constructed. Downs found a value of 91.4° while Reidel found a value of 93.5°.

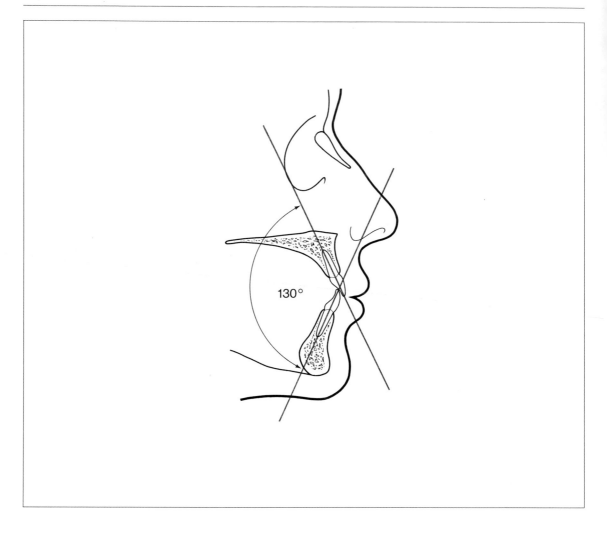

1 to 1

The procumbency of the incisors can be measured by the angle formed by their long axes. Downs gives a value of 135.4° with a range of 130° to 150° for Caucasians. This angle changes greatly in different racial groups[1, 5].

Other methods of assessment

Cephalometrics can be validly used to study skeletal morphology and skull growth as well as the relations between the component parts. The problem of selecting registration areas that are stable and change least during growth has been considered by many investigators. To overcome this problem, several investigators have developed analytical methods, each with its own advantages but also with its own bias.

The evaluation of relations between areas cannot always be related to other areas of the face and often a study of these relations is of diagnostic significance.

Enlow, et al.[9] developed an equivalent balance concept of the facial architecture in which the different bony parts or equivalents should match in order to produce a harmonious balance. Growth areas are compared since somatic and genetic factors interplay causing variation in individual or segmental dimensions but the end result should be in balance. This method introduces a new evaluation tool. However, ethnic differences must still be taken into consideration when this method is used since studies demonstrate that the measurements differ between different populations[13]. The emphasis in Enlow's method is not on individual landmarks but on the combination of individual anatomical and development characteristics.

The "Wits" (abbreviation for the University of Witwatersrand) appraisal is a diagnostic aid for the study of the degree of anteroposterior disharmony between maxillary and mandibular bone without the use of the ANB angle. This method is useful in cases where Nasion is placed in such a manner as to make its use as a diagnostic tool suspect[11]. The "Wits" method consists in drawing perpendicular lines from point A and B onto the occlusal plane. The point of intersection on the occlusal plane is labeled AO (in the maxilla) and BO (in the mandible). The "Wits" reading is the distance between these two points projected on the occlusal plane. Jacobson[12] found this reading to be O in females, that is, the AO and BO lines coincided, whereas in males point BO was approximately 1mm ahead of AO (giving a −1.0mm reading for normal males.

References

1. Altemus, L. A.:
   Cephalofacial relationships. Angle Orthod. *38*:175-184, 1968.

2. Broadbent, B. H.:
   A new X-ray technique and its application to orthodontia. Angle Orthod. *1*:45-46, 1931.

3. Broadbent, B. H.:
   The face of the normal child. Angle Orthod. *7*:183-208, 1937.

4. Brodie, A. G.:
   On the growth patterns of the human head from the 3rd month to the 8th year of life. Am. J. Anat. *68*:209-262, 1941.

5. Chan, G. K.:
   A cephalometric appraisal of the Chinese (Cantonese). Am. J. Orthod. *61*:279-285, 1972.

6. Cohen, M. M., Sr.:
   Minor tooth movement in the growing child. Philadelphia, Saunders, 1977.

7. Downs, W. B.:
   Variations in facial relationships: their significance in treatment and prognosis. Am. J. Orthod. *34*:812-840, 1948.

8. Enlow, D. H.:
   Handbook of facial growth. Philadelphia, Saunders, 1975.

9. Enlow, D. H., R. E. Moyers, W. S. Hunter and J. A. McNamara, Jr.:
   A procedure for the analysis of intrinsic facial form and growth. Am. J. Orthod. *56*:6-23, 1969.

10. Hofrath, H.:
    Die Bedeutung der Röntgenfern- und Abstandsaufnahme für Diagnostik der Kieferanomalien. Fortschr. Orthodont. *1*:232-257, 1931.

11. Jacobson, A.:
    The "Wits" appraisal of jaw disharmony. Am. J. Orthod. *67*:125-138, 1975.

12. Jacobson, A.:
    Application of the "Wits" appraisal. Am. J. Orthod. *70*:179-189, 1976.

13. Klami, O. and K. Koski:
    The application of the "equivalent-balance concept" to a cephalometric study of two age groups. Proc. Finn. Dent. Soc. *71*:201-206, 1975.

14. McWilliam, J. S. and U. Welander:
    The effect of image quality on the identification of cephalometric landmarks. Angle Orthod. *48*:49-56, 1978.

15. Oka, S. W. and H. J. Trussel:
    Digital image enhancement of cephalograms. Angle Orthod. *48*:80-84, 1978.

16. Reidel, R. A.:
    The relation of maxillary structures to cranium in malocclusion and in normal occlusion. Angle Orthod. *22*:142-145, 1952.

17. Steiner, C. C.:
    Cephalometrics for you and me. Am. J. Orthod. *39*:729-755, 1953.

18. Walker, G. F. and C. J. Kowalski:
    On the growth of the mandible. Am. J. Phys. Anthropol. *36*:111-118, 1972.

Chapter 9

Interceptive Orthodontics

The purpose of interceptive orthodontics is the achievement of normal and satisfactory development of functionally and morphologically harmonious occlusion and interception of any local factors which would induce malocclusion. Fullfillment of that purpose requires frequent evaluation of the developing dentition until the permanent dentition is satisfactorily in place.

Not all malocclusions can be prevented. In some instances a skilled and well trained dentist can, with the help of the patient and parents, treat malocclusion early and intercept worsening of the condition. Extensive diagnostic and therapeutic skill is required and such procedures should not be initiated by the untrained practitioner. These procedures involve the use of chin caps, activators and other special appliances which alter development of bony parts to achieve better occlusion. Some patients with malocclusion, particularly those in whom the malocclusion is caused by local etiological factors rather than a basic genetic skeletal discrepancy, can benefit greatly by interceptive measures. Several different means of interception may be necessary to enhance development of a full and adequate jaw relationship.

The most common problems which require careful evaluation, analysis and interceptive orthodontic treatment are:

A. Crossbite, either of individual teeth or of arch segments

B. Prolonged retention of primary teeth and ectopic eruption of the permanent teeth

C. Ankylosis of one or more teeth or loss of arch space because of abnormal position of the other teeth in the arch, or both

D. Loss of arch space because of premature loss of primary or permanent teeth or inadequate restorative dental care

E. Abnormal oral habits, including finger sucking, mouth breathing, tongue thrusting, or lip or cheek biting

F. Abnormal frenulae, including the upper labial frenum and other frenulae found in some pathological conditions

G. Congenitally missing or supernumerary teeth

H. Malformed teeth

I. Structural pathologic conditions with associated dental and oral abnormalities, such as cleft palate, cleidocranial dysostosis, endocrine disturbances, ectodermal dysplasia, etc.

J. Systemic pathologic conditions such as frequent episodes of upper respiratory disease that may condition the patient to become a mouthbreather and may then interfere with facial development.

Of great importance in the diagnosis of incipient malocclusion likely to be responsive to interceptive orthodontics is distinguishing between conditions essentially dentoalveolar in origin and those which are skeletal. In diagnosing anterior crossbite, for example, it is necessary to distinguish a pseudo Class III from a true Class III malocclusion. In cases of pseudo Class III malocclusion (in reality Class I occlusion with lingually malpositioned upper incisors and a functional displacement of the lower arch), correction at an early age is necessary to prevent the later development of a more severe problem.

The masticatory apparatus is formed by a tooth component and a bone component. The former is made up of the teeth and the alveolar process which connects the teeth to the basal bones. Teeth, alveoli, and alveolar ligaments appear and develop together and do not exist independently. Teeth and bones develop in different rhythms because the genes involved in skeletal development and in tooth development are independent of one another. Further, bones and teeth react to exogenous and pathologic conditions in unique patterns. Some pathologic conditions affect the skeleton but not the teeth, and vice versa.

Facial skeleton type is determined genetically, and the shape, size, and inter-relation of the jaws are prenatally established with hereditary tendency to Angle Class I, Class II or Class III. However, individual variations in external factors influence the developmental process. Various forces act on predetermined development in different ways. Teeth and jaws are under the influence of muscular forces, normal and abnormal, and any deviation of the muscular equilibrium will influence tooth positioning and induce migration, inclination, or even rotation.

Eruptive forces play an important part in facial development. The first mandibular permanent molar erupts in a mesiolingual direction until it meets the second primary molar, when it begins to straighten. The maxillary first molar, however, erupts distovestibularly, changing direction when it encounters muscular resistance and straightening to enter into occlusion. Changes in direction are also responsible for

closing the diastemata developed during the eruption of the teeth. The size of the teeth and bone discrepancies also play roles in the persistence of diastemata after eruption of all the teeth. Because certain abnormal habits interfere with normal occlusal development, it is important to alter these habits when such effects are still reversible. Occlusal forces also act during mastication. Primary teeth have longitudinal axis in vertical positions but permanent teeth have a mesial inclination of the longitudinal axis. Therefore, particularly when continuity of the arch is interrupted by premature removal of tooth elements, such occlusal forces can cause a shift of the remaining elements.

Establishment and timing of the necessary therapy is a complex diagnostic problem. Skilled acquisition of data and understanding of the mechanisms involved in growth and development are required. Data include determination of the type of problem, the treatment possibilities and prognosis, and careful study of timing of treatment. For best results, the following data must be evaluated:

A. Facial configuration and profile

Evaluation of the profile is a long established anthropologic method. While it lacks precision, it gives the clinician a rapid impression as to whether the patient is orthognathic, retronathic or prognathic and his potential to an Angle Class I, II or III occlusion. Evaluation of the profiles of other members of the family is of assistance in determining genetic tendencies. In true Angle Class III malocclusion, a prognathic mandible usually will be noticeable at all times but a pseudo Class III at rest is characterized by a normal profile. A pseudo Class III is the result of an anterior accommodation shift of the mandible after a few teeth enter into premature contact. If the pseudo Class III patient is asked to bite, his anterior teeth usually come to an edge to edge incisal relationship and then the mandible slides forward and the posterior teeth occlude as the jaw goes into crossbite. In a true Class III, the closure is smooth and without premature contacts and the teeth move directly into a crossbite relationship. In pseudo Class III at rest, the molar relationship and the terminal plane will appear normal and the incisors are usually inclined and show some spacing. However, if the patient is unable to place the incisors into an edge to edge relationship, a true Class III jaw relationship should be suspected and consultation with a specialist is advisable.

B. Intraoral examination

Knowledge of age-related changes of growth and development is necessary for accurate data collection. Flush terminal plane is a normal finding in younger patients, as is flaring of the incisors during the period of eruption called the "ugly duckling" stage. Diastemata between the maxillary incisors may be self-correcting at this stage but correction after eruption of the canines may require surgery and orthodontic treatment.

C. Radiographic survey

Observation of the sequence of tooth eruption as well as prediction of tooth size and absence of tooth development are needed in the diagnosis and prognosis of space discrepancies. Supernumerary teeth, ankylosis, and ectopic eruption are important factors to be noted. While tooth size of unerupted teeth cannot be determined completely because of rotations that cannot be fully visualized and because of X-ray angulations which may give false impressions, an attempt at measuring other erupted teeth on the radiograph and calculation of the possible size of the unerupted teeth may improve the validity of space analysis.

D. Space analysis

The best way to study space during mixed dentition is with the aid of study models. While measurements must be analyzed carefully, clinical judgment is very important, especially in patients with protrusion and disharmonies. Space analysis is absolutely necessary to evaluate the potential need for space when there is premature loss of primary molars. If there is any doubt about the space available, a space maintainer should be placed. Further orthodontic consultation may be indicated when analysis of the mixed dentition and arch length and the tentative measurement of the unerupted teeth provide an impression of future space inadequacies.

Several methods are used for evaluation of the amount of space available and its adequacy for proper tooth alignment. A number of radiographic methods have been used, but, because of the possible different directions of the central beam and tooth rotations in the crypts, this type of analysis is often inadequate and unreliable.

The mixed dentition analysis method developed by Moyers[13] is easy to perform and has proven to be usually reliable. Because good correlation has been found to exist between the size of the different teeth in the arch, the relationship between the size of the incisors, canines and premolars is used in this analytic method. The mesiodistal widths of the mandibular incisors are measured as accurately as possible and the size of the canines and premolars predicted according to a probability chart (Table 9-1a and b). Various types of work sheets to record the measurements have been developed to facilitate calculations (Table 9-2).

Table 9-1a **Probability chart for predicting the sum of the widths of maxillary canine and premolars from mandibular incisors** (Upper)

Sum of Mandibular Incisors =	19.5	20.0	20.5	21.0	21.5	22.0	22.5	23.0	23.5	24.0	24.5	25.0	25.5	26.0	26.5	27.0	27.5	28.0	28.5	29.0
95%	21.6	21.8	22.1	22.4	22.7	22.9	23.2	23.5	23.8	24.0	24.3	24.6	24.9	25.1	25.4	25.7	26.0	26.2	26.5	26.7
85%	21.0	21.3	21.5	21.8	22.1	22.4	22.6	22.9	23.2	23.5	23.7	24.0	24.3	24.6	24.8	25.1	25.4	25.7	25.9	26.2
75%	20.6	20.9	21.2	21.5	21.8	22.0	22.3	22.6	22.9	23.1	23.4	23.7	24.0	24.2	24.5	24.8	25.0	25.3	25.6	25.9
65%	20.4	20.6	20.9	21.2	21.5	21.8	22.0	22.3	22.6	22.8	23.1	23.4	23.7	24.0	24.2	24.5	24.8	25.1	25.3	25.6
50%	20.0	20.3	20.6	20.8	21.1	21.4	21.7	21.9	22.2	22.5	22.8	23.0	23.3	23.6	23.9	24.1	24.4	24.7	25.0	25.3
35%	19.6	19.9	20.2	20.5	20.8	21.0	21.3	21.6	21.9	22.1	22.4	22.7	23.0	23.2	23.5	23.8	24.1	24.3	24.6	24.9
25%	19.4	19.7	19.9	20.2	20.5	20.8	21.0	21.3	21.6	21.9	22.1	22.4	22.7	23.0	23.2	23.5	23.8	24.1	24.3	24.6
15%	19.0	19.3	19.6	19.9	20.2	20.4	20.7	21.0	21.3	21.5	21.8	22.1	22.4	22.6	22.9	23.2	23.4	23.7	24.0	24.3
5%	18.5	18.8	19.0	19.3	19.6	19.9	20.1	20.4	20.7	21.0	21.2	21.5	21.8	22.1	22.3	22.6	22.9	23.2	23.4	23.7

Table 9-1b **Probability chart for predicting the sum of the widths of mandibular canine and premolars from mandibular incisors** (Lower)

Sum of Mandibular Incisors =	19.5	20.0	20.5	21.0	21.5	22.0	22.5	23.0	23.5	24.0	24.5	25.0	25.5	26.0	26.5	27.0	27.5	28.0	28.5	29.0
95%	21.1	21.4	21.7	22.0	22.3	22.6	22.9	23.2	23.5	23.8	24.1	24.4	24.7	25.0	25.3	25.6	25.8	26.1	26.4	26.7
85%	20.5	20.8	21.1	21.4	21.7	22.0	22.3	22.6	22.9	23.2	23.5	23.8	24.0	24.3	24.6	24.9	25.2	25.5	25.8	26.1
75%	20.1	20.4	20.7	21.0	21.3	21.6	21.9	22.2	22.5	22.8	23.1	23.4	23.7	24.0	24.3	24.6	24.8	25.1	25.4	25.7
65%	19.8	20.1	20.4	20.7	21.0	21.3	21.6	21.9	22.2	22.5	22.8	23.1	23.4	23.7	24.0	24.3	24.6	24.8	25.1	25.4
50%	19.4	19.7	20.0	20.3	20.6	20.9	21.2	21.5	21.8	22.1	22.4	22.7	23.0	23.3	23.6	23.9	24.2	24.5	24.7	25.0
35%	19.0	19.3	19.6	19.9	20.2	20.5	20.8	21.1	21.4	21.7	22.0	22.3	22.6	22.9	23.2	23.5	23.8	24.0	24.3	24.6
25%	18.7	19.0	19.3	19.6	19.9	20.2	20.5	20.8	21.1	21.4	21.7	22.0	22.3	22.6	22.9	23.2	23.5	23.8	24.1	24.4
15%	18.4	18.7	19.0	19.3	19.6	19.8	20.1	20.4	20.7	21.0	21.3	21.6	21.9	22.2	22.5	22.8	23.1	23.4	23.7	24.0
5%	17.7	18.0	18.3	18.6	18.9	19.2	19.5	19.8	20.1	20.4	20.7	21.0	21.3	21.6	21.9	22.2	22.5	22.8	23.1	23.4

From Moyers, R. E., Handbook of Orthodontics, Year Book Publishers[13]

Table 9-2 **Mixed dentition analysis (75 percentile)**

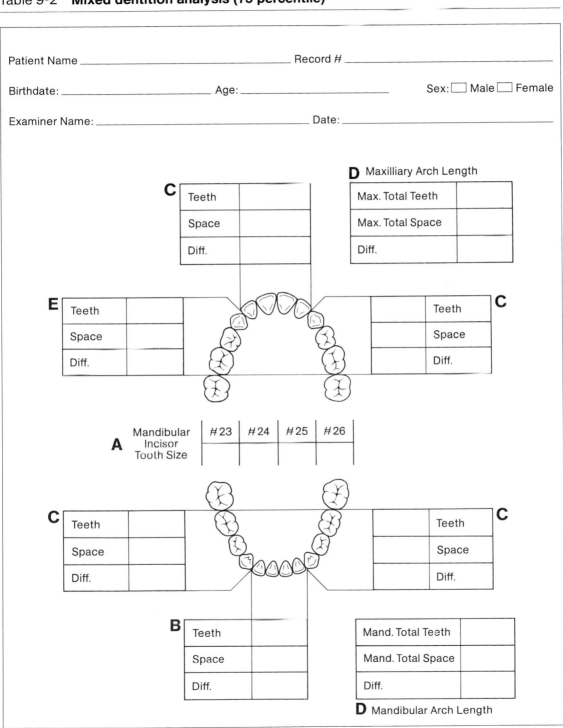

Patient Name _____ Record # _____

Birthdate: _____ Age: _____ Sex: ☐ Male ☐ Female

Examiner Name: _____ Date: _____

D Maxilliary Arch Length

C

Teeth	
Space	
Diff.	

Max. Total Teeth	
Max. Total Space	
Diff.	

E

Teeth	
Space	
Diff.	

C

Teeth	
Space	
Diff.	

A Mandibular Incisor Tooth Size

	# 23	# 24	# 25	# 26

C

Teeth	
Space	
Diff.	

C

Teeth	
Space	
Diff.	

B

Teeth	
Space	
Diff.	

Mand. Total Teeth	
Mand. Total Space	
Diff.	

D Mandibular Arch Length

The mesiodistal width of each mandibular incisor is measured individually and the values are summed (Table 9-2 A) (antimeres may be used if one of the incisors is still absent or is malformed). The sum of the tooth sizes is compared to the actual space available in the anterior region (Table 9-2 B). This proportion indicates the difference between the total tooth size and space available for anterior teeth.

Using the sum of the sizes of the mandibular incisors as a basis, the space required for the canines, premolars, and maxillary incisors can be predicted (Table 9-1a and b). While the upper limit of the 95% prediction interval is desirable, in practice the upper limit of the 75% prediction interval is generally used. This means that we can predict the maximum requirement of needed space in 75% of the cases.

Calculations are performed by the following method: The values based on the columns of Table 9-1a and b are recorded in the appropriate space of Table 9-2 C. The space available for the teeth on each side is measured on the model (as the arch is curved, measurements should be made in small segments to assure accuracy).

Comparison between the two values for each of the different parts of the arch indicates whether there is enough space available for all permanent teeth. In section D of Table 9-2 the total maxillary and mandibular arch length is noted for each arch and the difference between them indicates space adequacy or lack thereof. As primary molars are larger than their permanent premolars, lack of space in the anterior segment may be compensated in the posterior segment. To be of diagnostic value, the mixed dentition analysis must be supplemented by good study model analysis.

Crossbites

A crossbite may involve one or more teeth in the anterior or posterior segment or both. In some instances it may interfere with the closing of the mandible and cause a mandibular shift at the end of the closure. As crossbites may induce shift of mandibular movement, they should be corrected. Since correction in the primary dentition does not assure that permanent teeth will erupt in proper alignment, some clinicians do not advocate correction at an early age[6]. However, early correction can create a more favorable development and allow a better growth pattern by reestablishing proper muscle balance before deterioration becomes well established. These conditions, when they arise, must be correctly analyzed.

Simple dental anterior crossbite involving a single tooth or localized malocclusion such as prolonged retention of primary teeth as the etiological factor is easy to diagnose. There are cases, however, in which the differentiation between an Angle Class III malocclusion involving skeletal abnormality from a pseudo Class III is difficult because of functional protraction of the mandible. In these subjects a precise evaluation is required. Profile examination may supply some additional data, and examination of lateral cephalometric head films may permit an accurate evaluation of dental and skeletal structures and their relationship.

Anterior crossbite

Anterior crossbite caused by lingual eruption of a maxillary incisor should be corrected before space loss can result from the migration of the other teeth or trauma can be created by the abnormal position of the occluding teeth. Anterior crossbite may be associated with a skeletal discrepancy and be caused by a true Class III malocclusion. It may be an acquired muscular reflex pattern of mandibular closure to a pseudo Class III malocclusion. Alternatively, it may be a simple lingual shift of one or more maxillary anterior teeth caused by an abnormal inclination of the maxillary incisors. This abnormal inclination is sometimes related to abnormal eruption patterns caused by prolonged retention of primary teeth or the presence of a supernumerary tooth. It may also be an idiopathic lack of space in the dental arch.

Failure of the primary teeth to exfoliate at the appropriate time may cause the permanent teeth to erupt in abnormal positions (Fig. 9-1) with overretention of the primary teeth. The permanent teeth may be in crossbite. If the condition persists, the opposing teeth may be extruded or adjacent teeth may tip into the space, making later correction more difficult.

The abnormal position of the maxillary lateral teeth may adversely affect the mandibular incisor with the consequent development of traumatic occlusion and clear apical migration of the periodontal tissues, usually vestibular in direction. In severe cases this may cause periodontal pathology and even result in loss of the mandibular incisor. Maxillary anterior crossbite usually forces the patient's mandible into a malposition which can affect growth and function of the maxilla and mandible. Also it can cause a functional posterior crossbite and undesirable muscular changes.

Where there is ample space in the arch for the involved tooth to be brought into correct alignment, correction of a simple anterior crossbite is a short and easy procedure. Several methods are available from which to select.

Tongue blade correction

In early cases, when the maxillary incisor is still erupting, with no major overbite and

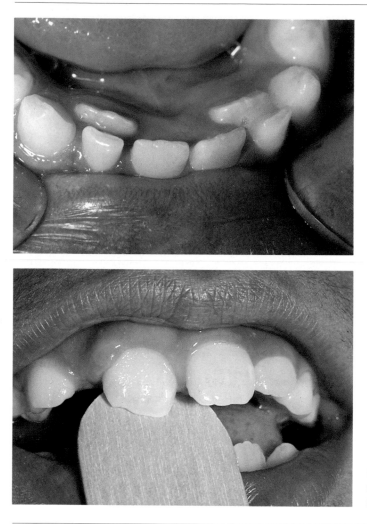

Fig. 9-1 Eruption of permanent teeth with primary teeth still in place.

Fig. 9-2 Tongue blade correction can be attempted in cases of good spacing and not fully erupted teeth.

adequate space in the arch for the misaligned tooth, a tongue blade may be sufficient for crossbite correction (Fig. 9-2). The patient is instructed to insert the tongue blade at an angle between the teeth and bite firmly, maintaining the pressure for 5 seconds, then interrupt and repeat for 25 times, 3 times a day. If the tongue blade exercise is not successful after two weeks or if tooth eruption is too advanced, a bite plane is more satisfactory. The major disadvantages of the tongue blade method are the complete dependence on the patient for both frequency of performance and accuracy of placement. This makes the technique somewhat unreliable.

Bite plane for correction of anterior crossbite

The bite plane should have sufficient inclination to produce a definite forward sliding motion of the maxillary incisor on closure (Figs. 9-3a to c). The acrylic bite plane should not impinge on soft tissue of the mandibular teeth to avoid food impaction. The acrylic part of the bite plane should in-

Fig. 9-3a to c   Anterior crossbite correction using a fixed acrylic appliance.

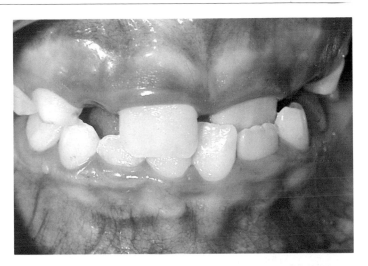

Figure 9-3a

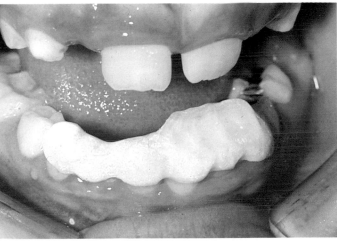

Figure 9-3b

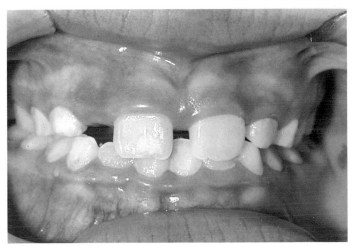

Figure 9-3c

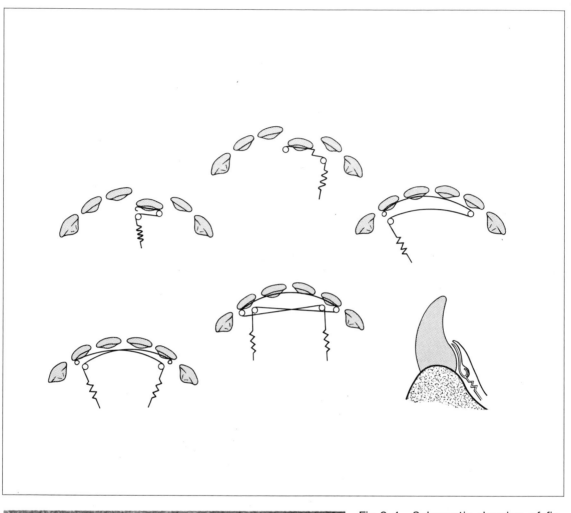

Fig. 9-4 Schematic drawing of finger springs suitable for incorporation in appliance for tooth movement (Courtesy of Drs. R.S. and J. Bodenham, Dent. Pract. 20:52-58, 1969 with permission from J. Wright & Sons).

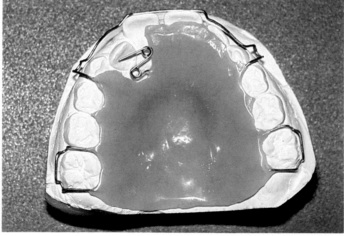

Fig. 9-5 Appliance with finger spring for correction of position of tooth 7.

clude more teeth than the ones for which correction is sought. If the maxillary central incisor requires correction, the bite plane should include all four mandibular incisors for adequate support.

The appliance is cemented with a temporary cement. The posterior teeth will be slightly out of occlusion but the discomfort is minimal as the appliance is used for no longer than two weeks. If no improvement has taken place by then, the original diagnosis should be reviewed. The major advantages of this appliance are its ease of manufacture and insertion and its rapid action. It requires careful supervision because if it is not removed after a short period of time, a posterior open bite and speech problems may develop. In the absence of adequate root formation dilaceration can become a problem.

Hawley retainer with auxiliary springs

The Hawley retainer is a palatal acrylic plate with finger springs placed lingually to the malpositioned tooth and with acrylic on the occlusal surfaces of the molars. This is a very useful appliance when the overbite is small, but because the patient must wear the appliance full time, maximal cooperation is essential. The major disadvantage of this technique is the need for cooperation. Because the corrective movement is slow, if cooperation is not forthcoming, the tooth will consistently be "locked back" into its abnormal position whenever the appliance is not in use. The appliance requires careful construction with the proper retention since there is displacement of the active anterior component by the appliance. Posterior bite planes should be placed over all the occlusal surfaces of the posterior teeth and should be thick enough to allow the anterior teeth to barely clear each other. Large anterior separation is not necessary, and would actually make the treatment more difficult. Usu-

ally the incisors respond in a few weeks and frequently cooperation is easily attained. If it cannot be obtained, a fixed appliance is necessary.

The finger spring used is a function of personal preference and the number of teeth involved in the malocclusion (Figs. 9-4 and 9-5).

Instead of springs, some clinicians use pegs or screws partially imbedded in the acrylic. While some patients complain of discomfort in fitting such appliances and of the bulk of acrylic needed to imbed the screw, others enjoy the fact that the screw requires adjustment at regular intervals and enjoy being active participants in the therapy.

Use of a retainer after correction of anterior crossbite is unnecessary. The opposing arch prevents relapse.

In patients with crowding as the etiological factor of incisor malpositioning, it is useless to attempt to move the incisors until space has been created into which the tooth can move. Frequently a palatally inclined maxillary lateral incisor has its roots in close proximity to the unerupted permanent canine. This must be ascertained before any movement is initiated so that the canine does not damage the incisor root.

Posterior crossbite

The etiology of posterior crossbites has been widely studied. According to Moyers[1] there are three different types to be considered: dental, muscular, and osseous. Dental crossbite involves only the tipping of teeth, muscular crossbite involves the muscular alterations caused by tooth interference, and osseous crossbite is related to skeletal disharmonies. Day and Foster[5] studied 2,441 patients in Birmingham, England and found 400 with posterior crossbite. Of these, 35% were associated with skeletal Class III malocclusion. In 11% the molar crossbite was associated with cuspal interferences and in

50% the crossbite was associated with finger sucking and abnormal tongue swallowing habits.

In diagnosing a posterior crossbite, the most important point is determining whether it is unilateral or bilateral. The majority of posterior crossbites are bilateral. However, most affected patients develop a convenience bite that may lead to the hasty diagnostic conclusion that the problem is unilateral only.

In patients with bilateral crossbite, the maxillary and mandibular midlines coincide with the middle of the upper half of the face and the middle of the chin, respectively. These midlines approximate each other when the mouth is partially open but do not align when the teeth are closed. If the arch midlines coincide with their respective parts of the face but not with each other when the teeth are open, the discrepancy is not the result of a lateral shift of the teeth in one of the arches but that of a unilateral crossbite.

Treatment for posterior crossbite should be initiated as soon as the condition is diagnosed, because it is not self-correcting. Delay in treatment may lead to further abnormal growth and abnormal neuro-muscular patterns. A crossbite in the primary dentition usually will be present in the permanent dentition as well. If corrected in the primary dentition, it may not reappear in the permanent dentition. Untreated functional posterior crossbites gradually bring about compensatory structural changes of the mandible and sometimes of the condyle.

Occasionally, elimination of the interfering factors may be achieved by occlusal equilibration alone but more often appliances are needed. Treatment is accomplished either with a removable or fixed appliance. Retainers should be worn after correction to assure permanent position as relapse occurs frequently.

In some cases, only light tooth tipping forces are needed. In simple cases involving one tooth, only 2 bands and an S-elastic may be effective. A number of appliances have been designed for the purpose of correction of posterior crossbite. All use reciprocal intra-arch anchorage which effects a symmetrical arch width enlargement.

One of the most frequently used fixed appliances is the "W" appliance (Fig. 9-6). It is convenient for patients who tend to be uncooperative, is self-limiting in action, and requires few adjustments. The appliance consists of 2 bands for each of the posterior molars (one on each side, soldered to a 0.036" stainless steel "W"-shaped wire). Activation by opening the loops of the wire permits lateral movement of the tooth surfaces contacting the wire. The opening of the wires should be slow. A final slight overcorrection is desirable at the end of the treatment. The appliance should be removed for activation and remain as a retainer for a time after completion of the treatment.

Fixed appliances for the purpose of suture opening also can be constructed by using bands on the posterior teeth. These are united by an acrylic palatal plate which has a jack-screw in the midline (Fig. 9-7).

Where a dental base rather than a dental arch width correction is indicated, mid-palatal suture opening is desirable to increase the maxillary width (Fig. 9-8a and b)[7].

Among removable appliances, the most frequently used is a modification of the Hawley retainer with a jack-screw which is opened at regular intervals until the necessary width is obtained. The patient is instructed to turn the screw very slowly weekly or biweekly, until the desired correction is obtained. The appliance then can be used as a retainer.

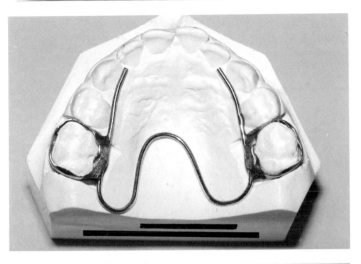

Fig. 9-6   Appliance for correction of posterior crossbite.

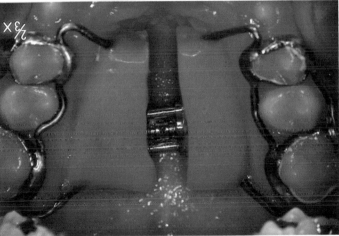

Fig. 9-7   Fixed appliance for correction of posterior crossbite and opening of midsagital suture.

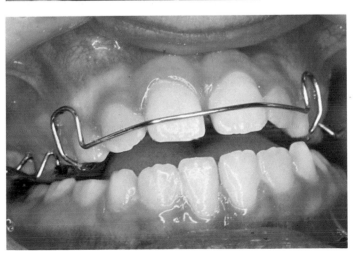

Fig. 9-8a   Removable appliance for correction of posterior crossbite.

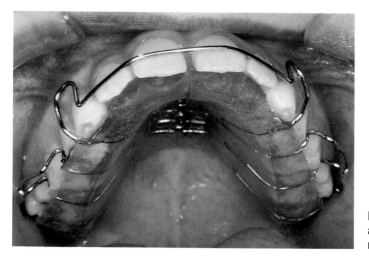

Fig. 9-8b Intra-oral view of removable appliance for correction of posterior crossbite.

Open bite

Causes of open bite include one or a combination of the following:

A. Finger sucking habits
B. Enlarged tonsils or adenoids interfering with proper tongue position, creating upper respiratory problems
C. Mouth breathing associated with tonsil and adenoid pathology, or allergies
D. Macroglossia or abnormal tongue position
E. Muscular defects of the tongue or lips
F. Abnormal tongue habits with tongue thrust and cheek biting
G. Constricted, narrow upper arch with or without crossbite
H. Hemifacial atrophy.

If the etiology is evaluated and properly handled at an early mixed dentition stage, the condition can be corrected in some children. However, severe bone problems may need more extensive correction by either orthodontic or surgical means.

Oral habits

Damaging oral habits that may interfere with growth and development of the face and the position of the teeth must be recognized and treated early, otherwise the problem becomes progressively worse and more difficult to manage. Further, other habits may be initiated to complicate the deformity and to add to the difficulty of treatment. Early recognition of undesirable habits requires discussion of the problems with alerted parents.

Finger sucking

Thumb or finger sucking is the most frequent habit producing abnormal jaw relationships. Thumb sucking is a spontaneous activity that may develop soon after birth. Some research evidence indicates that it may be present prenatally[11]. Between birth and age 3 months, its intensity increases until age 7 months and then usually it decreases with the development of other motor activities[3]. Sometimes it is possible to attempt a substi-

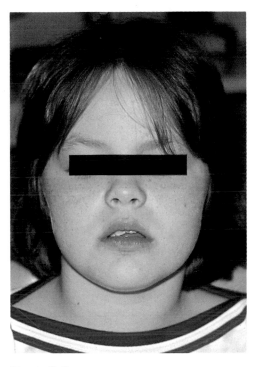

Figure 9-9a

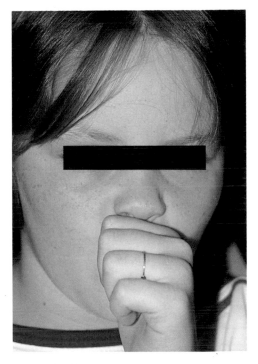

Figure 9-9b

Figure 9-9c

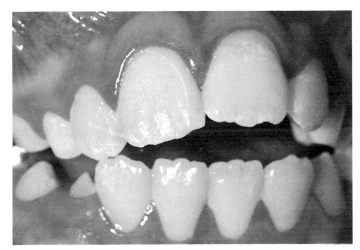

Fig. 9-9a to c   Open bite caused by finger sucking habit.

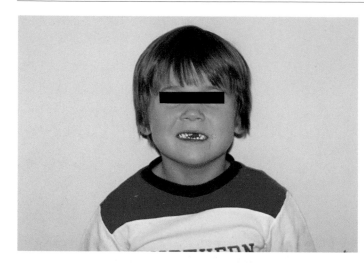

Fig. 9-10 a to c   Open bite caused by finger sucking habit.

Figure 9-10 a

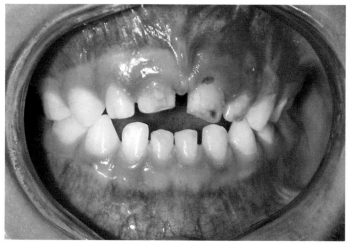

Figure 9-10 b

Figure 9-10 c

Fig. 9-11a and b   Self-correction of crossbite after the patient stopped finger sucking habit.

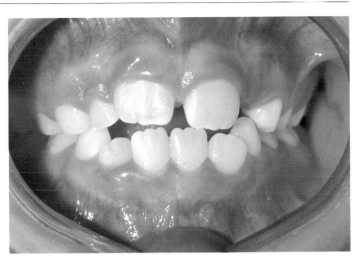

Figure 9-11a

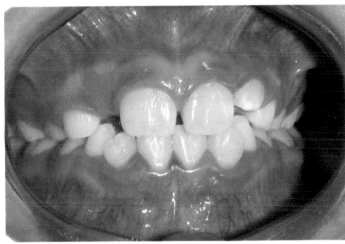

Figure 9-11b

tution of the finger by a properly designed pacifier[14] that may be less damaging. However, the habit frequently is established by the time the dentist sees the child for the first time. Often the habit is dropped before the appearance of the permanent teeth when the child starts school because of peer pressure. Open bite is in many instances associated with an unbroken, constant and persistent thumb sucking habit, often with displacement of the anterior bony structures. Even when the finger sucking habit is no longer present, the tongue or the lip may intrude in the open gap, leading to development of malocclusion and speech problems. The speech defects are particularly noticeable in the use of words containing the letters "S" or "Z", when the sound becomes more that of "th" with the tongue filling the space between the teeth. If the habit is discontinued before appearance of the permanent teeth, the open bite usually is self-correcting. If the finger sucking habit persists, occlusal problems frequently develop.

In management of a thumbsucking habit, the age of the child and the type of malocclusion

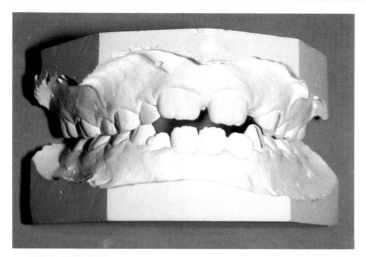

Fig. 9-12 a Models before patient stopped sucking.

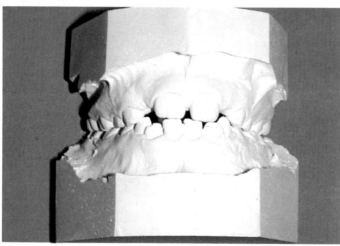

Fig. 9-12 b Models made three months later.

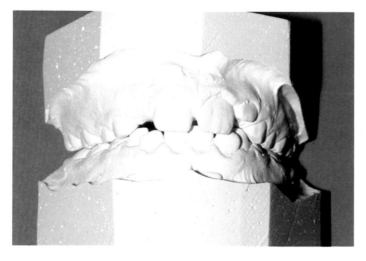

Fig. 9-12 c Models made five months after the first ones.

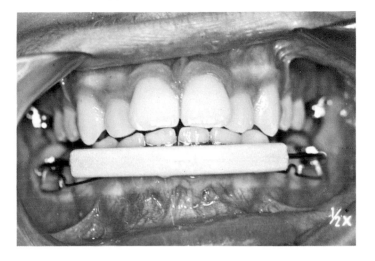

Fig. 9-13   Lip bumper for correction of lip biting habit (Courtesy of Dr. J. G. Crawford).

present are of primary importance. The duration, intensity, and frequency of the habit must be assessed. If the child is willing to stop thumbsucking, several aids and reminders are available to help him. It is important that the family stop scolding, nagging, and ridiculing. When severe emotional problems are involved, it is wiser to wait and correct the dental problem orthodontically later. Without the child's readiness to cooperate, a relapse of the habit is likely or the level of anxiety will be such that other deleterious habits may develop (Figs. 9-9a to c and 9-10a to c).

Aids that can be used include both simple home "reminders" such as taped bandages, mittens or solutions with unpleasant taste, and specially constructed devices, fixed or removable such as oral screens, Hawley appliances, etc.

Most such devices use the maxillary teeth for anchorage and some form of wire as a deterent to finger positioning. Some clinicians go so far as to recommend sharp prongs to "remind" the tongue and finger to stay back; many question the possible psychological damage of such measures[9].

As most affected patients have suffered considerably from peer pressure, they will try to cooperate as soon as they understand the damage to the dentition, even if stopping the habit is not easy. If the child decides to want a "reminder" such as a glove, a finger tape, or an oral screen, it is acceptable. However, it is the child who should want the reminder. If the child is cooperative, keeping a diary of a sucking habit is often enough to transform an unconscious act into a conscious one and stop it (Figs. 9-11a and b, 9-12a to c).

Abnormal lip habits

Abnormal lip habits usually involve the lower lip. The force exerted by the lower lip caught between the maxillary and mandibular teeth may move the maxillary incisor labially and the mandibular incisor lingually. As the abnormal lip habit may also include mentalis hyperactivity and may result in the collapse of the anterior segment of the arch, a supporting lingual arch is indicated in some patients as a preventive measure at the same time other measures are instituted.

Barber[1] advocates the construction of a lip bumper as a means of inhibiting muscular pressure of the orbicularis oris and mentalis

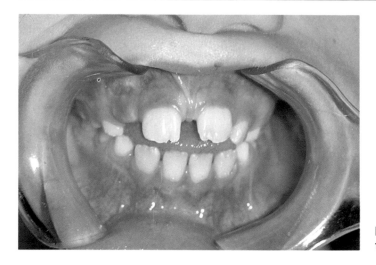

Fig. 9-14 Open bite caused by tongue thrusting.

on the teeth. Bands with tubes are placed on the molars, a labial arch wire (0.040″) is shaped appropriately, and acrylic is placed on the wire away from the teeth and without occlusal interference. Two stops are soldered to the wire. Care is taken to make the acrylic bumper flat and broad to avoid any irritation to the soft lip mucosa (Fig. 9-13).

The arch can be inserted or removed at will by the patient. Because the major function of the appliance is to retain the musculature by making an unconscious habit uncomfortable, the child's cooperation is necessary.

When muscle exercises are needed, simple measures are preferred, such as placing a large button attached to a string in the vestibule and asking the patient to pull with closed lips for a period of time, several times each day. Lip "ballooning" by holding air in the vestibule and making sure the lips are closed tight may also help some children.

Cheek biting

Cheek biting usually is accompanied by cheek sucking. The patient places the buccal fat pad between the maxillary and mandibular teeth with a lingual tipping of the teeth in the posterior region. Unilateral pos-

terior open bite may result. Treatment consists in altering the habit by placing a device to separate the cheek from the teeth. If patient cooperation can be obtained, frequently only a properly constructed shield is necessary.

Tongue thrusting

In tongue thrusting, the tongue takes an abnormal anterior position during swallowing. It may cause protrusion and diastema formation of the maxillary teeth (Fig. 9-14). Abnormal tongue habits such as tongue thrusting are difficult to correct. In more severe cases, the tongue protrudes between the maxillary and mandibular anterior teeth during swallowing. The incidence of tongue thrusting reported varies according to the parameters and definitions used[8]. There seems to be a normal decrease of the habit with increase in age. If correction is needed, the most common exercise is placement of an orthodontic elastic or a sugarless candy lozenge at the tip of the tongue and asking the patient to place the tip of the tongue in correct position on the palate for a certain length of time several times each day. Myofunctional therapy may be required for some children and

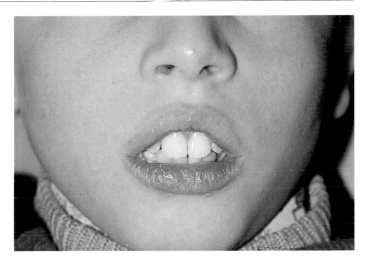

Fig. 9-15   Characteristic appearance in mouth breathing.

appropriate consultations may be indicated to evaluate the need for such therapy.

Mouth breathing

In evaluating the patient for this problem it is important to keep the patient unaware of the evaluation. Most patients, if asked, are capable of nose breathing. A mouth breather, when asked to close his lips and take a forced deep breath, will not change the size and shape of the external narcs appreciably (Fig. 9-15). An habitual nose breather usually has good control over the alar muscles and will dilate the nostrils when breathing deeply.

Another diagnostic device is placement of a small wisp of cotton or thin piece of tissue paper alternately in front of the nose and the mouth. The cotton or tissue paper will move according to the air movement of the nostrils or the mouth. This test is more accurate when the child is asleep, because the child should be unaware that a test is being made. Parents can be instructed to perform the test at home. A cold mirror also can be used to evaluate the location of hot air fogging. Several etiological factors may be involved in producing mouth breathing:

1. naso-pharyngeal deformity and obstructions
2. enlarged adenoids or tongue
3. frequent irritation of nasal mucosa and Waldeyer ring, caused by frequent upper respiratory problems or allergies
4. systemic disturbances leading to abnormal muscular control such as nerve dysfunctions, etc.
5. abnormally short upper lip preventing proper lip seal.

It is obligatory in some instances of open bite to request an otorhinolaryngologic examination to determine whether conditions requiring treatment are present in tonsils, adenoids, or nasal septum. As mouth breathing may continue in some children even after correction of the pathologic conditions, it is necessary first to diagnose and then to correct the problem.

Correction of the mouth breathing habit first involves the removal of any anatomical or functional cause. If there is no physiologic cause, the patient should be instructed in breathing and lip exercises and an oral screen may be fitted. Breathing and lip exercises consist of deep inhaling and exhaling for 5-10 minutes, 3-4 times daily with the lips

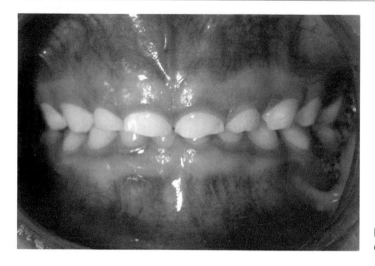

Fig. 9-16 Loss of tooth structure due to bruxism in a 5-year-old boy.

closed, before a mirror. Various methods can be used to remind the patient to breathe through the nose. The patient, but not the parent, can apply a tape or adhesive bandage to the mouth for a few minutes several times each day (at least 5 minutes and at least 3-4 times a day). An oral screen can be placed by the patient. The oral screen has the advantage that it can be activated by increasing the thickness of acrylic selectively in some areas and may help reposition the teeth. However, if adequate labial tonus is re-established this will take care of a greater part of the tooth problem. The oral screen can be constructed of any material compatible with oral tissues which does not irritate the vestibular mucosa. Care must be taken to avoid overextension of the acrylic to protect this rather delicate tissue.

Bruxism

Bruxism is a habit not infrequent in children. It is usually done during the sleep but can occur during the day. The etiology of this tooth grinding is still controversial. Attrition, sometimes severe, can be found in young children and is sometimes associated with bruxism. Some patients with cerebral palsy show extensive attrition caused by muscular reflex bruxism (Fig. 9-16).

Several investigators believe that there is an emotional basis for the habit as many of the children who brux are irritable; however, more research in this question is needed. With some children it may be advantageous to consult the pediatrician. If the habit is damaging to the temporomandibular joint a splint can be constructed but it is not always effective in children.

Space management in the mixed dentition

Loss of arch length during development may be caused by loss of tooth substance from caries or trauma or by premature loss of teeth from caries, trauma, or root resorption resulting from abnormal eruption patterns of the permanent teeth other than the succedaneous ones.

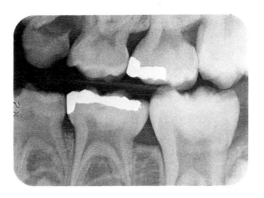

Fig. 9-17 Ectopic eruption of tooth 14 is responsible for the resorption of the distal area of tooth J.

Ectopic tooth eruption

In some instances the permanent first molars erupt ectopically and their pathways interfere with the distal surfaces of the primary second molar causing pathologic resorption of areas of that tooth. In addition to damage to the primary second molar which may be irreparable, this eruption path will lead to loss of arch length, and should be monitored and corrected as necessary. In many cases, the first permanent molar is prevented from assuming its full occlusal contact. In other cases the molar may be deflected and continue erupting, pathologic resorption being noted only incidentally during routine dental examination (Fig. 9-17).

The mesial eruption of the permanent first molar may be a purely local eruption problem or may be indicative of a major arch length deficiency that requires further consideration. No treatment is necessary if the permanent molar erupts and the primary molar can be held in position until eruption of the second premolar. If the first molars have not been able to "jump" the resorption area, treatment to change the eruption pathway is necessary. The treatment consists in distalizing the tooth with the aid of a brass ligature wire (Fig. 9-18 a to c). The brass ligature wire (0.032″ gauge) is threaded between the maxillary permanent first molar and the maxillary primary second molar and the ends are twisted. This wedging of the wire will distalize the molar and will, hopefully create enough space for the correct path for the full eruption of the permanent molar. When the damage to the primary molar is such that the wire cannot remain in place, it may be necessary to place a band with a small vertical extension to guide the eruption path of the permanent molar. When damage to the distal surface of the primary second molar includes pulp involvement, the tooth must be removed and a space maintainer placed to prevent mesial drift of the maxillary permanent molars.

According to Cheyne and Wessels[4], 5 stages of ectopic eruption patterns can be distinguished:

Stage I – The marginal ridge portion of the mesial surface of the first permanent molar is lodged in close vicinity to the cervical portion of the second primary molar and a small area of radiolucency can be seen on the cervical region of the second primary molar. The interseptal bony crest shows slight or

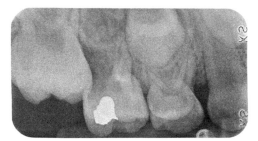

Figure 9-18a

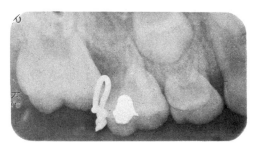

Figure 9-18b

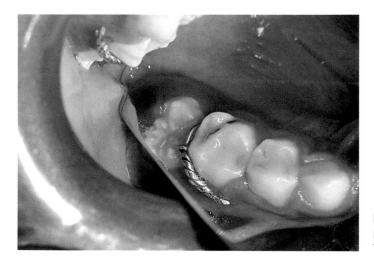

Fig. 9-18a, b and c   Radiograph and photograph of the brass ligature wire to separate teeth 3 and A.

moderate compression. No treatment is necessary at this stage but careful follow-up is needed.

Stage II – Definite resorption can be noted on the distal cervical aspect of the root of the primary molar. The first permanent molar is lodged in the concavity of the resorption area or shows signs of having passed the "lock" and is now continuing eruption. If the first permanent tooth has freed itself from the resorption site, only re-evaluation of the primary molar is necessary. If the permanent molar is still lodged, separation should be attempted.

Stage III – Nearly all the distal root structure of the primary molar is lost with the resorption of both the tooth structure and the supporting bone. If the permanent tooth is still

unerupted and lodged in the resorption area, loss of arch space is evident. If the permanent tooth shows indication of being able to overcome the interference, separating wires may be used. Alternatively, the primary tooth may have to be removed and a space maintainer placed.

Stage IV – The primary tooth shows progressive resorption involving its cervical region. If the permanent tooth has remained in the unerupted position, several millimeters of space may be lost from the tipping of the first permanent molar. The primary tooth will have to be removed and the position of the permanent molar will require correction.

Stage V – The primary molar has tipped and drifted into the region formerly occupied by the primary second molar. Orthodontic evaluation of the first permanent molar and the first premolar is necessary as the second premolar may be crowded into a lingual or buccal position.

Diastema

Diastemata in the primary dentition are quite normal and desirable for proper alignment of the larger permanent teeth (see Fig. 3-19). In the mixed dentition, physiologic spacing between incisors also is normal because of the eruption pattern of the permanent teeth. When the canines erupt, all the spaces will close. Abnormal diastemata may result from supernumerary or missing teeth, oral habits, macroglossia, frenulae, excessive midline bone development, or systemic conditions such as some endocrine disturbances. Accurate diagnosis is necessary before treatment can be initiated. No treatment should be initiated if there is a possibility that a diastema is physiologic or if the canines have not erupted. Treatment when necessary includes surgery or orthodontics, or both.

Serial extraction

Spacing in the primary dentition is commonly found in the young patient and is desirable because the permanent anterior teeth are larger. If such space is absent, a moderate to severe temporary space discrepancy may result. During normal development of the permanent dentition, additional space also is provided by the position of the eruption and inclination of the permanent teeth and the smaller size of the premolars as compared to primary molars (See page 61).

It is important that the sequence of eruption and normal development of the occlusion be monitored closely so that any undesirable occurrences are noticed. Usually root re-

sorption proceeds normally allowing for spontaneous exfoliation of the primary teeth. Occasionally the permanent incisors will erupt without the resorption of the primary teeth (see Fig. 9-1). As growth progresses, the teeth will in most cases move labially into normal occlusion after removal of interferences. Occasionally, when adequate space is lacking, the lateral incisors erupt lingually and ectopic resorption may affect the primary canines. However, the indiscriminate premature removal of primary canines to permit eruption of the lateral incisors may seriously compromise favorable tooth positioning in the arch. Orthodontic consultation is indicated, and treatment coordination will become necessary when lack of space does not permit proper alignment of the teeth. Slight irregularities of the mandibular incisors evidenced by a somewhat lingual eruption pathway or slight tooth rotation should not be corrected by removal of the primary canine. Sometimes slight disking of the primary canines may alleviate the problem. The extraction of the canine under these conditions may allow the lateral shift distally and possibly lingually of the incisor. It also may lead to an anterior closed bite and loss of space with encroachment of the lateral on the space of the erupting canine. There are, however, conditions in which a true tooth-bone discrepancy can be diagnosed and when removal is indicated. This discrepancy may be the result of oversized mandibular lateral incisors or premolars or a basal bone deficiency and will require later removal of premolars.

If the irregularity is sufficiently severe to justify removal of the canines, this should be done bilaterally to avoid midline shift and only after a full analysis of the problem to ascertain that serial extraction is the indicated procedure. In any event, removal of the first primary molars must be timed to allow eruption of the permanent canines in a more distal position. Early loss of a primary canine on one side because of root resorption caused by an erupting lateral incisor usually required removal of the other primary canine to maintain arch symmetry.

Serial extraction is a valid, important therapeutic measure which must only be used judiciously. Its indiscriminate use may lead to concave profiles or to open spaces in the arch which may be the cause of periodontal and prosthetic problems in later life. Serial extraction should not be used in instances of severe overbite or lingual inclination of incisors, or when the large size of the primary first molars indicates that some space will be available in the posterior segment of the arch after their substitution by the smaller permanent premolars. It should also not be used in cases where malocclusion problems are caused by skeletal dental discrepancies that will require orthodontic correction. Serial extraction can be considered when there is indication of a full face, when the lateral incisors are very nearly in contact with the primary first molars, and when the anterior teeth do not show major overbite. Serial extraction in most instances will have to be followed by orthodontic treatment. If the procedure is carried out correctly the orthodontic treatment will be faster and easier with reduced danger of relapse.

Ankylosed teeth

Patients whose primary teeth have failed to erupt properly, remaining below the level of the other teeth in the arch and causing the adjoining teeth to tip into the space or over-erupt should have the ankylosed teeth extracted and the space maintained with a suitable appliance. If the ankylosed teeth have no permanent successors, it is possible to fit crowns to restore proper occlusion until a more suitable prosthesis can be constructed or possibilities of orthodontic treatment have been analyzed. Careful consider-ation of the mesiodistal width is important since the succeeding tooth may be smaller mesiodistally than the primary tooth.

Space maintenance

The problem of early loss of primary teeth and possible harmful effects on the developing occlusion is of great importance in pedodontics. The loss may be from caries, trauma, or ectopic eruption of the permanent teeth. The seriousness of space loss varies according to age, type of tooth lost, the timing and type of molar relation, and the eruption pattern of the patient. A clear understanding of the problems associated with space loss will benefit the patient and will be of value in future treatment, even if orthodontic therapy is required.

Space maintenance is the process of maintaining the space previously occupied by a tooth, several teeth or tooth structure before the eruption of the permanent tooth. The best space maintainer is the tooth with proper mesiodistal diameter. Therefore all procedures – including pulp therapy – should be used to retain teeth. The objectives of space maintenance are the preservation of primate space, the integrity of both dental arches and of normal occlusal planes.

Space maintainers may be fixed or removable and can be constructed by direct or indirect techniques. Each type has advantages and disadvantages. A removable space maintainer requires good cooperation of the patient, close supervision by the dentist, and good understanding among the child, the parent, and the dentist. Fixed appliances require periodic reevaluation and may require recementation to prevent decalcification of the abutment teeth.

A space maintainer should have a simple design permitting easy construction and placement. It should be hygienic so that caries susceptibility is not increased. It should be durable, corrosion resistant, easily adjustable, and require minimal supervision. It must prevent abnormal tooth position pattern of occluding and adjacent teeth, and must not hamper normal growth pattern in the area in which it is being used. Moreover, the appliance should be reasonable in cost and in time required for fabrication. While no space maintainer at present fulfills all of these requirements, adequate devices exist to permit proper therapy in most instances.

Space maintainers are contraindicated when the permanent teeth are about to erupt and when careful analysis has demonstrated that there will be no space loss after removal of the tooth. Moreover, oral hygiene and dental care standards too poor to permit proper care of the appliance are also a contraindication.

Congenital absence of a permanent tooth after premature loss of the primary teeth is not a contraindication for a space maintainer. The jaw relationships have to be considered carefully to determine whether a permanent prosthesis substituting for the nonformed element is desirable for the patient's occlusion. Congenital absence of the maxillary lateral incisors frequently requires space maintenance for proper development of maxillary width and therefore the whole maxillary configuration should be considered.

The orthodontic problem that may result from the congenital absence of the teeth must be evaluated early. Often, orthodontic closure of the space may be indicated and may result in adequate functional occlusion. Early interceptive treatment may preclude need for prosthetic replacement. Early extraction of the primary second molar and subsequent orthodontic positioning of the permanent first molar and first premolar can achieve an acceptable occlusal relationship[12].

If radiographs show that there is an appreciable amount of bone above the erupting tooth, space loss is likely to occur. Then usually it will be necessary to use a space maintainer when the primary second molars are lost and the permanent second premolars have not reached the region of bifurcation of the roots of the permanent first molars. If careful study indicates that the space available is adequate to accommodate the permanent tooth without the use of an appliance, a period of observation with short intervals is needed[2]. Brauer[2] found that loss of space occurred in only 36% of instances of premature loss of primary first molars and in 62% of loss of primary second molars.

Eruption sequence is also an important consideration in space maintenance. Careful assessment of the development of permanent dentition is essential. If the diagnosis indicates that major orthodontic treatment may be necessary later, an orthodontic consultation is indicated before space maintainers are placed. If the planned therapy indicates need for extraction and space closure, the space maintainer is unnecessary or even undesirable.

A difficult and controversial problem is the preservation of space when the primary second molars are lost before the eruption of the permanent first molars. An intra-alveolar fixed space maintainer has been advocated[10] but major complications can make its use undesirable. These complications include difficulty in accurate construction, the presence of a constant foreign body in a sensitive area in the mouth, introduction of a possible route of infection between intraoral and submucosal areas, need for periodic reevaluation for correct positioning, possible breakage of the appliance *in situ,* and subsequent trauma and infection.

The placement of a removable appliance (Fig. 9-19) at such an early age requires major patient and parent cooperation which is very difficult to attain for a period of many years. It is therefore more desirable to place

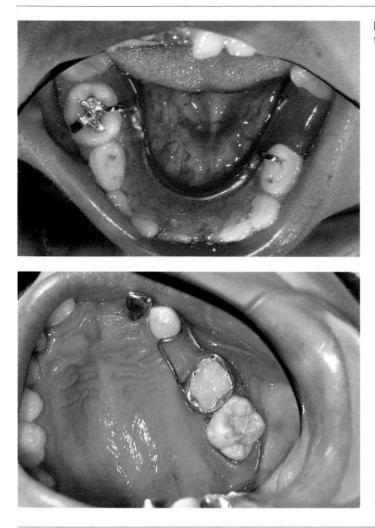

Fig. 9-19 Removable space maintainer.

Fig. 9-20 Band loop space maintainer.

a space maintainer at the time of eruption of the permanent first molar.

The construction of a space maintainer to prevent loss of arch length caused by the removal of a primary first molar is a different problem and requires a device easy to construct and to place. A proper prefabricated stainless steel band is selected and a wire (usually a 0.040″ gauge) is bent into a loop. Care should be taken that the final width of the loop is sufficient to permit the premolar to erupt inside the loop and not be deflected by the wire. The distal parts of the wire should contour the buccal and lingual surfaces of the band by approximately 1/3 to allow adequate adaptation for proper soldering. Occasionally a stainless steel crown on the primary second molar is necessary. Some clinicians solder the bent wire directly to the stainless steel crown. In the long run it is easier to adapt a stainless steel band around the crown, as the space maintainer may dislodge and require removal and adjustments. Moreover, once the permanent incisors have erupted a lingual arch is preferable.

Fig. 9-21a and b   Space maintainer that was not properly controlled and embedded in the tissues.

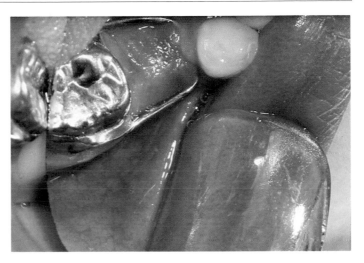

Figure 9-21a

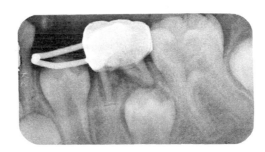

Figure 9-21b

The axial inclination and the degree of inter-cuspidation between opposing teeth as well as super eruption of opposing teeth into the edentulous region may prevent space loss and mesial tooth tipping. In such cases, only periodic monitoring is necessary.

Early loss of primary first molars may result in mesial shift of the primary second molar and permanent first molar. If the loss occurs before complete eruption of the permanent tooth or if the cusp relationship is end-to-end, a space maintainer is indicated, either as a band-loop (in unilateral cases) (Figs. 9-20, 9-21a and b) or a lingual arch (in cases of bilateral loss) (Figs. 9-22 and 9-23) but the appliance must be controlled regularly to assure no interference with erupting teeth (Fig. 9-24). If the loss of the primary first molar occurs after the permanent first molar has erupted and the primary second molar is present in the arch, close observation is usually sufficient.

If the primary second molar is lost prematurely, there may be a mesial drift of the permanent molar and a distal tipping of the permanent premolar (Fig. 9-25). A space main-

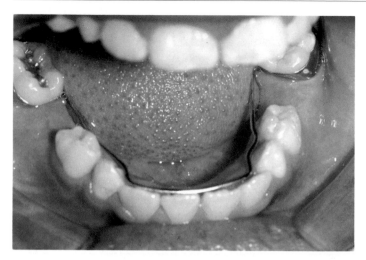

Fig. 9-22 Lingual arch as space maintainer for lower arch.

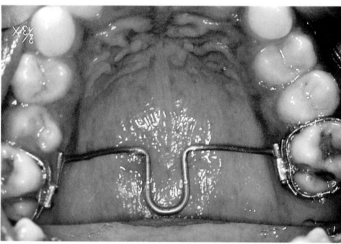

Fig. 9-23 Fixed space maintainer for upper arch.

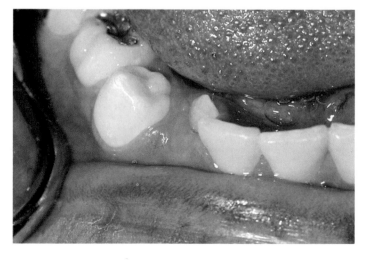

Fig. 9-24 Deflected eruption pattern of tooth 27 due to lingual arch interference.

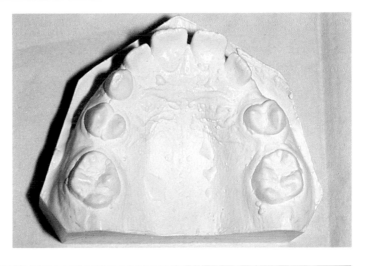

Fig. 9-25 Loss of space due to premature loss of second primary molar.

tainer therefore is indicated. A transpalatal arch in the maxilla and a lingual arch in the mandible are the recommended appliances.

In the anterior region, no space maintainer is required if the primary incisor is lost after eruption of the primary canines. Replacement of the lost anterior teeth is then simply an esthetic measure which also facilitates speech. Loss of anterior teeth may influence the development of deleterious finger and tongue habits, and anterior appliances may be useful to prevent their development. Appliances for anterior space maintenance may be fixed or removable. Removable appliances usually are made of acrylic plates to which anterior teeth are attached which are retained through bilateral retention clasps on the molars. Since these appliances have major esthetic value, they will be used by children who are interested in their appearance (Fig. 9-26a to c).

Fixed anterior appliances also have been described. Steffen et al.[15] describe an anterior space maintainer consisting of a plastic tooth processed onto a lingual arch attached to molar bands. An attachment post is soldered to the lingual arch in the middle of the site of the missing tooth or teeth. An artificial tooth is prepared and processed on the post with fast setting acrylic.

Space regaining procedures

It is often advisable to correct space loss resulting from a mesial drift of the permanent first molar in the absence of timely space maintenance. Procedures for space regaining are indicated in cases where there is otherwise normal dental and skeletal relationship and favorable tooth size, and where analysis indicates that distalization will allow normal eruption and occlusal pattern.

Sometimes space can be regained by uprighting a tipped tooth. The construction of appliances for this purpose has to take anchorage into consideration. It is important to assure proper anchorage, lest the wrong tooth be inadvertently moved. Timing is also a very important consideration since the regained space may have to be maintained a long time to allow eruption of the permanent tooth. In general, distalization of the permanent first molar when the permanent second molar is erupted requires major correction of

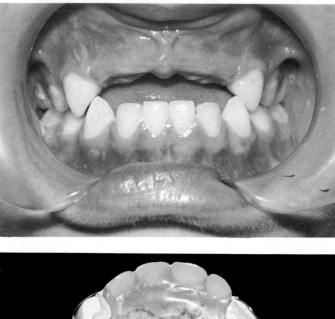

Fig. 9-26 a, b and c   Removable appliance for replacement of anterior maxillary teeth (Courtesy of Dr. L. Morton).

Figure 9-26 a

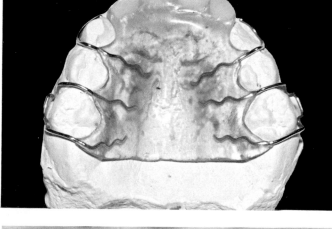

Figure 9-26 b

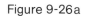

Figure 9-26 c

both teeth with orthodontic appliances (head gear, usually). Any device which is not anchored properly will displace the anterior segment. Before treatment is initiated the region of space loss must be evaluated. In some subjects the premature loss of a tooth has caused over eruption of the antagonist, arresting further tipping of the teeth adjacent to the space. Here the timing of the regaining procedure should be such that it coincides with the loss of the antagonist. If, however, the space loss continues progressively, regaining procedures should be initiated quickly and a space maintainer should be placed afterwards.

Many different types of removable and fixed appliances have been designed for the purpose of regaining space through the use of simple tipping forces by means of different types of springs. The removable types use an acrylic surface with embedded wire springs that may be opened until the tooth is tipped back into the correct position. These appliances require patient cooperation and should not be used when buccolingual rotation has taken place in addition to tipping. The action corrects only simple axial tipping. If coupled forces are required and the tooth needs to be rotated as well as to be uprighted, or if there is lack of patient cooperation, a fixed appliance is indicated. Anchorage is obtained through bands and a fixed lingual arch with a broad base required for anchorage. The tooth to be uprighted is also banded and the movement is achieved by use of coil springs.

References

1. Barber, T.K.:
   Lip habits in preventive orthodontics. J. Prev. Dent. 5:30-36, 1978.

2. Brauer, J.D., L.B. Demeritt, I.B. Higley, M. Massler and I. Schour:
   Dentistry for children. 3rd Ed. London, Kimpton, 1952.

3. Brazelton, R.B.:
   Finger sucking in infancy. Pediatrics 17:400-404, 1956.

4. Cheyne, V.D. and K.E. Wessels:
   Impaction of permanent first molar with resorption and space loss in region of deciduous second molar. J. Am. Dent. Assoc. 35:774-787, 1947.

5. Day, A.J.W., and T.D. Foster:
   An investigation into the prevalence of molar crossbite and some associated aetiological conditions. Trans. Brit. Soc. Study Orthod. 57:18-26, 1970-71.

6. Gianelly, A.:
   Rationale of orthodontic treatment in the primary and mixed dentition. J. Acad. Gen. Dent. 20:41-44, 1972.

7. Haas, A.J.:
   The treatment of maxillary deficiency by opening the midpalatal suture. Angle Orthod. 35:200-217, 1965.

8. Hanson, M.L., L.M. Barnard and J.L. Case:
   Tongue-thrust in preschool children. Am. J. Orthod. 56:60-69, 1969.

9. Haryett, R.D., F.C. Hansen, P.O. Davidson and M.L. Sandilands:
   Chronic thumb-sucking: the psychologic effects and the relative effectiveness of various methods of treatment. Am. J. Orthod. 53:569-585, 1967.

10. Hicks, E.P.:
    Treatment planning for the distal shoe space maintainer. Dent. Clin. North Am. 17:135-150, 1973.

11. Humphrey, T.:
    The development of mouth opening and related reflexes involving the oral area of human fetuses. Ala. J. Med. Sci. 5:126-157, 1968.

12. Joondeph, D.R. and R.W. McNeill:
    Congenitally absent second premolars: an interceptive approach. Am. J. Orthod. 59:50-66, 1971.

13. Moyers, R.E.:
    Handbook of orthodontics for the student and general practitioner. 3rd Ed. Chicago, Year Book, 1973.

14. Rutrick, R.E.:
    Crossbite correction with a therapeutic pacifier. J. Dent. Child. 41:442-444, 1974.

15. Steffen, J.M., J.B. Miller and R. Johnson:
    An esthetic method of anterior space maintenance. J. Dent. Child. 38:154-157, 1971.

Chapter 10

Management of Traumatic Injuries

Traumatic injuries to the teeth and supportive structures occur frequently in children, particularly in those who are learning to walk and in children 7-10 years old. In a study conducted in Scotland, 6% of 17,831 children 4 to 18 years of age had traumatized anterior teeth[11].

In the deciduous dentition, the teeth most frequently traumatized are the maxillary incisors. The nature of the alveolar bone in very young children is such that a blow to the maxillary incisors will often result in a displacement of the teeth. In older children, the heavier alveolar bone does not yield so easily and fractures are more likely to occur.

Traumatic injury to the mouth of a child is an emergency which requires immediate attention, not only because of the damage to the dentition but also because of the psychological effect of the trauma to the child and his parents. A complete and adequate history must be obtained, and the magnitude of the injury must be evaluated. In cases of major injuries involving possible bone fractures or extensive damage to soft structures, appropriate consultants should be called in to assure adequate treatment of all aspects of the damage.

The clinical examination (extraoral and intraoral) should include:

1. examination of the child's ability to open the mouth and an evaluation of the temporomandibular joint function
2. identification of lacerations and bruises of the soft tissues of the area
3. location of tooth mobility, which can be indicative of root fractures
4. identification of tenderness to gentle percussion
5. traumatized teeth, avulsions, intrusions, etc.

A good radiographic survey is essential and will indicate possible fracture sites as well as displacements and stages of tooth development. When root fracture is suspected, the position of the X-ray cone is extremely important for evaluation of the extent and type of fracture. Inappropriate angulation of the cone can give the impression of a multiple fracture where it does not exist or miss the presence of multiple fractures (Fig. 10-1). Subsequent examination may reveal tooth discoloration as well as fistulous formations indicating pulp degeneration. Vitality tests in young children are not always reliable, especially in the first 3 months after trauma[5]. Light tapping of the tooth and slight apical pressure to the region with the fingers will demonstrate possible site of root fracture. As a fractured buccal alveolar plate will permit mobility simulating a fractured root, palpation along the vestibular sulcus while attempting to move the tooth will help in differential diagnosis of this condition.

The most common etiologic factor in tooth fracture is injury by falling. A major predis-

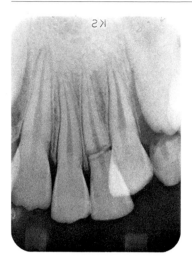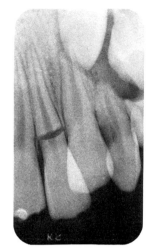

Fig. 10-1   Change in angulation disclosed the double fracture in root of tooth 25.

posing factor is increased overjet with maxillary protrusion accompanied by lip incompatibility. There is a higher incidence of fractured incisors in children with protrusion[15]. A study in Ireland[17] demonstrated that 12.8% of the 2,792 children examined had one or more injured incisors. In permanent teeth a higher percentage of children with Angle Class II division I occlusion had fractured anterior teeth than children with other occlusal patterns. The incidence of fractured incisors was slightly higher in children with inadequate lip tonus and coverage, but this difference was significant only in those under 12 years. No correlation between fractured incisors and organized contact sports was demonstrated.

Injuries to the anterior teeth are usually classified in 8 categories[7] (Figs. 10-2 to 10-8, Table 10-1).

Table 10-1   **Categories of anterior tooth injury**[7]

Class I	Simple fracture of crown involving little or no dentin
Class II	Extensive fracture of crown involving considerable dentin but not the pulp
Class III	Extensive fracture of crown involving considerable dentin and exposing the pulp
Class IV	The traumatized tooth which becomes nonvital, with or without loss of crown structure
Class V	Teeth lost as a result of trauma
Class VI	Fracture of the root with or without loss of crown structure
Class VII	Displacement of tooth without fracture of crown or root
Class VIII	Fracture of the crown en masse and its replacement.

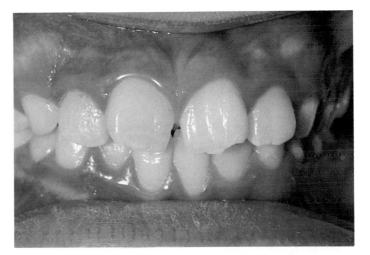

Fig. 10-2   Class I fracture.

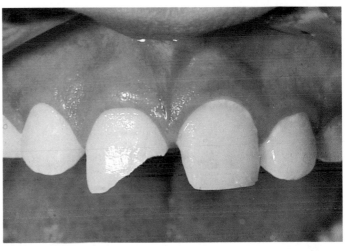

Fig. 10-3   Class II fracture.

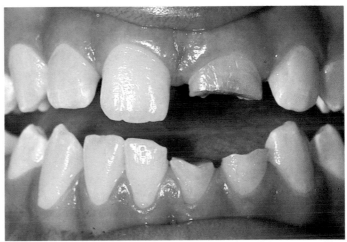

Fig. 10-4   Class III fracture.

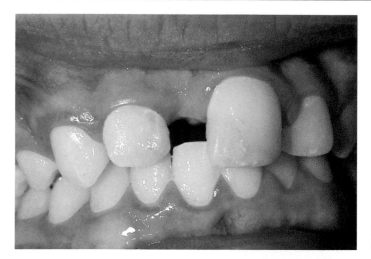

Fig. 10-5　Class V. Tooth lost as result of trauma.

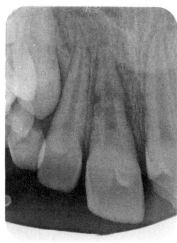

Fig. 10-6　Class VI fracture. Fracture of root.

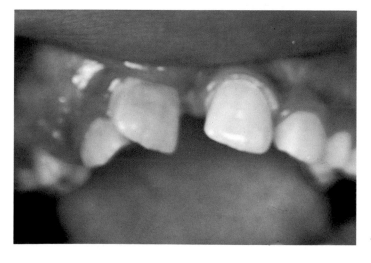

Fig. 10-7　Class VI. Displacement of tooth following trauma.

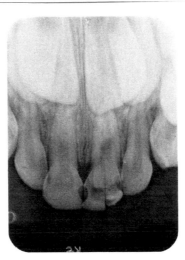

Fig. 10-8   Vertical fracture of tooth F.

Management of injuries to primary teeth

Trauma to primary teeth may result in discoloration with or without pulpal degeneration, crown fracture, or displacement. The teeth may be avulsed, luxated, or intruded.

Discoloration (Fig. 10-9) is caused by degradation of blood and migration and deposition of the degradation products into the dentinal tubules. While discoloration is not synonymous with pulp degeneration, this is frequently the case. Pulp degeneration is often accompanied by root resorption and when extensive root resorption occurs, extraction is the indicated treatment. Coronal fractures of primary teeth are rare. When fractures involve only the enamel, a smoothing of the edges with careful polishing of the enamel is adequate treatment. The parents, however, should be instructed to watch the appearance of the tooth and report any color change. If more than enamel has been fractured, the tooth is evaluated carefully for dentinal and pulpal involvement. When indicated, pulp therapy is initiated, and the tooth is restored with a polycarbonate (Fig. 10-10a and b) or stainless steel crown. Often a small amount of composite seal is preferable to grinding to minimize damage to pulp by heat.

The selection of the type of treatment of coronal fractures with or without pulp involvement also depends on the stage of development of the root and the extent of root resorption. According to Hawes[12], the success of a pulpotomy decreases if more than one-half of the root of a primary tooth has been resorbed, because root resorption will accelerate greatly after pulpotomy. Andreasen[1] advocates that teeth with root fractures without dislocation be preserved and reports exfoliation occurring at the normal time following such treatment.

When pulp therapy is indicated, the canal should be filled with a resorbable paste such as zinc oxide-eugenol or Ox-para. Gutta percha should not be used, as it may not be resorbed with the root and can interfere with the normal pathway of eruption of the permanent tooth.

An avulsed primary tooth should not be reimplanted if the primary canines have erupted as there is then little danger of severe loss of space. Many children welcome prosthetic appliances which will restore appearance and normalize speech.

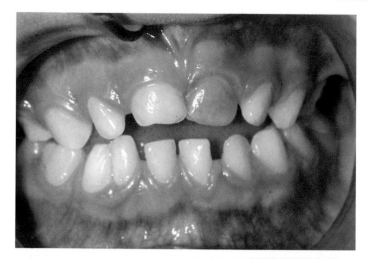

Fig. 10-9 Discoloration of primary tooth subsequent to trauma.

Fig. 10-10a and b Polycarbonate crown as restorative treatment.

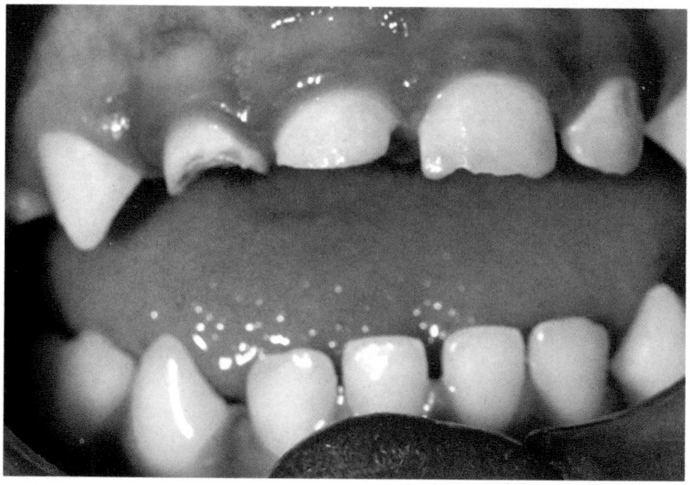

Figure 10-10a

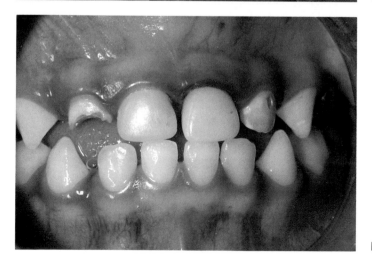

Figure 10-10b

Fig. 10-11a and b   Tooth intrusion in a 3-year-old boy immediately after trauma (a) and three weeks after the incident (b).

Figure 10-11a

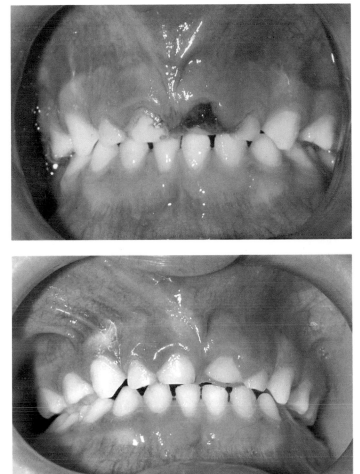

Figure 10-11b

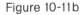

While an avulsed primary tooth should not be reimplanted because of likelihood of external resorption, a tooth displaced in a crossbite relationship should be repositioned in correct occlusion and loosely splinted.

While extruded primary teeth normally are extracted, intruded teeth should not be repositioned mechanically because they will usually re-erupt. In the very rare instances where no re-eruption takes place, the tooth should be extracted. The major problem here is the possible injury to the developing tooth buds of the permanent teeth. A preliminary study of the problem has not demonstrated a significantly different rate of complications when intruded teeth were allowed to re-erupt spontaneously, as compared to the rate when the teeth were extracted[4]. Therefore when clinical and radiographic evaluation demonstrate the dislocation of the primary tooth to be vestibular to the germ of the permanent tooth, no further immediate action is necessary. The patient, however, should be re-evaluated at regular intervals to follow the progress of re-erup-

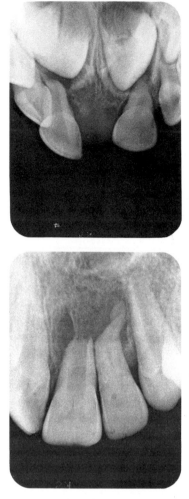

Fig. 10-12 Intrusion of tooth E in a 3.5-year-old girl. Note the proximity of the intruded tooth to the developing tooth 8 (Courtesy of Dr. H. Freudenthal).

Fig. 10-13 Several traumas to the upper incisor region caused dilaceration, necrosis and obliteration of canal (Courtesy of Dr. H. Freudenthal).

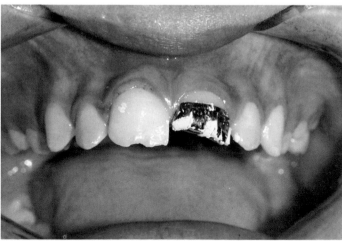

Fig. 10-14 Isolation of exposed dentin after trauma with a band and an additional band strip.

tion of the primary tooth (Fig. 10-11a and b). Total re-eruption should not be expected and pulpal necrosis may necessitate pulp therapy.

Influence of trauma to primary teeth on permanent tooth buds

The crowns of permanent incisors develop lingually and very close to the roots of the primary teeth during the entire development period (Fig. 10-12). The permanent tooth follicle is separated from the apex of the primary tooth only by a thin layer of alveolar cancellous bone and is vulnerable to injury if the primary tooth is intruded apically and medially. As calcification of the crown is completed only in approximately the 5th year of life, apical displacement of the primary tooth may be damaging in the very young child. The age of the patient at the time of the trauma, the direction of the force and the stage of development of the permanent tooth are each contributing factors in determining the possible adverse effects on the permanent tooth. The most common effects of trauma to primary teeth on the developing permanent teeth are dilacerations (Fig. 10-13) and enamel defects (hypoplasias and hypocalcifications)[18]. These defects usually are detected only when the primary teeth have exfoliated as standard radiographs may not demonstrate the abnormalities of the unerupted teeth. The position of certain defects may be masked by the direction of the central beam and specially directed films may be necessary for adequate diagnosis. In cases of dilaceration, the prognosis of the dilacerated tooth is not favorable, as this injury interferes with the pathway of normal eruption. In Van Gool's[29] series of trauma-induced dilacerations of anterior permanent teeth caused by trauma to primary teeth, the critical age at which the trauma occurred was between 1 and 3.5 years.

Ravn[18] demonstrated that the most common (15%) effect on the permanent successors of intrusion of primary teeth is hypoplasia of the enamel. Other rare abnormalities such as crown or root duplication, interference with root development, necrosis of the tooth germ, or development of odontomas have been reported[29].

Management of injuries to permanent teeth

The treatment of traumatized permanent incisors is directed to the maintenance of pulp vitality through protection of the damaged dentin or exposed pulp tissue, and fixation and reduction of mobility if necessary. The most favorable results are obtained with early treatment. Treatment also should allow subsequent normal development of the teeth and other oral structures. Emergency treatment can be one of the following:

1. maintaining vitality of the non-exposed pulp tissue by protection of the damaged region
2. treatment the exposed pulp tissue
3. reduction and fixation of the displaced tooth, or
4. reimplantation of the avulsed tooth.

If there is a risk of tetanus because of the site of the accident, the physician who has the record of the child's immunization history should be consulted.

Simple fractures involving enamel

Treatment of crown fractures that involve only the enamel require only limited and selected polishing of sharp angles to prevent damage to the tongue and lips. The tooth should be reevaluated 6-8 weeks after the accident to determine condition of the root

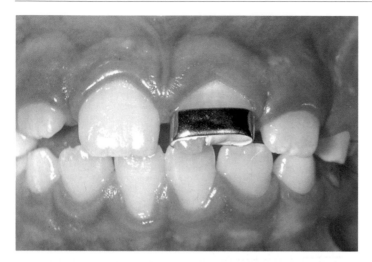

Fig. 10-15   Isolation of exposed dentin with orthodontic band a and b.

Fig. 10-16a and b   Angle repair with acid-etch technique. Same patient as in Fig. 10-14.

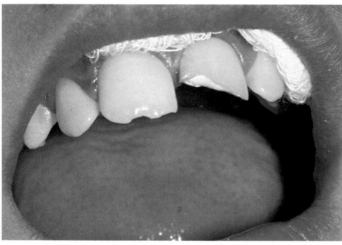

Figure 10-16a

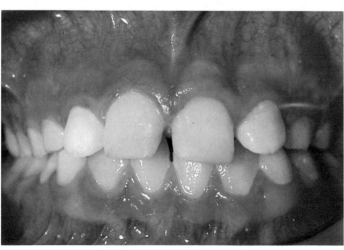

Figure 10-16b

and possible damage to the pulp not detected initially.

Fracture of the crown involving dentin without pulp exposure

Traumatized teeth with dentinal involvement should be treated for immediate pulp protection to establish optimum conditions for the pulp to form secondary dentin. A protective calcium hydroxide dressing is applied to the exposed dentin, and the region is isolated either with a stainless steel band (Figs. 10-14 and 10-15) or with a stainless steel crown cemented with zinc oxide-eugenol paste.

Restoration of fractured incisor crown angles

Several methods have been described for the restoration of fractured incisors. Repair of the incisal angles with composite resin is becoming more popular because esthetic results are obtained with minimal tooth preparation. Major mechanical preparations which can endanger an already traumatized pulp are not required. Further, gingival margins usually are not involved, which decreases the danger of gingivitis from irritation caused by the restoration. Several types of resins are available and improved products will probably be developed. At present, several problems of color stabiltiy remain. Over the years, color changes have been observed in individuals consuming large amounts of coffee or tea[20]. The results are such that the use of these materials is justified. The commitment of large amounts of tooth structure at a time when the tooth is not fully erupted and the pulp chamber is large is delayed by temporary restoration. The use of pin reinforcement to support these resins has been advocated[25]. Improvements in the cold-curing resins in most cases, seem to make this step unnecessary[19]. Starkey[26] advocates the use of a shoulder,

1mm wide, over half the depth of the enamel, and acid etching with a 50% aqueous phosphoric acid solution. The incisal angle can be repaired with a cold-curing resin applied in incremental layers with a 50% aqueous phosphoric acid solution. The incisal angle can be repaired with a cold-curing resin applied in incremental layers with or without a matrix crown, or by using a material cured by ultraviolet light. Alternatively, the enamel may be prepared in a gentle chamfer, since a thin layer of the composite resin at the outer border improves the appearance and reduces discoloration. The chamfer or the enamel serves to increase the surface area available for bonding (Fig. 10-16a and b).

Before restoration of the fractured incisal angle is undertaken, the exposed dentin and underlying pulp are protected with calcium hydroxide. A 50% phosphoric acid etch solution is used and the resin applied in accordance with manufacturer's instructions. Care is taken to wash the acid off completely before application of the resin. The occlusion is checked carefully when the preparation is complete, if cold-curing acrylic is used with preformed matrices. If ultraviolet light-curing resin is used, a layer of activated fissure sealant material is applied beneath the composite.

When the amount of tooth loss is not extensive, orthodontic treatment by selective extrusion of the fractured tooth and intrusion of the non-fractured tooth has been suggested. This can be considered in patients for whom orthodontic treatment is recommended for other reasons[14]. However, when orthodontic intrusive forces are used, the danger of root resorption should be considered.

When the fracture is too extensive for composite resins, veneer crowns or acrylic jackets can be used. Here the eruption pattern of the tooth must be considered, and esthetic problems as well as gingivitis may be anticipated[16].

Crown fractures involving the pulp

If only a small portion of the pulp is exposed and treatment is performed immediately after the accident, pulp capping before adaptation of a temporary crown can be attempted (Fig. 10-17). Several examples of positive results of this pulp capping have been reported [6, 8] but most investigators advise pulpotomy to treat pulp exposure, as the pulp chamber does not usually allow fast reversal of the inflammatory condition of the damaged pulp tissue [1]. Major pulp exposures are treated by pulpotomy or pulpectomy, depending on the development of the tooth apex.

Root fractures

In cases of crown fractures with associated root fractures the prognosis and treatment depend on the size of the lost coronal fragment. If the coronal fragment includes more than 4 mm of root structure the prognosis is unfavorable and the tooth may have to be extracted because prosthetic replacement may not be possible. If less root structure is involved, treatment with a post crown substitute can be initiated. Vertically fractured teeth require extraction. It is advisable to take a variety of periapical films and sometimes even occlusal films to obtain different views and angulations of the tooth to facilitate diagnosis of the type of root fracture.

The treatment of choice of root fractures without loss of coronal tissue depends on the location of the fracture. Studies have demonstrated that healing after root fracture can take place either by formation of calcified tissue or by the development of non-calcified connective tissue [1]. When the fracture line is in the coronal third of the root, the prognosis is poor. If the fracture is such that the remaining portion of the root cannot be used for adequate post crown preparation, extraction may be inevitable. If the frac-

ture line is in the middle third, the prognosis is guarded, but immobilization for 10 to 12 weeks may be effective in promoting healing and allowing functional use of the tooth for several years. If the fracture is located in the apical third of the root, a rare condition in children, the tooth should be checked regularly for vitality but no treatment should be initiated. If pulp death occurs, necessary pulp canal therapy should be initiated. Andreasen's research indicates that splinting of fractured teeth for about 2 months decreases incidence of pulp necrosis as compared to teeth without fixation [3].

Traumatic tooth avulsion

If a tooth is lost, a suitable space maintainer should be placed as a semi-permanent restorative treatment to prevent loss of space (Fig. 10-5). Radiographs of soft tissues of the head may be necessary to be certain that the tooth is really lost and not embedded in soft tissues. When the latter occurs, immediate surgical removal is necessary.

Tooth reimplantation

An extensive literature describes various techniques of tooth reimplantation, and many different approaches have been attempted, most with limited success. Despite poor prognosis, reimplantation efforts often are psychologically beneficial to the child as a temporary measure to provide proper alignment guidance in the arch for the erupting teeth, or as a temporary space maintainer until a permanent prosthetic substitute can be constructed.

In the last few years, it has become increasingly apparent that better results can be expected when the tooth has not been out of the mouth for a long period of time. Andreasen [1] found that in 90% of cases where reimplantation took place within 30 minutes, no root resorption was observed. The incidence of root resorption was directly proportional to the length of time the tooth had been out of the oral cavity[2, 9]. Intact periodontal ligament also is a factor in improving success. Sterilization of the tooth surface and chemical treatment of the periodontal tissue with caustic agents is no longer an accepted treatment. If cleaning of the root is necessary, it is done gently with physiologic saline solution with as little damage as possible to the periodontal tissue because damaged periodontal ligament may contribute to ankylosis[10]. Re-establishment of the vascular supply in the pulp seems to be facilitated in very immature pulp by the condition of the tissue and the large communicating apex. Difficulty in obtaining an adequate apical seal is a major factor in cases of failures; retrograde apical fill sometimes is used[23].

When stabilization is necessary to maintain luxated or avulsed teeth, it is important to splint atraumatically and quickly. Numerous methods, including interdental wiring, acrylic incisal splints and direct bonding with self-curing materials have been described[22-24]. The method selected depends on the number of teeth present for anchorage, the type of occlusal interferences on the tooth to be stabilized, and the shape and spacing of the teeth. Any quick but secure method of tooth immobilization that will last a few weeks is acceptable for stabilizing the avulsed tooth. Stabilization and splinting are important aspects in the treatment of the avulsed tooth, as it is necessary to retain a desirable occlusal relation and to enhance periodontal reattachment. The splints should be light so that they do not overload the tissues. They may be of light wire and include several teeth in a figure-8 ligature. Alternatively an acid etch technique and a resin are used over the labial surfaces of the affected tooth and its neighbors.

A method has been described recently using mesh-backed stainless steel orthodontic brackets attached to a piece of stainless steel wire. The orthodontic brackets with the inserted wire are bonded into position with an acid etch and composite resin technique to hold the luxated tooth in position to allow alignment[13].

If endodontic treatment becomes necessary, it should be initiated only after the tooth has been reimplanted. The sooner the tooth is returned to the alveolus, the better the chances that the treatment will be successful. Endodontic treatment before reimplantation lengthens the time the tooth is out of the oral cavity and increases the possibility of damage to periodontal fibers and cells. If the tooth has been out of the oral cavity for several hours and has been allowed to dry, root canal therapy is necessary and may be performed before reimplantation. The prognosis in such instances is poor. Failure of reimplantation is frequently caused by external root resorption. In such instances, a simple space maintainer – either as a lingual arch, a temporary bridge, or a removable partial denture – may be constructed both for esthetic reasons and prevention of space closure and speech defects. In designing such an appliance, the position of the incisors and the habits of the patient must be considered.

Electrical burns of the lip commissure in children

Electrical burns of the mouth are accidents with grave consequences to the child. They are disfiguring and because they usually occur in very young children, the scarring process may alter the growth and development pattern of the face[21]. The most common cause of these burns is chewing on an electrical cord and the commissure of the lip is the most frequent site of injury. Usually the injury is unilateral[21]. Other regions that can be affected are the tongue, hard palate, and alveolar process. Plastic surgery procedures often are necessary to alleviate the scarring problem. To reduce the damage of the disfiguring wound healing process, appliances may be constructed that will prevent some of the tissue contraction at the level of the commissure. Wright *et al.*[28] describe two types of appliances, fixed and removable. In either case the appliance is anchored on the upper arch with two lateral posts that flare out of the mouth and fit the region of the commissures. These extension posts are constructed in such a manner as to keep the commissures equidistant and with as little retraction from the midline as possible. The appliance must be worn continuously for several months. Wright *et al.*[28] advocate the use of the fixed appliance for at least ten months or the removable appliance for six months followed in either case by the use of a removable appliance at night every day for another six months. Wood *et al.*[27] recommend the use of a removable appliance for six months followed by another 6 months in which the appliance is used for only 12 hours a day. Since these accidents usually occur in children younger than age three, a fixed appliance may have some advantages of patient and parent cooperation. The removable appliance is easier to adjust during the process of wound healing.

References

1. Andreasen, J.O.:
   Traumatic injuries of the teeth. St. Louis, Mosby, 1972.

2. Andreasen, J.O. and E. Hjørting-Hansen:
   Replantation of teeth. I. Radiographic and clinical study of 110 human teeth replanted after accidental loss. Acta Odontol Scand. 24:263-286, 1966.

3. Andreasen, J.O. and E. Hjørting-Hansen:
   Intraalveolar root fractures: radiographic and histologic study of 50 cases. J. Oral Surg. 25:414-426, 1967.

4. Andreasen, J.O. and J.J. Ravn:
   The effect of traumatic injuries to primary teeth on their permanent successors. II. A clinical and radiographic follow-up study of 213 injured teeth. Scand. J. Dent. Res. 79:284-294, 1971.

5. Barkin, P.R.:
   Time factor in predicting the vitality of traumatized teeth. J. Dent. Child. 40:188-192, 1973.

6. Dausch, H.:
   Weitere Erfahrungen bei der Vitalerhaltung der Pulpa mit Calcium-Hydroxyd-Preparaten. Dtsch. Zahnärztl. Z. 9:67-72, 1954.

7. Ellis, R.G. and K.W. Davey:
   The classification and treatment of injuries to the teeth of children; a reference manual for the dental student and the general practitioner. 5th ed. Chicago, Year Book, 1970.

8. Gaare, A., A. Hagen and S. Kanstad:
   Tannfrakturer hos barn. Diagnostiske og prognostiske problemer of behandling. Nor. Tannlaegeforen. Tid. 68:364-378, 1958.

9. Grossmann. L.I. and I.I. Ship:
   Survival rate of replanted teeth. Oral Surg. 29:899-906, 1970.

10. Hargreaves, J.A.:
    The traumatized tooth. Oral Surg. 34:502-515, 1972.

11. Hargreaves, J.A. and J.W. Craig:
    The management of traumatized anterior teeth of children. Edinburgh, Livingstone, 1970.

12. Hawes, R.R.:
    Traumatized primary teeth. Dent. Clin. North Am. 391-404, July, 1966.

13. Howland, E.J. and J.L. Gutmann:
    Atraumatic stabilization for traumatized teeth. J. Endodont 2:390-392, 1976.

14. Jensen, E.K.:
    Fractured incisors – A meeting point between operative dentistry and orthodontics. C.D.S. Rev. 71:37-40, 1978.

15. Lewis, T.E.:
    Incidence of fractured anterior teeth as related to their protrusion. Angle Orthod. 29:128-131, 1959.

16. Magnussen, B., A.K. Holm and H. Berg:
    Traumatized permanent teeth in children – follow up. II. The crown fractures. Svensk Tandlak, T. 62:71-77, 1969.

17. O'Mullane, D.M.:
    Some factors predisposing to injuries of permanent incisors in school children. Brit. Dent. J. 134:328-332, 1973.

18. Ravn, J.J.:
    Sequelae of acute mechanical traumata in the primary dentition. A clinical study. J. Dent. Child. 35:281-289, 1968.

19. Ripa, L.W. and Z. Sheykoleslan:
    Acid etch technique of fracture repair: description and current status. J. Pedodont 2:128-143, 1978.

20. Rule, D.C. and B. Elliott:
    Semi-permanent restoration of fractured incisors in young patients. A clinical evaluation of one "acid-etch" technique. Brit. Dent. J. 39: 272-275, 1975.

21. Savara, B.S. and Y. Takeuchi:
    A longitudinal study of electrical burns on growth of the oro-facial structures. J. Dent. Child. 44:369-376, 1977.

22. Senzamici, N.P.:
    Emergency fixation of traumatized anterior teeth using autopolymerizing acrylic resin. J. Pedodont. 1:255-260, 1977.

23. Shusterman, S., S. M. Meller and J. Kane:
Reimplantation of traumatically avulsed immature incisor: report of case. J. Dent. Child. *43*:49-52, 1976.

24. Skyberg, R. L.:
Stabilization of avulsed teeth in children with the flexible mouthguard splint. J. Am. Dent. Assoc. *96*:797-800, 1978.

25. Starkey, P. E.:
The use of self-curing resins in restoration of young fractured permanent anterior teeth. J. Dent. Child. *34*:15-29, 1967.

26. Starkey, P. E. and D. R. Avery:
The acid etched restoration for fractured anterior teeth. J. Ind. State Dent. Assoc. *52*:157-160, 1973.

27. Wood, R. E., R. M. Quinn and J. E. Forgey:
Treating electrical burns of the mouth of children. J. Am. Dent. Assoc. *97*:206-208, 1978.

28. Wright, G. Z., R. G. Cocleugh and L. K. Davidge:
Electrical burns to the commissure of the lips. J. Dent. Child. *44*:377-381, 1977.

29. Van Gool, A. V.:
Injury to the permanent tooth germ after trauma to the deciduous predecessor. Oral Surg. *35*:2-12, 1973.

Chapter 11

Pain, Anxiety, and Infection Control

Regional analgesic agents

While some patients require specific medication for control of anxiety and fear of dental treatment, the majority of patients are routinely treated in the dental office with only regional analgesia being used to control pain. Regional analgesia is a convenient, efficient, and generally safe method of pain control when used alone or in combination with other pharmacological agents. The term "local anesthesia," often used to describe this type of treatment, while widespread, is incorrect. The type of medication normally used in routine dentistry affects primarily the nerve fibers transmitting pain sensations. The fibers transmitting temperature, touch and proprioception sensation are usually affected later, but not completely. As a result patients may be able to feel pressure and touch but not pain.

Many different theories concerning pain impulses and perception of pain have been promulgated. Further elucidation is required. Two aspects must be considered: the pain pathway from the sensory end organs such as skin, mucosa, etc., to the central nervous system (CNS), and the reaction to pain. The pathway of pain perception depends on various neural conductive structures and understanding of the whole pathway requires more detailed studies. The pain reaction depends not only on neural pathways but also on individual factors which include pain threshold, personal attitudes, and inhibitions.

The aim of regional analgesia in dentistry is to reduce the perception of pain at the level of end organs and afferent sensory fibers[4]. In this manner the patient's reaction to pain is altered and better patient control is attained. Appropriate chemical substances are placed close to the sensory nerve ending to be depolarized. The success of the regional analgesia depends on the proximity of the substances to the nerve fiber and the size of the fiber as well as the particular condition of health or disease of the tissue receiving the chemical.

The temporary interruption of all afferent nerve impulse transmissions produces lack of sensation, or anesthesia. The interruption of the pain sensation only is analgesia. However, the term local anesthesia is in general use as meaning lack of pain sensation when drugs are injected locally. Since sensory fibers other than the pain fibers are also affected in many instances, the effect of analgesic drugs increases with increased time.

All local analgesics must have lipophilic and hydrophilic properties to diffuse properly through interstitial tissues which are rich in water and through the nervous tissues with lipid components. The ideal local anesthetic should be highly potent with no or minimal toxicity and no local irritating effect. Thus far, the pharmaceutical industry has not been able to produce such an ideal compound. An increase in potency is usually accompanied by an increase in toxicity. This is particularly important in children whose low body weight has to be considered. Once the anesthetic solution has been injected, it diffuses in all directions and is removed by absorption into the general circulation[9]. The duration of the local anesthetic action can be increased greatly by the addition of vasoconstrictors to the injection fluid, and these have already been added to most local anesthetic solutions on the market. Such vasoconstrictors, by delaying absorption of the local anesthetic into the general circulation, reduce the danger of systemic toxicity. Some local anesthetic solutions without vasoconstrictors are available which can be used in patients with systemic disorders in which vasoconstrictors are contraindicated, e.g., in patients taking monoamine oxidase inhibitors, but then the duration of the anesthesia is limited. Local anesthetic solutions should not be injected into a region of inflammation. If local anesthetic solution is deposited into infected tissue, the tissue pH may alter the ionization of the drug and prevent effective analgesia.

Injectable products currently available for local analgesia can be classified into two major groups[4]:

1. Ester group

    A. Benzoic acid esters, e.g. piperocaine
    B. Para-aminobenzoic acid esters, e.g. procaine
    C. Meta-aminobenzoic acid esters, e.g. metabutethamine
    D. Para-ethoxybenzoic acid esters, e.g. parethoxycaine.
2. Non-ester group

    A. Cyclohexylamino-2-propyl-benzoate, e.g. hexylcaine
    B. Anilides, e.g. lidocaine.

Regional analgesia is designated as *topical* when the chemical administered is placed on the surface area close to the free sensory nerve endings. The term *local* is used when the chemical solution is injected into the region of treatment to prevent pain impulses from stimulating the central nervous system. The term *nerve block* is used when the chemical solution is injected close to the nerve trunk to interrupt afferent impulses from traveling beyond that point.

If topical analgesia is used, the chemical should be placed in contact with the mucosal surface for an average of 2-4 minutes to be effective. The mucous membrane should be as dry as possible to avoid dilution of the drug. Many topical solutions are available and can be used in pedodontics. The solutions should be as pleasant tasting as possible and non-irritant. They should not be toxic or cause necrosis of tissue. In pedodontics it is not always possible to use a topical solution effectively because of the anxiety level of the patient. In some children topical solutions make the injection easier, but in others they are avoided as they predispose the child to a more antagonistic behavior by raising the anxiety level.

Vasoconstrictors are used in local analgesia because their action reduces the drug removal by the local circulation and therefore causes an increase in the duration of the drug effect. The amount of vasoconstrictor used in dentistry is so small that usually there are no side effects. However, it must be remembered that repeated injections of local anesthesic solution will increase the concentration of the vasoconstrictors in the patient and an intravascular injection may produce some toxic effects, characterized by tachycardia.

EPINEPHRINE.

The most commonly used vasoconstrictor is epinephrine (adrenalin).

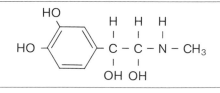

It is used in concentrations of 1:50,000 or 1:100,000 to 1:250,000. Bennett[4] recommends 0.2 mg as a safe maximum dosage of epinephrine. Most frequently used commercially available solutions have a concentration of 1:50,000 epinephrine. This is equivalent to 0.02 mg/ml and 10 ml of anesthetic solution therefore contains 0.2 mg of epinephrine. Other sympathomimetic amines used as vasoconstrictors for dental procedures are norepinephrine, phenylephrine, nordefrin and levonordefrin.

Routes of local infiltration include submucosal, supraperiosteal, intraosseous, and rarely, intrapulpal. The most frequently used route is submucosal. Injections into bone structure are difficult and painful. Such injections may also be dangerous, as the needles commonly used are not strong enough for such an approach even if the child's alveolar bone is more cancellous than that of adults. The technique for local infiltration of anesthetic solutions in children is the same as that used for adults. The smaller size of the bone reduces the amount of tissue that must be penetrated to permit the solution to reach the proper location. The reduced compactness of the bone tissue facilitates infiltration of the chemical substance and therefore less anesthetic may be used. Because children weigh less than adults, the amount of medication is reduced in relation to total body weight. The injection needle should be of small gauge to avoid discomfort. It is good technique to aspirate before initiation of the injection of material into the supraperiosteal area, but sometimes the child's lack of cooperation makes this difficult. The solution should be injected slowly to reduce pain and be deposited close to the apical foramen of the tooth to be treated. If more than one tooth is to be treated, it is often possible to inject one site, and by altering the direction of the syringe and the needle, inject at the other site without another puncture.

All maxillary teeth can be anesthetized by local infiltration technique by injecting at the level of the mucobuccal fold of the specific tooth. The palatal roots on the maxilla are anesthetized either by injecting a small quantity of anesthetic solution in the submucosal region of the corresponding root at the level of the apical foramen or by an interdental papilla injection[18]. Both methods are painful and must be done carefully.

The six anterior mandibular teeth can also be anesthetized by local infiltration. For molars, an inferior alveolar nerve block is preferred.

Only the inferior alveolar nerve block is used in pedodontics. While in adults the needle location for the inferior mandibular nerve block is at the level of the occlusal plane of the molars, in small children the level is slightly lower, as the mandibular foramen is located slightly below the occlusal plane[19]. It is important to explain to patients and to parents that the area has been anesthetized and that the child must be careful to avoid self-inflicted injury by biting, chewing, or damaging the non-sensitive area in some other manner.

The buccal nerve can be anesthetized by infiltration into the muccobuccal fold at the level of the tooth to be treated. McCallum[18] advises that this injection should be given only after the child has noticed the appearance of signs of inferior alveolar nerve block so that evaluation of the effectiveness of the injection will not be confused with the tingling sensation of the buccal nerve injection. Before administration, the child should be informed of the subjective symptoms associated with regional analgesia, such as tingling, numbness, and the feeling of a swollen tongue and lip. After the solution has been administered, the area should be tested with an explorer. It must be remembered that loss of sensation of the superficial layers does not necessarily mean full analgesia at deep layers.

PROCAINE

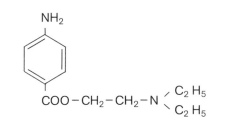

Procaine is one of the *p*-aminobenzoic acid esters and has been used in dentistry since its synthesis at the beginning of the 20th century. It has been used extensively as a local anesthetic in the form of a 2% solution of procaine hydrochloride with epinephrine added to prolong duration of the analgesia. It has been supplanted to a large extent by some of the non-ester drugs synthesized in the 1950's.

LIDOCAINE

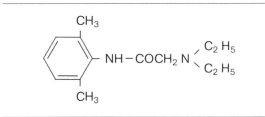

Lidocaine is currently used in dentistry as the hydrochloride salt. It is a very good analgesic, but its effect is usually of long duration. The anesthetic properties of several local anesthetic solutions were reviewed by Kramer[15] who found that a 2% lidocaine solution with 1:50,000 epinephrine as a vasoconstrictor was an excellent medication for children. However 1:100,000 epinephrine is also extensively used.

MEPIVACAINE

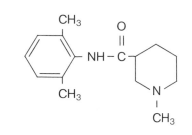

Mepivacaine is similar to lidocaine and is also a very good local analgesic drug. Like lidocaine, it is compatible with all vasoconstrictors and can be sterilized by boiling and autoclaving.

Premedication for anxiety control

When a child does not respond to routine behavior management, premedication has to be considered. Selection of the drug to be used will depend not only on the effects desired but also on avoidance of side effects with attention to possible interaction with other drugs being taken. While premedication is not intended to impair reflexes, the dentist must know how to handle basic emergencies including cardiopulmonary resuscitation. While it may be convenient to have medication administered at home so that the child may be transported without difficulty, it is safer to give the medication in the office. Administration of premedication in the office also has the advantage of better dosage control and better evaluation of the drug effects. The reaction of a small child to a drug is often difficult to predict, and if administered at home, optimal drug response may occur while the child is still in transit. Premedication should not be administered in the presence of upper respiratory infection, gastrointestinal disturbances, or other acute disease.

Once premedication has been administered, the child should not remain unattended. It is advisable to have a trained assistant available in the room as parents are not trained to note the reactions during premedication and may try to keep the child active instead of allowing him to relax. Premedication should not be a substitute for the use of correct local anesthesia since many of the drugs used for premedication do not eliminate perception of pain stimuli.

Many premedication agents remain in the body for some time. The parent therefore must be instructed to put the child to bed after returning home. Since adverse effects of premedication include emesis, dizziness, and irritability, stressful situations should be avoided while the medication is wearing off.

General conditions that determine dosage include age, weight, general health of the child, and route of administration. Tables of required dosage based on clinical experience for different age groups are usually provided for each drug. Occasionally Young's rule for adjustment of dosage according to age or Clark's rule for weight may be used:

Clark's rule: $\dfrac{\text{weight x adult dosage}}{150}$

Young's rule: $\dfrac{\text{age x adult dosage}}{\text{age} + 12}$

However, it is usually preferable to rely on clinical experience and the dosage recommended for a given age.

Several drugs, alone or in combination, can be used to modify children's behavior to obtain cooperation for dental treatment. An understanding of some of the pharmacologic aspects of the major categories of drugs enables the dentist to select the drug most adequate for each requirement.

Patients receiving tranquilizers such as prochlorperazine or chlorpromazine may be sensitive to epinephrine. Patients who have had prolonged treatment with corticosteroids usually have some degree of atrophy of their adrenal cortex, and therefore a reduced ability to secrete additional corticosteroids in response to stress. This predisposes the patient to stress-induced adrenal insufficiency. These patients may require additional steroid therapy before dental treatment and the child's physician should be consulted.

Well controlled diabetic patients taking insulin usually can undergo dental treatment including elective surgery. Many children, however, are not well controlled. Insulin medication should be adjusted before dental treatment. Diabetic patients also may have decreased healing ability as well as decreased resistance to infection; therefore, antibiotic coverage may be desirable in more extensive procedures.

A prominent drug interaction involving antibiotics involves the ability of tetracyclines to chelate with metal ions (Ca^{++}, Mg^{++}, Al^{+++}, etc.) found in dairy products and antacids. Because the tetracycline-metal ion complexes are insoluble, gastrointestinal absorption of the tetracycline is reduced. Antibiotics are also allergenic. Although an allergic reaction is difficult to predict, certain factors should be remembered. Any route of administration may produce allergic reaction. The probability of allergy is increased if the patient has demonstrated allergy to other drugs, foods, or pollens. The highest incidence of allergy is seen with the penicillins. Patients allergic to penicillin are occasionally also allergic to cephalosporins.

Sedation

Sedation is a conscious state induced by drugs characterized by reduction of anxiety but without abolishing protective reflexes. It may be accompanied by amnesia. Local

251

anesthesia is still required. Sedation should not be confused with general anesthesia which renders the patient unconscious, even though the drugs used in sedation are often capable of inducing general anesthesia in larger doses. A sedated patient can respond to instructions. Sedation should not be used without medical consultation for patients suffering from systemic disease.

Premedication with orally, intramuscularly, or intravenously administered drugs is used for anxious patients who will otherwise not permit the use of local anesthetic and in patients who will not accept the machinery required for nitrous oxide. In some cases, to reduce the anxiety level further and despite the disadvantages, the drug is administered at home. The major problem, particularly in children, is titration of the drug dose. A dose that may produce sedative effects in one child may be of little effect in another; retarded patients may react differently to premedication. If the drug must be administered at home, parental cooperation is essential to assure correct dosage at the proper time. In some instances intramuscular sedation may be necessary in the management of an emergency in an uncooperative child. Authors differ in the recommendation of particular drugs, combinations of drugs, and even the desirable amount of sedation.

In 1973 Wright and McAulay[24] conducted a survey of 409 members of the American Academy of Pedodontics and found that 64% of pedodontists used premedication only 10% of the time. Another 15% did not use premedication. Pedodontists with hospital training used premedication more frequently than those without hospital training, either because hospital trained dentists have more practical experience with respiratory and cardiac monitoring and emergency measures or because such pedodontists get more referrals of patients who cannot be treated without sedation. According to the survey, the drugs most frequently used alone were secobarbital, hydroxyzine, chloral hydrate, promethazine, and meperidine. The drugs most frequently used in combinations, according to the pedodontists surveyed were meperidine, promethazine, hydroxyzine, chloral hydrate, and alphaprodine hydrochloride.

Many different classifications have been proposed for the various chemical agents which can be used to reduce anxiety and considerable confusion exists in the field. In recent years[2], these agents have been classified as:

antianxiety agents
barbiturate sedatives and hypnotics
non-barbiturate sedatives and hypnotics
nitrous oxide-oxygen psychosedation.

Antianxiety agents

A number of compounds have been developed which have some antianxiety effect. These drugs previously were called "tranquilizers". Many of these drugs were synthesized because of their antihistaminic properties. Later it was found that some antihistamines, many of them chemically related, also had antianxiety properties[10]. Some of the drugs have been tested in children in dental situations and found to be effective in reducing anxiety.

MEPROBAMATE

$$H_2N-\overset{\overset{O}{\|}}{C}-OCH_2-\overset{\overset{C_3H_7}{|}}{\underset{CH_3}{C}}-CH_2O-\overset{\overset{O}{\|}}{C}-NH_2$$

Although classified as an antianxiety agent, meprobamate also causes sedation. In addition, it possesses central muscle-relaxing properties. Thus, meprobamate is not a simple drug, but displays a variety of effects at therapeutic doses. While safer then barbiturates, acute overdosage of meprobamate may produce loss of consciousness, shock, respiratory depression, and even death. Meprobamate is readily absorbed from the gastrointestinal tract and is effective after oral administration. If the drug is given in a single dose before dental treatment, the indicated dose for children is 12.5 mg/kg of body weight. The drug is contraindicated in children under 6 years of age. Lund and Anholm[17] used meprobamate as a premedication in children before dental extractions and found it effective as an antianxiety agent in 32 of 39 patients. Chambiras[6], however, found that the drug alone or in combination with secobarbital was effective in only 20% of his patients.

DIAZEPAM

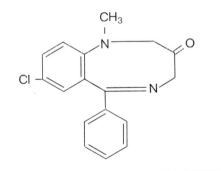

Diazepam is used as one of the drugs administered before general anesthesia because of its psychotropic and amnesia effects. It is also used in certain anxiety situations and in some patients with cerebral palsy, particularly in patients with spasticity and athetosis. Diazepam also increases seizure threshold, and thus is useful for terminating convulsions associated with local anesthetic toxicity and *status epilepticus*. For termination of convulsions the drug is administered intravenously. Following intra-

venous administration the drug reaches high concentration in the brain, but is rapidly distributed to other tissues. The central effects develop rapidly but are of short duration. In contrast, oral administration results in maximal effects after 1 to 2 hours. Paradoxical reactions such as increase in anxiety have been found. While toxicity is low, the drug can produce confusion, nausea, vertigo, ataxia, and incoordination. Since small children are very sensitive to the drug, it should not be used in children under 6 months of age. Circulatory and respiratory depression also may result from the use of diazepam and it is incompatible with meperidine and pentobarbital. Diazepam is available in tablets, suspension and injectable preparations. Kurland[16] used 15 mg of diazepam one hour before treatment for children aged 6 to 12 years with good results. Hargreaves[11] recommends 0.5 mg q.i.d. as a tranquilizing agent for children 1 to 5 years old and 1.0 mg q.i.d. for children 6 to 12 years old.

HYDROXYZINE

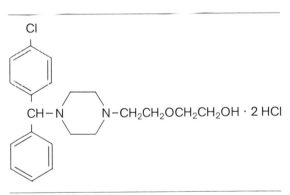

Hydroxyzine is used frequently in pedodontics by those who prefer to employ a single drug for sedation[23]. Hydroxyzine is an antihistamine but advantage can be taken of its prominent side effects, e.g., CNS depression (sedation), anticholinergic action (bronchodilatation and antisialogue effect), antispasmodic, and antiemetic effects. The drug can be administered orally as a solid or liquid preparation, or intramuscularly. Like most CNS depressants, it potentiates the action of narcotics. In children the dosage ranges from 50 to 100 mg daily, but if given in combination with barbiturates or narcotics the dosage should be reduced. Stewart[20] recommends 10-20 mg 45 minutes before dental treatment. Kopel[14] recommends 50 mg two hours before treatment and another 50 mg one hour before treatment. Kopel also used the drug in combination with meperidine for some extensive operative treatment and in combination with chloral hydrate in other such patients. Chambiras[6] found the drug effective only in 10% of the children medicated with administration of 1 mg/lb body weight.

Barbiturate sedatives and hypnotics

Barbiturates produce drowsiness and sleepiness. They also cause a general depression of many tissues including the CNS and cardiovascular systems.

Barbiturates are effective sedatives and hypnotics, depending on the dose used, and are sometimes used to decrease apprehension or induce sleep before treatment. In these instances they are used in combination with other drugs. At low doses they are useful as sedatives. At higher concentrations they may produce anesthesia or even coma and death. Toxic doses depress the respiratory centers and cardiovascular centers in the brain and also directly affect the heart and vascular smooth muscle, leading to a lowered blood pressure, hypoxia and a shock-like syndrome. Barbiturates, particularly phenobarbital, may be used as an antiepileptic. Barbiturates are not analgesics and do not relieve pain.

Barbiturates can be administered orally, rectally, intramuscularly, or intravenously. Usually they are given orally as they may be damaging to the tissues because of their alkalinity. Intravenous injection, while possible, is not without risks and can lead to respiratory and circulatory distress including respiratory arrest or a major drop in blood pressure. Barbiturates are absorbed through the stomach and intestine and circulate in the blood stream. Metabolism takes place for the most part in the liver, but some activity may be present in the kidney and brain tissues. Barbiturates are eliminated primarily by the kidney. Some patients have a paradoxical reaction, to barbiturates and may become excited instead of sedated[13]. If a history of adverse reaction to barbiturates is known or if the patient has kidney, liver, or lung damage, these drugs should not be administered. There is no specific antidote for barbiturate poisoning. Acute barbiturate poisoning is treated by maintaining circulatory and respiratory function and removing the barbiturate from the patient's gastrointestinal tract.

Barbiturates can be classified as:

Long acting (mephobarbital, phenobarbital)
Intermediate acting (amobarbital, sodium butabarbital)
Short acting (pentobarbital, secobarbital)
Ultrashort acting (sodium methohexital, sodium thiamylal, sodium thiopental)

Of the large number of barbiturates available, the most commonly used are pentobarbital sodium and secobarbital. Both are available as elixirs, capsules, and injectable solutions. Dosage is 2 mg/kg when given as a sedative before dental treatment.

Non-barbiturate sedatives and hypnotics

As barbiturates tend to be habit forming, the need for development of non-barbiturate sedatives has long been apparent. Several alternate drugs have been developed but in general they are less potent sedatives than barbiturates. Among these drugs are chloral hydrate and the phenothiazines. Promethazine, frequently used at present, is 10-(2-dimethylaminopropyl)phenothiazine hydrochloride. The phenothiazines are useful not only because of their sedative effect but also because of their antiemetic properties.

PROMETHAZINE

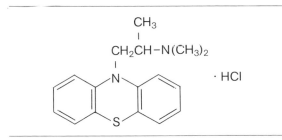

Promethazine is a potent antihistaminic often used as an antiemetic. It shares with other antihistamines a number of side effects including involvement of the central nervous system. The intensity of these side effects varies among the antihistamines, and those with prominent CNS effects are frequently used for the CNS actions and not for their ability to block the actions of histamine. Promethazine can be given orally, rectally, intramuscularly, or intravenously and is used frequently in combination with other drugs to potentiate their effects. Adverse reactions to the drug include paradoxical reactions in some patients, as well as nausea, emesis, and dizziness; dryness of the mouth occurs in some patients. A young child may have some mild jerking movements during sleep after being medicated with promethazine. This must be explained to the parents before administration to avoid concern that the child is convulsing.

The product is available as tablets, syrup, and rectal suppositories. Stuebner and Sadove[21] found that 0.5 mg/lb weight in combination with scopolamine administered 45 minutes before surgery was effective as sedation. Promethazine is usually used in combination with other drugs for its synergistic effects[1].

CHLORAL HYDRATE

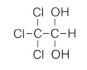

Chloral hydrate is used frequently for sedation. It has been known for over 100 years and has been found to be useful in dental treatment. The primary effect of chloral hydrate seems to be depression of the central nervous system in a manner similar to barbiturates. Sleep of 4-5 hours duration is induced one hour after administration, but the patient can be aroused easily.

Chloral hydrate is usually administered orally, as an elixir, a syrup, or in capsules. Suppositories also are available. The unpleasant taste of the drug can be disguised with juices or soft drinks or by administering capsules followed by a large amount of liquid. Chloral hydrate is absorbed from the gastrointestinal tract and is excreted by the kidneys. It is irritating to the skin and mucosa and therefore should not be given as an injection. Because it is metabolized in the liver and kidneys, it is contraindicated in patients with hepatic and renal disease, nor should it be given to patients with severe heart problems. Signs of chloral hydrate poisoning include emesis, depressed respiration, hypotension, and coma. Treatment of accidental poisoning includes supportive respiratory therapy and removal of the drug from the gastrointestinal tract. Czarnecki and Binns[7] reported improvement in the management of 80 of 100 children both above and below 6 years of age after administration of chloral hydrate.

The drug may cause laryngospasm if aspirated; therefore rectal suppositories are indicated for handicapped patients. As a sedative, chloral hydrate is usually given 10-20 mg/kg/24 hr. More than 1,500 mg a day should not be given.

Nitrous oxide-oxygen psychosedation

One of the most frequently used methods of sedation is inhalation of a nitrous oxide-oxygen mixture[23]. This technique has increased in popularity in recent years with the improvement of anesthetic machines. Its aim is to create a pleasant (sometimes euphoric) state of relaxation in the anxious patient but without acting as a general anesthetic. The drug has several adverse effects such as nausea and vomiting, and oxygen must be delivered in adequate amounts as reduced oxygen supply may lead to hypoxia. It is a relatively safe sedative when used with equipment that shuts off the nitrous oxide automatically if the flow of oxygen is interrupted for any reason. (Modern equipment is set in such a manner that oxygen flow cannot be decreased below 2.5 liters/minute.)

Nitrous oxide is a gas, stored in cylinders as a liquid. It is tasteless and has no marked odor. It is not explosive or flammable under normal conditions. It causes depression of the cerebral cortex, does not combine with hemoglobin, and is excreted through the lungs.

The primary advantage of nitrous oxide is the production of a mild sedation, calmness, and even euphoria with reduction of anxiety and apprehension and development of general state of relaxation. In combination with behavior guidance it is highly effective as a management technique.

Low concentrations of nitrous oxide (10-25%) usually produce a sensation of tingling and numbness of the extremities and a reduction of anxiety. Maximal analgesic properties together with mild drowsiness, euphoria, and increased sleepiness are usually achieved at 25-50% concentration. In most patients a 35% concentration of nitrous oxide is sufficient to obtain good analgesia and patient cooperation.

Nitrous oxide should always be administered with at least 20% oxygen. At the time of induction a 70% to 80% concentration of nitrous oxide may be administered although 40% to 60% is usually adequate[5, 8]. There are no major adverse reactions to nitrous oxide, but some patients report unpleasant dreams. Houck and Ripa[12] reported vomiting in some patients, but some of those evaluated had a previous history of vomiting during dental treatment even without nitrous oxide.

Nitrous oxide is carried in solution in the blood plasma but it does not compete with oxygen or carbon dioxide for hemoglobin. It replaces the nitrogen in the bloodstream. Initial uptake of nitrous oxide takes place in the brain tissue, heart, liver, and other organs. If nitrous oxide is continued for a long period of time, muscle, fat, and other body tissues will take it up. As soon as administration stops, nitrous oxide is eliminated via the lungs, but since the body has a high content of accumulated nitrous oxide at the end of administration, several liters of oxygen should be administered to flush the nitrous oxide.

Before a decision is made to use nitrous oxide, a good medical history is essential. The child should be told what kind of sensations he will perceive and the equipment should be demonstrated in the usual "tell, show, do" approach. The breathing bag should be filled before the inhaler is placed and the inhaler should fit snugly. The child is instructed to breathe through the nose. Initially a 2-3 minute inhalation of oxygen is provided. After nitrous oxide-oxygen inhalation is initiated the child should be questioned about his sensations. At the end of the treatment a 3-5 minute period of oxygen without nitrous oxide must be provided.

After proper oxygenation the child may be discharged to the parents[22].

Not all children experience the sensations commonly associated with nitrous oxide. Low concentrations of nitrous oxide usually produce a tingling sensation of hands and feet, numbness of the tongue, mild sleepiness. Moderate doses, about 30%-40%, produce euphoria, analgesia, numbness of the extremities, and sometimes sweating, but the patient is able to follow verbal commands. Doses around 50% may produce amnesia, sleepiness, dreams, laughing, uncoordinated movements, sluggishness in response to verbal commands, and general inability to remain awake. Doses of 60% may produce nausea and vomiting, sleepiness, sometimes unconsciousness, and light general anesthesia[3]. The sedative effect of other drugs which the patient is taking can add to the depression caused by N_2O-O_2 inhalation.

The equipment used to deliver nitrous oxide varies. The gas supply may be portable or central. Without regard to the source, by convention the cylinders and all the buttons and tubing associated with nitrous oxide are color-coded blue and the ones for oxygen green. Most machines are adjusted to deliver at least of 3-5 liters of oxygen per minute. To compute the amount of nitrous oxide, the following formula is used:

$$\frac{\text{Nitrous oxide being administered (l/min.)}}{\text{Total nitrous oxide + oxygen gas flow (l/min.)}}$$

If for example 2 liters/min. of nitrous oxide are used this is computed:

$$\frac{2N_2O}{2N_2O+4O_2} = \frac{2}{6} = 33.3\% \text{ } N_2O \text{ concentration.}$$

Contamination of the operatory atmosphere with nitrous oxide may be harmful to the personnel in the operatory.

Other drugs

Other drugs used occasionally as sedatives in dentistry but used also as premedication for general anesthesia include meperidine hydrochloride and scopolamine.

MEPERIDINE

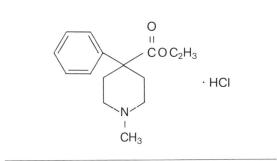

Meperidine is a narcotic analgesic and shares the following actions with other narcotics: analgesia, drowsiness, euphoria and other mood changes (sometimes dysphoria), emesis, constipation, and respiratory or cardiovascular depression. As a premedication in dental surgery, it is often given in combination with other drugs. It is less potent than morphine and has a much shorter duration of action. The drug may be administered orally, intramuscularly, or intravenously. The intramuscular and intravenous injections are much more effective. It is metabolized in the liver and excreted as a conjugate in the urine.

Meperidine is contraindicated in patients with increased cerebrospinal fluid pressure. It may also precipitate convulsions in patients with seizure disorders and may aggravate the convulsions. The drug can have a respiratory depressant effect, particularly in patients with sensitivity to the drug.

The commercial preparation is available as a solution, in tablets, and as an elixir. The recommended dosage for children is 1.1 to 2.2 mg/kg body weight.

SCOPOLAMINE

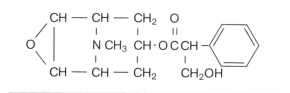

Scopolamine is an anticholinergic agent which blocks the action of acetylcholine at the postganglionic parasympathetic nerve endings. It is used in dentistry primarily in general anesthesia to reduce secretions, but it also produces drowsiness, sleep, and amnesia. Therefore it is often used in oral surgery. Its use before anesthesia reduces not only gastrointestinal tract secretions, but also those of the respiratory tract. For this reason it reduces the danger of laryngospasm.

Scopolamine can be administered orally, topically, or by subcutaneous, intramuscular or intravenous injection. It is rapidly absorbed and is excreted in the urine. Adverse effects include rash, hallucinations, excitement, inadequate respiration, coma, and death. Physostigmine can be used to counteract scopolamine action. Dosage is 6 μ/kg of body weight per dose.

Management of infections (Table 11-1)

Acute infections of dental origin require proper local as well as systemic care. Antibiotics also may be indicated. The dentist should ascertain whether pus is present, and drainage should be established. Factors to be taken into consideration are duration of the infective process, temperature of the patient, and clinical and radiographic appearance of the infected region. In many instances, administration of antibiotics will avoid both spread of the infection and the need for extraoral drainage. A decision must be made as to whether the involved tooth can be saved. The condition of the pulp tissue must be evaluated, and if indicated, the pulp chamber must be opened for drainage. If the tooth has been destroyed beyond repair, extraction is necessary.

Antimicrobial agents are indicated in severe cellulitis, bacterial infections of bone and salivary glands, and other types of severe infection. Indiscriminate use of antibiotics in situations in which they are not specifically indicated should be avoided because of possible development of sensitization to the antibiotic and development of bacteria resistant to antibiotics. In acute infection, pericementitis, or abscess the patient may be febrile and toxic. In these cases, care should be taken to prevent dehydration.

Antibiotics are of great value in the treatment of dental infections encountered in childhood. Most of these infections are caused by gram positive bacteria which are sensitive to commonly used antibiotics.

The principal group of antibiotics employed are the *penicillins* which are bactericidal against gram positive organisms. Penicillin G, benzylpenicillin, the basic penicillin preparation, is indicated for most of these infections. The drug can be administered orally, intravenously, or intramuscularly. The blood level of aqueous penicillin G is only sustained for a short time after intramuscular injection. For this reason repository forms of penicillin G, which prolong the action of penicillin after intramuscular injection have been developed. The repository forms of penicillin G commonly used are procaine penicillin G and penicillin G benzathine. An intramuscular injection of procaine penicillin G maintains effective blood levels for 24 hours. An intramuscular injection of benzathine penicillin G maintains blood levels for some 26 days but the levels obtained are too low for treatment of acute dental infection. An important congener is penicillin V, the phenoxymethyl analog of penicillin G. The advan-

Table 11-1 **Principal antibiotic agents employed in pediatric dentistry**

Antibiotic	Route of Administration	Dose	Indication
Penicillin G	oral	25,000 units/kg/24 hrs. divided q. 4 or 6 hours administered 1/2 before or 2 hours after a meal	common gram positive bacterial infections
Penicillin V	oral	15-30 mg/kg/24 hours divided q. 6 to 8 hours	common gram positive bacterial infections
Procaine Penicillin G	intra muscular	30,000 units/kg/24hours single dose	severe dental infection caused by common gram positive bacteria
Erythromycin	oral	30-50 mg/kg/24 hours divided q. 6 hours	sensitivity to penicillin
Dicloxacillin	oral	25-100 mg/kg/24 hours divided q. 6 hours	infections with penicillin resistant staphylococci
Cephalexin	oral	25-50 mg/kg/24 hours divided q. 6 hours	alternative for penicillin G or V
Nystatin	topical		*Candida* infections

tage of penicillin V is great stability in acidic media so that better absorption can be achieved after oral administration. Neither penicillin G nor penicillin V are resistant to the action of penicillinase.

Semi-synthetic penicillins resistant to degradation by penicillinase have been developed. These preparations are indicated for treatment of penicillin resistant staphylococci. Methicillin, the first drug of this group to be developed, is administered as methicillin sodium either intravenously or intramuscularly, although the need for frequent painful injections makes this route of administration undesirable. Methicillin cannot be administered orally because of poor absorption and destruction by gastric fluid. Several other related semi-synthetic penicillins also resistant to penicillinase are available. These

include oxacillin, cloxacillin, dicloxacillin and nafcillin. Oxacillin can be given orally, intramuscularly, or intravenously. Cloxacillin and dicloxacillin are available for oral use only. These preparations can be used for the treatment of infection by penicillin-resistant staphylococci. Nafcillin is available for parenteral or oral use. Because of difficulty in absorption it should not be administered orally for severe staphylococcal infections. Nafcillin also is not a good substitute for penicillin against organisms sensitive to penicillin.

Ampicillin and its congeners *amoxocillin* and *hetacillin,* are semi-synthetic compounds which have broader spectrum of antibacterial activity. Most strains of *H. influenza* type b are sensitive as well as many strains of *E. coli* and *Proteus.* With widespread use of these compounds, more resistant strains of bacteria have emerged. Because ampicillin and its congeners are inactivated by penicillinase they are not useful against staphylococci which produce penicillinase. Ampicillin is available for oral and parenteral use. Amoxicillin is available only for oral use.

Carbenicillin is a penicillin congener which is effective against many strains of *Pseudomonas* and *Proteus* organisms. It must be administered parenterally and rapid development of resistant organisms is a problem. Carbenicillin is inactivated by penicillinase.

All forms of penicillin may produce hypersensitivity reactions. These may be expected to occur in 5% of patients. Reactions include skin rash, glossitis, stomatitis, fever, interstitial nephritis, diarrhea, angioedema, serum sickness, and anaphylaxis. Before penicillin is prescribed a history of sensitivity to the drug must be ascertained.

Since in pediatric dentistry most infections are caused by penicillin-sensitive organisms, penicillin G can be administered orally or intramuscularly. Penicillin V can be administered orally. For some infections treatment is started intramuscularly and then continued orally. Treatment should ordinarily be given for about 7 days. Occasionally when infection with resistant staphylococcus organisms is suspected, use of one of the penicillinase resistant penicillins should be considered. Sometimes one of the broad spectrum penicillins may be of value.

Patients with rheumatic heart disease run the risk of developing subacute bacterial endocarditis and must be premedicated because dental procedures may produce transient bacteremia. A mixture of penicillin G (30,000 units/kg to a maximum of 1,000,000 units) mixed with penicillin procaine G (600,000 units) 30 to 60 minutes before dental intervention, followed by a complete course of antibiotic treatment with oral doses of penicillin V is indicated. If the patient is allergic to penicillin, 20 mg erythromycin/kg (maximum of 1 gram), may be administered 1.5-2 hours before the procedure, followed by erythromycin treatment for several days.

For patients who are sensitive to penicillin, *erythromycin* is frequently used in pediatric dentistry. Erythromycin is an antibiotic with an antibacterial spectrum similar to that of penicillin G. The drug is administered orally because intramuscular administration is painful. Intravenous administration is reserved for severe infections. Hypersensitivity reactions to erythromycin are uncommon but are known.

Cephalosporins, antibiotic agents produced semi-synthetically, have activity against both gram positive and gram negative bacteria. These antibiotic agents can be administered orally or parenterally. Cephalosporins commonly used include the original preparation, cephalothin, cefazolin, and cephalexin. Cephalexin is acid-stable and can be given orally. Patients who are hypersensitive to penicillin also may be sensitive to the cephalosporins.

The *tetracyclines* are a group of antibiotic compounds which include chlortetracycline, oxytetracycline and tetracycline. These antibiotics are bacteriostatic, and therefore generally not as efficacious against bacterial infections as penicillin. In addition, the tetracyclines can cause permanent discoloration of developing teeth. These drugs are no longer used in pediatric dentistry.

The *sulfonamides,* bacteriostatic chemotherapeutic agents, were used in the past against pediatric dental infections. Since these agents are not as effective as the antibiotics currently used, and as reactions are not uncommon, sulfonamides are not presently recommended for use in pediatric dentistry.

A number of other antibiotics are used in pediatric medicine, such as gentomycin and tabamycin. These agents rarely have indications in pediatric dentistry.

Candidiasis (moniliasis) is occasionally found in pediatric dentistry patients, particularly in those who have been treated with broad spectrum antibiotics. In the treatment of candidiasis of the oral cavity, it is helpful to discontinue antibiotic agents when possible. *Nystatin*, an antifungal agent, is used for topical treatment.

References

1. Album, M.M.:
   Meperidine and promethazine hydrochloride for handicapped patients. J. Dent. Res. *40*:1036-1041, 1961.

2. American Dental Association Council on Dental Therapeutics.
   Accepted dental therapeutics. 37th edition. Chicago, American Dental Association, 1977.

3. Bennet, C.R.:
   Conscious-sedation in dental practice. St. Louis, Mosby, 1974.

4. Bennett, C.R.:
   Monheim's local anesthesia and pain control in dental practice. St. Louis, Mosby, 1978.

5. Berger, D.E., G.D. Allen and G.B. Everett:
   An assessment of the analgesic effects of nitrous oxide on the primary dentition. J. Dent. Child. *39*:265-268, 1972.

6. Chambiras, P.G.:
   Sedation in dentistry for children: selective medication. Aust. Dent. J. *14*:245-254, 1969.

7. Czarnecki, E.S. and W.H. Binns:
   Use of chloral hydrate for the apprehensive child. Penn. Dent. J. *30*:40-42, 1963.

8. Emmersten, E.:
   The treatment of children under general analgesia. J. Dent. Child. *32*:123-124, 1965.

9. Goldberg, A.F. and M.S. Sadove:
   Further studies in the spread of local anesthesia. J. Oral Surg. *19*:232-236, 1961.

10. Goth, A.:
    Medical pharmacology. 8th ed. St. Louis, Mosby, 1976.

11. Hargreaves, J.A.:
    Pharmacotherapeutic approaches to behavior management. III. Diazepam in behavior management in dentistry for children. G. Z. Wright (ed). Philadelphia, Saunders, 1975.

12. Houck, W.R. and L.W. Ripa:
    Vomiting frequency in children administered nitrous oxide-oxygen in analgesic doses. J. Dent. Child. *38*:404-406, 1971.

13. Jones, K.F.:
    Preoperative medications in operative dentistry for children. J. Dent. Child. *36*:93-101, 1969.

14. Kopel, H.M.:
    Pharmacotherapeutic approaches to behavior management. II. Hydroxyzine in behavior management in dentistry for children. G. Z. Wright (ed). Philadelphia, Saunders, 1975.

15. Kramer, W.S.:
    A comparative clinical evaluation of some commonly used local anesthetic compounds. J. Am. Dent. Assoc. *56*:820-830, 1958.

16. Kurland, P.:
    Diazepam. Brit. Dent. J. *125*:524, 1968.

17. Lund, L. and J.M. Anholm:
    Clinical observations on the use of meprobramate in dental procedures. Oral Surg. *10*:1281-1286, 1957.

18. McCallum C.A. Jr.:
    Oral surgery for children in clinical pedodontics. S.B. Finn (ed). 4th ed. Philadelphia, Saunders, 1973.

20. Stewart, J.G.:
    Routine preoperative medication for children. J. Dent. Child. *28*:209-212, 1961.

21. Stuebner, E.A. and M.S. Sadove:
    The use of promethazine for premedication. J. Am. Dent. Soc. Anesth. *5*:12-18, 1958.

22. Trieger, N., W.J. Losbota, A.W. Jacobs and M.G. Newman:
    Nitrous oxide – a study of physiological and psychomotor effects. J. Am. Dent. Assoc. *82*:142-150, 1971.

23. Wiedeman, M.:
    Premedication and sedation of the child dental patient. Part. I. J. Nebraska Dent. Assoc. *50*:11-28, 1974.

24. Wright, G.Z. and D.J. McAulay:
    Current premedicating trends in pedodontics. J. Dent. Child. *40*:185-187, 1973.

Chapter 12

Dental Materials – Use, Properties and Limitations

Sally J. Marshall, Ph.D.*

Many dental materials are used in pedodontic treatment. The most common are restorative materials, particularly amalgam, silicate and composite materials. Pit and fissure sealants are used for caries prevention.

Amalgam

Amalgam is one of the oldest and remains the most popular material for the restoration of a single tooth. Compounds containing mercury were used as early as the 16th century, with compositional variations until 1895, when G.V. Black introduced the alloy composition which remains in use today[12]. The next major change in composition came in the 1960's with the development of copper-rich amalgam formulations. G.V. Black's composition was adopted as the standard when American Dental Association (ADA) Specification No. 1 was established more than 50 years ago.

Components

The major phase in conventional, Black type alloys, is γ-Ag_3Sn, which is 73.15% Ag and 26.85% Sn. To enhance the properties of the amalgam, Cu and Zn are also present. Typi-

cally, conventional amalgam alloys contain 67-71% Ag, 24-28% Sn, 1-5% Cu and 0-2% Zn[14]. Copper substitutes primarily for silver in Ag_3Sn, but if the copper content is greater than 5%, Cu_3Sn also forms. The silver provides adequate strength and reactivity with mercury. It also helps to minimize creep and flow. If the silver content is greater than 70%, there will be increased setting expansion. Tin improves and increases the rate of amalgamation, which is why it was originally added to silver. However, it also causes increased contraction, creep and corrosion, as well as decreased strength and hardness. Copper in conventional alloys increases strength and hardness while decreasing creep and flow. It also causes increased tarnish and setting expansion. Zinc is present mainly as an oxygen scavenger during ingot production, but it also increases the plasticity of the amalgam mix. It is responsible for delayed expansion if the amalgam is contaminated by water during trituration or condensation.

High copper or copper-rich alloys contain up to 30% Cu. The increased copper content has been associated with reductions in marginal breakdown[22], creep[22] and corrosion[11]. The first commercially available copper-rich amalgam utilized a blend of conventional amalgam alloy particles and spheres of 71.9 Ag, 28.1 Cu[16]. Figure 12-1 shows the γ and Ag-Cu particles in the alloy powder of a blend system. In this system three parts of silver-copper spheres are added to five

* Associate Professor of Biological Materials at Northwestern University, Chicago, IL.

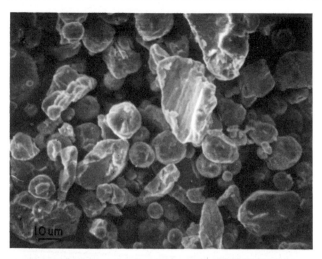

Fig. 12-1   Alloy particles of a blended copper rich amalgam system. The irregular particles are primarily γ and the spherical particles are Ag-Cu[23].

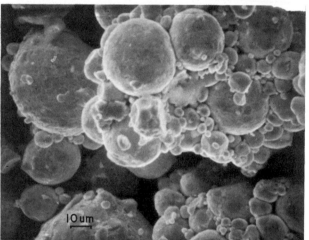

Fig. 12-2   Alloy particles of a single particle copper rich amalgam system[23].

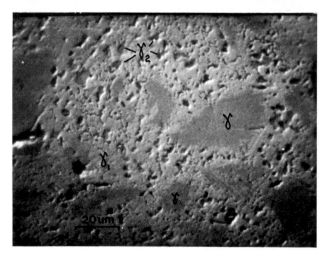

Fig. 12-3   Set microstructure of a conventional amalgam, showing γ, γ_1, and γ_2 phases (Courtesy of Dr. Grayson W. Marshall).

parts of conventional filings, yielding a copper content of about 13%. The copper content of the copper-rich particle, and thus of the alloy, varies among brands. The other method of incorporating increased copper in the alloy is to formulate spherical or spheroidal particles of a single composition containing up to 30% copper. An example of this type of alloy is shown in Fig. 12-2. The copper content of this alloy is also about 13%.

Ingots of conventional amalgam alloy are lathe-cut or milled to produce irregularly shaped particles which can be ball milled to finer sizes. Conventional composition alloys also are available in spherical shape, prepared by atomization. The spherical shaped alloys feel more plastic and require less mercury for trituration because they amalgamate more readily. They yield amalgams with a characteristic feel during condensation and carving[23]. Most copper-rich amalgams of the single particle type are spherical in shape, while the blended systems utilize conventional alloy filings and copper-rich spheres.

The manufacturer controls the composition of the alloy, the particle size and shape, and the rate of reaction with mercury. However, each dentist controls the choice of alloy, trituration and condensation techniques, alloy to mercury ratio, and finishing techniques. The selection of alloy is based on its composition, particle characteristics, and individual preference for handling qualities.

Mixing and setting reaction

When the alloy particles are triturated with mercury they form a plastic mass which can be readily condensed into the prepared cavity. The alloy particles absorb mercury which causes a slight contraction. Crystals of γ_1 and γ_2 form, resulting in an increase in volume and thus an expansion of the restoration. This expansion overcomes the initial contraction at about one hour and continues for about six hours after condensation in a conventional amalgam. The major setting reaction which occurs in conventional amalgam is:

$$\gamma\,(Ag_3Sn) + Hg \rightarrow \gamma_1\,(Ag_2Hg_3) + \gamma_2\,(Sn_3Hg) + \gamma\,(Ag_3Sn)\ (unreacted)$$

The stoichiometric compositions of the phases are only approximate for the phases as they occur in amalgam. From the reaction it can be seen that more alloy and less mercury will result in more unreacted γ and less γ_1 and γ_2 in the set amalgam. Fig. 12-3 is a scanning electron micrograph of the set structure of a conventional amalgam. The amalgam contains the unreacted particles surrounded by a γ_1 matrix and areas of γ_2. Copper rich amalgams set in a similar manner. The γ_1 matrix phase is virtually the same as in conventional amalgams. Residual alloy particles also remain in the structure. In the two particle blend systems these are γ particles and copper rich particles which are surrounded by a reaction zone of γ_1 and Cu_6Sn_5. In the single particle systems the residual alloy particles are also surrounded by a reaction zone of γ_1 and Cu_6Sn_5 in a γ_1 matrix. The major setting reaction for copper rich amalgams can be written as[26]:

$$\gamma + Ag\text{-}Cu + Hg \rightarrow \gamma_1 + Cu_6Sn_5 + \gamma\ (unreacted) + Ag\text{-}Cu\ (unreacted)$$
or
$$Ag\text{-}Cu\text{-}Sn + Hg \rightarrow \gamma_1 + Cu_6Sn_5 + Ag\text{-}Cu\text{-}Sn\ (unreacted)$$

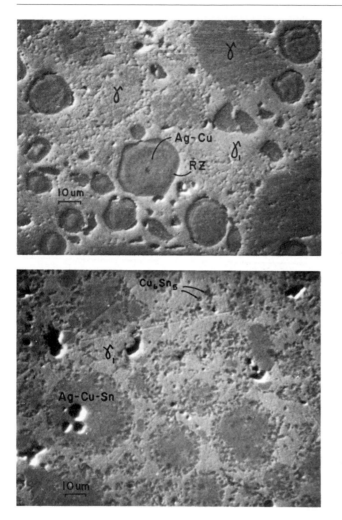

Fig.12-4 Set microstructure of a blended copper rich amalgam, showing γ and γ_1 phases and Ag-Cu spheres surrounded by reaction zones (RZ) of γ_1 and Cu_6Sn_5 phases[23].

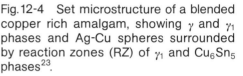

Fig.12-5 Set microstructure of a single composition particle amalgam, showing γ_1 and Cu_6Sn_5 phases and residual Ag-Cu-Sn particles. Note that the γ_1 and Cu_6Sn_5 phases are distinguishable around the residual particles[23].

Gamma-two has been shown to form initially in all these systems, but disappears quite rapidly in most copper-rich amalgams[26]. Thus, they are sometimes referred to as γ_2-free amalgams. The microstructures of a blend system and a single particle system are shown in Figs. 12-4 and 12-5.

The alloy to mercury ratio should be as high as possible and still produce a coherent mass which can be condensed properly. Most conventional amalgams should have about 50% mercury in the final restoration. Most amalgams begin with 48 to 51% mercury, but some are triturated with 60% mercury and the excess mercury is removed with a squeeze cloth during condensation. Increased mercury content leads to the formation of more of the phases containing mercury, γ_1 and γ_2. As these phases are weaker than γ the strength of the amalgam will be lower. The expansion and creep will be increased, as will marginal breakdown. The compressive strength drops precipitously at 55% mercury[34]. Because the mercury content of the margins tends to be several per cent higher than in the bulk of the restoration, the bulk mercury content should be kept near 50% to insure adequate strength in the margins.

Spherical alloys require only about 48% mercury for adequate plasticity of the mix and thus have higher early strength. Copper-rich amalgams utilize alloy to mercury ratios of 1:1 or more. Even though little γ_2 phase forms, it is desirable to minimize the mercury, because the other major phases are all stronger than the mercury containing γ, phase.

Manufacturer's instructions should be followed initially for alloy to mercury ratio but individual preference may cause adjustments to be made. Pre-weighed alloy pellets and a mercury dispenser yield more consistent results than alloys in the powdered form. Mercury dispensers should be calibrated periodically and kept at least half full for best results. Pre-capsulated amalgams offer the best control over alloy to mercury ratio but do not allow for any variations for personal preference.

The major purpose of trituration is the amalgamation of the alloy and mercury to form a plastic mass. In the process, the oxide film on the alloy particles is also removed, making the particles more reactive. Trituration is usually done in a mechanical amalgamator using a capsule with a pestle. Trituration time is critical with respect to handling characteristics and properties of the set amalgam. Manufacturer's instructions should be followed initially with small variations for operator preference. Under trituration yields a grainy mix which may harden too quickly with excessive expansion. Such an amalgam contains excess mercury which may result in decreased strength, increased roughness, and increased corrosion[31]. Over trituration may yield an amalgam mass which is difficult to handle and which sticks to the capsule. It will exhibit excessive contraction and will be weaker than one triturated properly[31]. Mulling, the trituration of the amalgam for an additional few seconds after the removal of the pestle, helps in the removal of the amalgam from the capsule in a single piece.

Condensation of the amalgam is also very important to its final properties. An amalgam should be condensed as soon as possible after trituration, but definitely within a few minutes. If crystals of γ_1 have already formed when condensation is done, they will be fractured, resulting in a weakened amalgam. For the best adaptation to the cavity, amalgams are usually condensed in small amounts and from the center of the cavity towards the walls. Loads of 1.4 to 1.8 kg are typical in practice. High condensation pressures are desirable to increase strength and decrease setting expansion and flow. The pressure can be increased by increasing the applied load or decreasing the size of the condenser tip.

A condensed amalgam should be carved to reproduce the lost anatomy. This can usually be done five minutes after it is placed, but the amalgam must be hard enough so that it does not pull away from the margins. Burnishing is controversial. It can result in a smooth surface with good margins[18] or it can result in increased marginal deterioration and a mercury-rich layer on the surface, depending on the amalgam alloy and technique used[20].

All amalgams should be polished, but not before 48 hours after condensation. Polishing reduces surfaces roughness, which minimizes tarnish, corrosion and trapping of food debris. A wet paste should be used to minimize the generation of heat. If an amalgam is overheated during polishing it will appear glossy for a short time because of the formation of a mercury-rich layer on the surface[13]. If an amalgam is polished too early the setting structure will be disturbed.

Properties

The mechanical and physical properties of any restorative material should match those of the surrounding tooth structure. A restoration must be strong enough to withstand the forces of mastication without fracture. The compressive strength of amalgams is required by revised ADA Specification No.1 to be 80 megapascals (MPa) at one hour[7]. Most amalgams have compressive strengths of over 300 MPa when set. This is adequate compressive strength, but there are also tensile forces at edges and margins. The tensile strength of amalgam is 15% of the compressive strength or less, which is not as high as desirable. The strengths at oral temperature also will be less than at room temperature. Thus the cavity should be designed to minimize tensile forces on the restoration and the amalgam should be manipulated to maximize its strength. As the phases containing mercury are weaker than the original alloy particles, strength will be increased by using a high alloy to mercury ratio. Proper trituration and condensation techniques should be used to maximize strength. The early strength of amalgam is considerably less than the set strength, so patients always must be cautioned to avoid biting on an amalgam for several hours. At 20 minutes after condensation, the strength is less than one-tenth of its set strength, increasing to about one-fourth at one hour and three-fourths at 8 hours.

Creep and flow are measurements of the change in dimensions of amalgam specimens. Flow measures the changes during setting, while creep measures the resistance to deformation of set amalgam specimens. Reduction in creep has been correlated with improved marginal integrity for some amalgam types[22]. The revised ADA Specification No. 1 requires less than 5% creep, but most conventional amalgams have creep values in the range of 2 to 4%, while values for copper-rich amalgams are in the range of 0.02-1.5%[9]. Creep and flow can be minimized by the choice of a copper-rich alloy, high condensation pressure, and a

minimum of mercury in the amalgam. Thermal properties of amalgam are both good and bad. The thermal expansion coefficient is approximately twice that of tooth, which is not ideal but is better than most polymeric restoratives. Amalgam is a good thermal conductor so a base is used to protect the pulp in a deep cavity.

Problems and failures

Many failures in amalgam restorations result from operator error or poor cavity design. Material failures fall into several categories: marginal breakdown, dimensional change, and corrosion. Gross fracture is usually the result of improper cavity design, poor carving or not protecting the fresh amalgam from masticatory stresses.

Marginal breakdown can be caused by a high mercury content at the margin, overheating during burnishing or polishing, creep, other dimensional changes which can cause the amalgam to extrude out of the cavity, or corrosion of the amalgam. High mercury content of the margins can be prevented by using a high alloy to mercury ratio, adequate condensation, removal of any excess mercury, and proper carving. Overheating can be avoided easily by using wet pastes, and creep can be minimized as described earlier.

Dimensional change on setting is limited in the revised ADA Specification No. 1 to no more than ±0.20%. Too much expansion can cause the amalgam to extrude out of the cavity or can cause pressure on the pulp and result in postoperative sensitivity. Too much contraction will cause the amalgam to pull away from the cavity walls, resulting in leakage. Some expansion on setting may be desirable to ensure that the restoration stays firmly in the cavity. A properly manipulated amalgam should show no clinically significant dimensional changes after one day.

Fig. 12-6a and b Microstructures of amalgams after clinical use showing Sn, Ca, and P containing corrosion products near the wall of the cavity. a) Conventional amalgam. b) Copper rich amalgam[24]. (Copyright by the American Dental Association. Reprinted by permission.)

Figure 12-6a

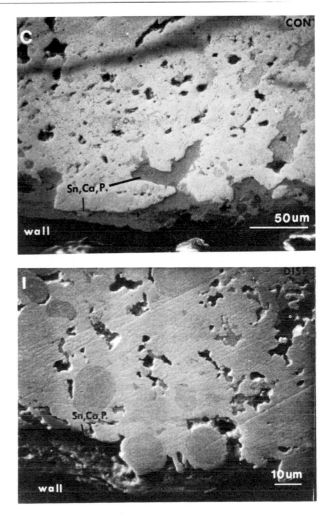

Figure 12-6b

Delayed expansion can be a major problem in amalgams containing zinc which are contaminated by moisture. Moisture contamination is caused by saliva, condensation on instruments, or moisture on the dentist's hands. The zinc reacts with water to form zinc oxide and hydrogen gas. If this reaction occurs near the surface, the gas bubbles escape, leaving a rough surface. If it occurs in the interior of the amalgam the gas pressure causes pain or the expansion of the amalgam. Delayed expansion can occur anytime from a few days after placement until several months later. Therefore, care should be taken to keep the amalgam dry until condensation is finished. In areas which are particularly difficult to keep dry, a zinc-free amalgam should be used.

As long as the amalgam is kept dry and properly manipulated, marginal leakage should not be a major problem. Use of a cavity varnish will help to seal the margins. Some studies have shown a decrease in leakage with time; the explanation is given that corrosion products fill the margin and 'seal' it[32]. Filled margins can be seen in

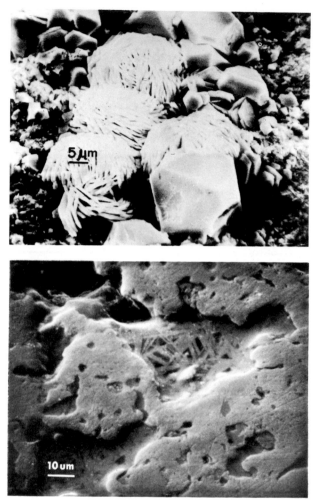

Fig. 12-7   Corrosion products of conventional amalgam; (a) SnO polyhedra and $Sn_4(OH)_6Cl_2$ plates grown in vitro on the surface of an amalgam. (From Marshall, N. K. Sarkar, and E. H. Greener: Detection of oxygen in corrosion products of dental amalgam. J. Dent. Res. 54, 904 [1975]); (b) $Sn_4(OH)_6Cl_2$ plates in a pore of an amalgam retrieved after clinical use[27].

Figure 12-7a

Figure 12-7b

Fig. 12-6 for conventional and copper-rich amalgams[24].

Corrosion and tarnish are problems associated with amalgams. Tarnish is esthetically undesirable and also provides a rougher surface for plaque adhesion. Corrosion can destroy a restoration. An amalgam in the mouth is an example of a galvanic cell. Saliva is a good electrolyte and the non-homogeneous nature of an amalgam provides the mixed metals and necessary contact. The γ_2 phase of conventional amalgams is the most corrosion prone phase. As γ_2 corrodes it releases mercury which can react with γ particles to form γ_1 and γ_2 and thus perpetuate the reaction. This reaction can be accompanied by mercuroscopic expansion[17]. The Sn which is released forms several compounds in the oral environment, including $Sn_4(OH)_6Cl_2$ and SnO[27]. These products are found in areas which have the morphology of the γ_2 phase and in pores as shown in Fig. 12-7.

Polishing reduces corrosion by providing a smooth surface. Copper-rich amalgams have greatly decreased corrosion tendencies. In these amalgams the tin is present primarily as Cu_6Sn_5 instead of γ_2. Copper-rich amalgams show less marginal deterioration than conventional amalgams. A number of reasons could account for this phenomenon, including the decreased creep and increased corrosion resistance.

There is considerable concern about the hazards of mercury. Because it is a liquid with a high vapor pressure at room temperature it must be handled carefully. Mercury and amalgam scrap should always be kept in tightly closed, unbreakable containers. Mercury should be used only over smooth surfaces, including floors, and any spills cleaned up immediately. It should be handled minimally and should be used only in well ventilated areas. Tight fitting capsules help prevent any unnecessary vaporization. All personnel involved in use of mercury should be educated about safety procedures, and mercury levels should be measured in the personnel as well as in the dental office[6].

Silicates

Silicate is one of the oldest tooth-colored restorative materials and remains the material of choice for an anterior restoration in the caries-prone child. Silicate restorations initially have good esthetic properties but dissolve and stain readily in oral fluids. As the material dissolves, fluoride ions are released which inhibit caries formation by the same mechanism as topical fluoride applications[28]. However, the average life of a silicate restoration is less than that of a composite restoration, and thus the use of silicates has decreased considerably since the development of composites.

Components

Most silicates are supplied as a powder and a liquid. The powder is an acid soluble alumino-silicate glass consisting primarily of silica, alumina, lime, cryolite (Na_3AlF_4), and fluorine-containing glass formers, such as sodium or calcium fluoride. The powders contain up to 15% fluorides and are available in a variety of shades to match the surrounding tooth structure. The liquid is phosphoric acid with about 40% water and is buffered with aluminum, zinc, or magnesium phosphates. The ratio of constituents in the liquid is critical and care must be taken to avoid evaporation or uptake of water as well as other contaminants. Even when the operator is careful there is ample opportunity for exposure of the liquid to the atmosphere and subsequent change in the water content, so the last 20% of the liquid in any container should be discarded. Liquids should also be discarded if they become discolored or have crystals growing in them.

Mixing and setting reaction

The powder to liquid ratio is very important to the properties of the set silicate restoration. A powder to liquid ratio of 4 to 1 yields the maximum strength and minimum solubility[31]. The reasons for this high powder to liquid ratio become evident when the mechanism of setting is considered.

When the powder and liquid are mixed the acid attacks the glass particles and dissolves the surface layers. A gel structure forms around each particle and further reaction is limited by the diffusion of acid through the gel reaction zone. The gel is very weak so only enough of it should be present to coat the particles and bind them together. As the glass particles are the strongest part of the material as well as the least soluble in oral

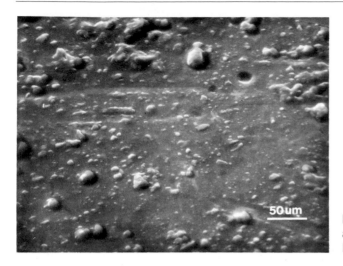

Fig. 12-8   Surface of a silicate restoration as finished (Courtesy of Dr. Grayson W. Marshall).

fluids, a maximum quantity of powder should be incorporated. The upper limit on powder content is that all powder particles must be wetted by the liquid. If the powder to liquid ratio is too high, the mix will be granular and the restoration weak and soluble. A powder to liquid ratio which is too low not only yields a weak and soluble end product, but the pH is also lower, thus having more potential for pulp damage. The set structure of a well proportioned and well mixed silicate consists of about 70-80% unreacted glass particles surrounded by a gel matrix[13,19].

Attainment of the high powder to liquid ratio which yields the optimum properties requires proper mixing. Mixing should be done on a cool, dry slab, allowing a slow reaction in which all the powder is incorporated. Usually about half the powder is mixed with the liquid for 30 seconds, followed by one-fourth portions mixed for an additional 15 seconds each. One minute is the optimum mixing time. As it is desirable to incorporate as much powder as possible, an excess of powder is generally dispensed and any not incorporated is discarded. Mixing is done with plastic, agate, or cobalt-chromium spatulas. A stainless steel spatula should not be used because the glass particles will abrade

it and the metallic particles will discolor the mix.

Avoiding moisture contamination in the preparation of a silicate is of the utmost importance since such contamination may result in the swelling of the restoration[30]. As soon as the required quantities of powder and liquid are dispensed the containers should be closed to prevent atmospheric contamination. Mixing should be confined to a very small area on the slab to minimize contact with any moisture. Another method to avoid moisture and other contamination is the use of pre-capsulated silicates. The capsules are similar to those for pre-capsulated amalgams and the silicate is mixed for about 10 seconds in a mechanical triturator. The advantages of such packaging are that the silicate components are not handled, the proportions of powder and liquid are always the same, thus giving reproducible mixes, and a homogeneous mix is easily obtained. There are also several disadvantages. Mechanical trituration generates more heat, so the silicate may set faster and care must be taken not to overtriturate; the fixed powder to liquid ratio may not meet operator preference; and this mode of packaging is expensive. Regardless of the mixing method, the mixed cement should be thick and the consistency of putty.

The mixed cement should be placed directly into the prepared cavity, covered with a matrix strip, and held in place for at least three minutes. The restoration should be contoured as well as possible while the matrix strip is in place, immediately after placement. The surface which sets against the matrix strip will be smoother than that obtained by other finishing techniques because the structure is abraded readily and the glass particles tend to fall out, leaving a rough surface and holes (Fig. 12-8). If finishing is necessary it is done carefully after several days of setting and with a good lubricant.

Gel formation is not complete for hours after the restoration is set, so the surface of the restoration must be covered with cocoa butter, cavity varnish, or other suitable material which can protect the restoration from the oral environment for 24 hours[35]. Silicates contract somewhat on setting, which makes marginal leakage very common. Because of the gel structure the silicate must be hydrated when fully set and remain hydrated to prevent shrinkage, cracking and crazing[35]. For this reason, silicates are not recommended as anterior restorations in mouth breathers.

ADA Specification No. 9 for silicates requires a setting time of 3 to 8 minutes at 37°C[14]. Most commercial products, when properly prepared, set in 3 to 6 minutes. A number of variables can be used to control setting time to individual operator preference. Setting time can best be increased by using a cool, dry mixing slab and selecting a product with a large average particle size. It is also increased if the mixing time is increased slightly, if less water is present in the liquid, or if the powder to liquid ratio is reduced. However, any of the last three methods may cause a degradation in the properties of the set silicate.

Silicates are acidic, having a pH of 3 or less when placed and about 5 after one month[30]. The pulp must be protected from this acidity so a cavity varnish is necessary on all dentin surfaces and a base is needed in deep cavities.

Properties

A well prepared set silicate has many properties which closely approach those of the natural tooth. Color and translucence are excellent initially. The index of refraction of shaded silicate powders varies from 1.47 to 1.60, while that of the gel matrix is about 1.46[31]. The corresponding values for enamel and dentin are 1.60 and 1.56, respectively[31]. Silicates stain, discolor and lose translucence in the mouth over periods of a few months to ten years or more, depending on the conditions in the mouth and how well the silicate was prepared.

A major advantage of silicates over other restorative materials is in thermal properties, especially the thermal expansion coefficient. The value for silicate is the nearest of any restorative material to that of the tooth structure replaced[13]. Thus, percolation is minimized. Thermal conductivity also is low, which is desirable in a restorative material since thermal shock to the pulp will be minimized.

Some mechanical properties are not as good for silicates as those of other restorative materials. The compressive strength at 24 hours is typically 150 MPa, which is adequate[30]. However, its tensile strength is only about 4.3 MPa and it is brittle. The surface hardness is comparable to that of dentin, but well below enamel. Abrasion resistance is poor and abrasion usually leaves a rough surface because the gel matrix abrades away and the glass particles either protrude from the surface or fall out, leaving holes.

Problems and failures

The major cause of silicate failure is dissolution of the restoration leading either to complete failure or excessive staining, especially at the margins. Failure and staining occur at various rates, depending upon the operator's manipulation techniques and the patient's oral environment. A properly manipulated silicate will meet the requirement in ADA Specification No. 9 of not more than 1% solubility in 37°C distilled water at 24 hours[14]. However, dissolution occurs more quickly in an acidic environment, particularly when citric acid is present. The solubility will also increase if the powder to liquid ratio is decreased. If not kept wet, silicates suffer from syneresis, which leads to a loss of translucency and shrinkage as the gel dries, leaving a soft, chalky surface.

The dissolution does have a beneficial side effect which makes silicates useful in spite of their limitations. As the restoration gradually dissolves fluoride salts are released which behave similarly to a topical application of fluoride in preventing the development of caries in the surrounding tooth. Clinical studies have shown that the development of secondary caries around silicate restorations is much less than around amalgam, gold, resin, or composite restorations[21]. The fluorine content of the enamel adjacent to a silicate restoration has been found to be six times normal[28]. Thus, as the restoration is failing it is protecting the surrounding tooth structure from further decay, which is the reason why silicates are recommended for use in a child highly susceptible to caries.

Composites

The development of dental composite restorative materials occurred because of the shortcomings of polymethyl methacrylate (PMMA) resin restorations. Many of the problems were inherent in polymer systems, including: low strength, elastic modulus, proportional limit and hardness, high thermal expansion coefficient, large polymerization shrinkage, poor abrasion resistance, and pulpal irritation from monomer penetration through the dentin tubules. Addition of a glass or ceramic second phase helped alleviate these problems. The mechanical and physical properties of a composite are intermediate between those of the two components. Adding a glass or ceramic phase to a polymer will therefore increase the strength, elastic modulus, proportional limit, hardness, and abrasion resistance. The addition of a relatively inert glass or ceramic also reduces the thermal expansion coefficient and setting shrinkage. Total monomer content is also reduced because much of the restoration mass is filler.

Components

Early composites used PMMA as the resin, but more recent developments have utilized cyanoacrylates, polystyrene, polyamide, polyester, polycarbonate and polyurethane[29]. Most composites, however, utilize BIS-GMA, an aromatic dimethacrylate, as the base resin. The chemical structure of BIS-GMA monomer (Bowen's resin)[2] is:

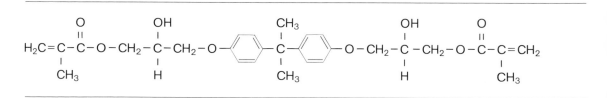

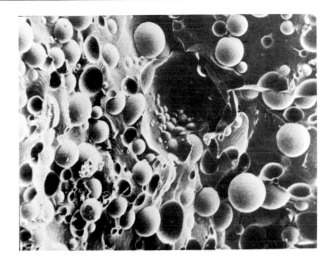

Fig. 12-9 Fracture surface of a composite showing spherical filler particles (Courtesy of Dr. Grayson W. Marshall).

The double bonds at the ends of the chain are broken to form the polymer. Many of the reasons making it the resin of choice are related to the complex structure of the molecule[2]. Its strength, elastic modulus, hardness, and abrasion resistance are greater than those of PMMA because of the complexity of the molecule and crosslinking which develops on setting. Similarly, the thermal expansion coefficient is reduced. The monomer is less likely to injure the pulp because it cannot travel down dentin tubules as a smaller molecule can, although bases are needed. Polymerization shrinkage is reduced because the number of double bonds available for polymerization per unit volume is reduced. BIS-GMA also hardens more rapidly in the mouth than PMMA.

A variety of fillers is used in composites, but most are chemically inert, hard, and have opacity and refractive index similar to teeth. Ceramic glasses are common fillers and include fused silica, quartz, lithium aluminium silicate, borosilicate glass, and barium fluoride glass. The barium containing glass renders the composite radiopaque. Recently colloidal silica has also been used. The particle shape, size, concentration, and distribution vary. Most composites have filler parti-

cles which are irregular in shape, although some are spheres and rods. Fig. 12-9 is a fracture surface of a composite with spherical fillers. Irregular particles are retained better than spheres or rods. Aside from the very fine colloidal fillers used in microfill composites, fillers vary in size in the 1 to 100 μm range, and some use graded sizes for better packing. Most composites are 70-80 weight percent filler, which is about 50 volume percent of the set restoration.

As fillers are generally glass or ceramic they have higher strength, elastic modulus, and hardness than the resin matrix. They also have significantly lower thermal expansion coefficients. Thus, the composite of the filler and resin matrix has higher strength, elastic modulus, and hardness, and a lower thermal expansion coefficient than the unfilled resin. The filler does not shrink as the resin polymerizes; therefore the overall polymerization shrinkage of the composite is considerably less than that of the unfilled resin. Similarly, the heat of polymerization and the water absorption of the composite are reduced.

In addition to the resin and filler a number of minor components are necessary to make a good composite. BIS-GMA is too viscous to

275

use alone as the base resin, so it is diluted with a low viscosity methacrylate monomer such as methyl or glycol methacrylate or an aliphatic dimethacrylate[3]. Sometimes a low concentration of methacrylic acid is added to increase the initial rate of polymerization. A major problem has been that the theoretical strength obtainable from a combination of the properties of the matrix and filler has not been achieved because of poor bonding between matrix and filler. Therefore a coupling agent to bind the inorganic filler to the organic matrix is usually present. The surfaces of the filler particles are coated with a silane for this purpose[29]. The coupling agent increases the strength and abrasion resistance of the composite.

An initiator to start the polymerization must be present. In chemically activated systems, organic peroxides, such as benzoyl peroxide, are usually used. Sulphinic acid is also used as an initiator. In these systems a chemical activator is used to break the initiator into free radicals. Typically an aromatic tertiary amine is used as the activator and setting is brought about by the same methods as in cold curing acrylic (PMMA)[3]. In ultraviolet light-activated systems the UV light breaks the UV-sensitive initiator molecules into free radicals. Aromatic ethers, such as benzoin methyl ether, are used as the initiators in these systems[5]. Similarly, in systems activated by visible light, the visible light breaks the diketone initiator into free radicals[1]. Once free radicals are formed, a chain reaction starts with the free radicals opening the acrylate double bonds and producing more free radicals which propagate the chain. Composites also contain a hydroquinone inhibitor to prevent spontaneous polymerization of the monomers and thus increase the shelf life of the product. In chemically activated systems utilizing the peroxide initiator and amine activator, a UV absorber is also present to minimize color changes in sunlight. Most composites come in a variety of shades which can be mixed to match tooth color.

Mixing and setting reactions

Retention of the composites to the tooth structure is by mechanical means. Frequently, the surrounding enamel is etched by 30-50% phosphoric acid for one to two minutes, followed by flushing with water and drying. The etching cleans any debris from the surface, thus enhancing the wetting of the tooth surface by the resin. The major retention mechanism occurs because the acid preferentially etches parts of the enamel rods, which allows the resin to penetrate into the rods, forming resin tags about 35 μm long. The dentin should not be etched and should be protected by a calcium hydroxide base during etching to prevent the penetration of the acid through the dentin tubules.

Most composites are supplied as two pastes, but can be supplied as a powder and liquid, as a paste and a liquid, or as a single paste. In the two paste chemically activated systems both pastes contain the resin and filler coated with a coupling agent, while one paste contains the initiator and the other contains the activator. Because the resin and filler are in both pastes in the proper proportions, the ratio of the two pastes is not critical and the quantities are estimated by the dentist. In powder and liquid or paste and liquid systems the proportions are more critical. In light-activated systems the proper proportions are in the single paste but the exposure time for curing is critical.

All composites should be mixed with a nonmetallic spatula on a non-absorbent mixing pad or slab. The filler particles are hard so they will abrade most spatulas and metallic particles will discolor the mix. A non-absorbent pad should be used so none of the resin is lost in the pad. Two paste, chemically activated systems are usually supplied with double ended spatulas, one end for each paste. Care must be taken to avoid contamination of the pastes with each other or polymerization will occur within the container. The two pastes must be mixed thoroughly to provide uniform curing. In all chemically activated composites, mixing time should be 30 seconds or less because the working time is usually slightly over a minute. All composites should be mixed and placed in dry areas because the polymerization will be adversely affected by water. Light activated systems have increased working time because polymerization does not begin until the composite is exposed to the light. These composites are inserted, contoured, and then exposed to the light for the recommended time. In large restorations they are inserted and cured in increments.

Chemically activated systems should be placed, covered by a matrix strip, and contoured by finger pressure. They should be cured under finger pressure to prevent the composite from pulling away from the walls as it cures. The matrix strip should be kept in place until polymerization is complete, because the resin is sensitive to air and, if exposed to air, the surface of most composites will be tacky and will set poorly. Contouring should be done before the composite is set because finishing most composites is very difficult. Some composites utilize glazes to cover the surface with a smooth layer. The glaze is a slightly filled or unfilled resin similar to pit and fissure sealants which gives a smooth surface initially but which abrades easily and quickly.

Properties

The mechanical properties of most composite systems are adequate for their use in non-

occlusal areas. Compressive strengths are about 220 MPa, which is more than for silicates or unfilled restorative resins, but less than for amalgam[8]. The tensile strength of composites is also intermediate. Elastic modulus values are about the same as for amalgam. Dimensional change on setting, water absorption, and solubility of composites are all less than for other non-metallic restorations. The thermal expansion coefficient is slightly larger than that of amalgam, or about two or three times that of tooth structure[8].

Problems and failures

Maintaining a smooth, clean surface after placement is one of the major problems in the use of composites. Because of the different natures of the two phases, filler and resin, they do not wear at the same rates. The resin matrix wears or abrades readily, leaving the filler particles either to protrude from the surface or fall out of it. This results in a rough surface which promotes the buildup of plaque and debris and promotes staining. The rough surface of an abraded composite is shown in Fig. 12-10 in contrast to the set surface before abrasion. The best surface which can be obtained on a composite is the one which sets against a matrix strip.

A new group of microfill composite restorative materials has been developed which uses a finer, softer filler and thus, should have a smoother surface following either finishing or wear. An abraded surface of such a composite is shown in Fig. 12-11. The change in filler also results in lower strength, higher dimensional change on setting, and an increased thermal expansion coefficient. There is increased wear because the concentration of filler must be reduced to incorporate the finer particle size, but the worn surface is smoother. It is apparent that there must be a compromise between the smooth-

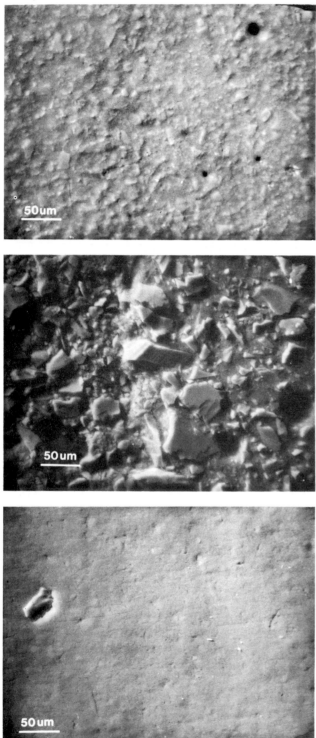

Fig. 12-10a and b Surface of a composite with irregular shaped filler particles; (a) set surface. (b) surface after 4000 strokes with a toothbrush and tooth paste (Courtesy of Dr. Grayson W. Marshall).

Figure 12-10a

Figure 12-10b

Fig. 12-11 Surface of a microfilled composite after 4000 strokes with a toothbrush and tooth paste (Courtesy of Dr. Grayson W. Marshall).

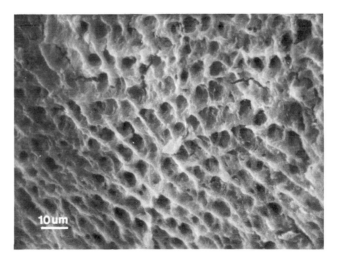

Fig.12-12 Pit and fissure sealant after penetration into etched enamel rods. Enamel was dissolved to reveal resin tags (Courtesy of Dr. Grayson W. Marshall).

ness of the surface and the other mechanical and physical properties.

Still another problem in the use of composites is the need for a cavity varnish and a liner in deep cavities. Liners containing eugenol should not be used because the eugenol may inhibit the polymerization of the resin.

Pit and fissure sealants

Pit and fissure sealants are the only truly preventive dental materials in use at present. They are used in children primarily to seal the pits and fissures on the occlusal surfaces of molars. Prior to the introduction of pit and fissure sealants, deep pits and fissures which were thought to be likely sites for caries were filled with amalgam or silicate restorations. However, those techniques required the removal of some healthy tooth structure. Current pit and fissure sealants require only acid etching of the tooth surface. To prevent the penetration of oral fluids, the resin must flow into the pits and

fissures and subsequently seal the region. The sealant provides a physical barrier to the penetration of oral fluids.

The resin in most pit and fissure sealants is primarily BIS-GMA, an aromatic dimethacrylate. BIS-GMA monomer is too viscous to flow into the pits and fissures, so it is usually diluted with methyl methacrylate or some other low viscosity methacrylate monomer. Cyanoacrylates and polyurethanes also have been used as the base resin. Most pit and fissure sealants are unfilled or only slightly filled.

Retention of pit and fissure sealants is by mechanical means. The tooth surface is usually etched with 30-50% phosphoric acid or other suitable acid, to provide micro-irregularities into which the resin can penetrate[4, 25]. Tags of resin form by polymerization; these retain the sealant on the tooth by mating with the acid etched enamel rod structure. Such tags are shown in Fig. 12-12, after dissolving the tooth structure. The surface must be free from debris and dry for this penetration to occur.

Polymerization of the sealant is accomplished by chemical initiator and activator, or by ultraviolet or visible light activation of a chemical initiator. In the chemically activated BIS-GMA systems the initiator is frequently benzoyl peroxide, which is broken up into free radicals by an amine activator. These systems are usually supplied as two liquids, each containing diluted BIS-GMA. One liquid contains the initiator, while the other contains the activator. The two liquids are mixed, sometimes directly on the tooth surface, and the resin cures in place. Ultraviolet light-activated systems usually utilize benzoin methyl ether as the initiator, which is easily broken up into free radicals by the UV light. Because little or no polymerization occurs before exposure to the UV light, these systems have an indefinite working time, but care must be taken to use a sufficient amount of sealant and proper UV exposure time to obtain adequate polymerization.

The visible light activated system is a urethane dimethacrylate polymer with a diketone initiator which is activated by blue light[1]. As with the UV activated systems, care must be taken to expose the polymer uniformly to the light to obtain proper polymerization. The major advantage is the indefinite working time.

The resin must be fluid enough to penetrate into the deep pits and fissures as well as into the etched enamel surface. Then it must polymerize in place, in intimate contact with the tooth surface, and form a seal against oral fluids. Pit and fissure sealants wear away readily, especially from occlusal surfaces. They must be checked regularly and reapplied if necessary. Some pit and fissure sealants are colored to make them more visible on the tooth surface. It is possible that some of the resin wears off the occlusal surface, while the portion in the pits and fissures remains intact, still providing an adequate seal. Clinical studies have shown continued caries reduction where the sealant was gone from the surface but was present in the pits and fissures[10,15]. Furthermore, even in areas where the sealant has apparently worn away, additional protection may occur through retention of resin tags which are not visible to the clinician. Other studies have shown that the progress of caries is significantly slowed in carious teeth where a sealant was applied[33]. The useful life of sealants varies, but sealants do inhibit caries formation and growth for significant periods of time.

References

1. Bassiouny, M. A. and A. A. Grant:
A visible light-cured composite restorative. Brit. Dent. J. *145*:327-330, 1978.

2. Bowen, R. L.:
Properties of a silica-reinforced polymer for dental restorations. J. Am. Dent. Assoc. *66*:57-64, 1963.

3. Bowen, R. L., J. A. Barton and A. L. Mullineaux:
Composite restorative materials. NBS Special Publ. 354, 1972.

4. Bozalis, W. G., G. W. Marshall and R. O. Cooley:
Mechanical pretreatments and etching of primary tooth enamel. J. Dent. Child. *46*:43-49, 1979.

5. Buonocore, M.:
Adhesive sealing of pits and fissures for caries prevention, with use of ultraviolet light. J. Am. Dent. Assoc. *80*:324-330, 1970.

6. Council on Dental Materials and Devices, ADA:
Recommendations in Mercury Hygiene. J. Am. Dent. Assoc. *88*:391-392, 1974.

7. Council on Dental Materials and Devices, ADA:
Revised American Dental Association Specification No.1 for Alloy for Dental Amalgam. J. Am. Dent. Assoc. *95*:614-617, 1977.

8. Dennison, J. B. and R. G. Craig:
Physical properties and finished surface texture of composite restorative resins. J. Am. Dent. Assoc. *85*:101-108, 1972.

9. Eames, W. B., and J. F. MacNamara:
Eight high-copper amalgam alloys and six conventional alloys compared. Oper. Dent. *1*:98-107, 1976.

10. Going, R. E., L. D. Haugh, D. A. Grainger and A. J. Conti:
Four-year clinical evaluation of a pit and fissure sealant. J. Am. Dent. Assoc. *95*:972-981, 1977.

11. Greener, E. H.:
Anodic polarization of new dental amalgams. J. Dent. Res. *55*:1142, 1976.

12. Greener, E. H.:
Amalgam: yesterday, today, and tomorrow. Oper. Dent. *4*:24-35, 1979.

13. Greener, E. H., J. K. Harcourt and E. P. Lautenschlager:
Materials Science in Dentistry. Baltimore, Williams and Wilkins Co., 1972.

14. Guide to Dental Materials and Devices, 6th Ed. Chicago, American Dental Association, 1972.

15. Horowitz, H. S., S. B. Heifetz and S. Poulsen:
Retention and effectiveness of a single application of an adhesive sealant in preventing occlusal caries: Final report after five years of a study in Kalispell, Montana. J. Am. Dent. Assoc. *95*:1133-1139, 1977.

16. Innes, D. B. K., and W. Youdelis:
Dispersion strengthened amalgams. J. Canad. Dent. Assoc. *29*:587-593, 1963.

17. Jørgensen, K. D.:
The mechanism of marginal fracture of amalgam fillings. Acta Odont. Scand. *23*:347-389, 1965.

18. Kato, S., K. Okuse and T. Fusayama:
The effect of burnishing on the marginal seal of amalgam restorations. J. Prosth. Dent. *19*:393-398, 1968.

19. Kent, B. E., K. E. Fletcher and A. D. Wilson:
Dental silicate cements. XI. Electron probe studies. J. Dent. Res. *49*:86-92, 1970.

20. Leinfelder, K. F., W. D. Strickland, J. T. Wall and D. F. Taylor:
Burnished amalgam restorations:
A two-year clinical evaluation. Oper. Dent. *3*:2-8, 1978.

21. Lind, V., G. Wennerholm and S. Nystrom:
Contact caries in connection with silver amalgam, copper amalgam and silicate fillings. Acta Odont. Scand. *22*:333-341, 1964.

22. Mahler, D.B., L.D.Terkla, J.Van Eysden and M.H.Reisbeck:
Marginal fracture vs. mechanical properties of amalgam. J. Dent. Res. *49*:1452-1457, 1970.

23. Marker, B.C., and G.W.Marshall:
Characteristics and handling of Cu-rich amalgam. Quintessence Int. *10*:125-132, 1979.

24. Marshall, Jr., G.W., B.L.Jackson and S.J.Marshall:
Copper-rich and conventional amalgam restorations after clinical use. J. Am. Dent. Assoc. *100*:43-47, 1980.

25. Marshall, G.W., L.W.Olsen and C.V.Lee:
SEM investigation of the variability of enamel surfaces after simulated clinical acid etching for pit and fissure sealants. J. Dent. Res. *54*:1222-1231, 1975.

26. Marshall, S.J., and G.W.Marshall:
Time-dependent phase changes in Cu-rich amalgams. J. Biomed. Mater. Res. *13*:395-406, 1979.

27. Marshall, S.J., and G.W.Marshall, Jr.:
$Sn_4(OH)_6Cl_2$ and SnO corrosion products of amalgams. J. Dent. Res. *59*:820-823, 1980.

28. Norman, R.D., R.W.Phillips, and M.L.Swartz:
Fluoride uptake by enamel from certain dental materials. J. Dent. Res. *39*:11-16, 1960.

29. Paffenbarger, G.C., and N.W.Rupp:
Composite restorative materials in dental practice: A review. Int. Dent. J. *24*:1-17, 1974.

30. Paffenbarger, G.C., I.C.Schoonover and W.Souder:
Dental silicate cements: Physical and chemical properties and a specification. J. Am. Dent. Assoc. *25*:32-87, 1938.

31. Phillips, R.W.:
Skinner's Science of Dental Materials. 7th Ed. Philadelphia, W.B. Saunders Co., 1973.

32. Phillips, R.W., H.W.Gilmore, M.L.Swartz and S.I.Schenker:
Adaptation of restorations in vivo as assessed by Ca^{45}. J. Am. Dent. Assoc. *62*:9-20, 1961.

33. Silverstone, L.M.:
Fissure sealants: The susceptibility to dissolution of acid-etched and subsequently abraded enamel in vitro. Caries Res. *11*:46-51, 1977.

34. Swartz, M.L., and R.W.Phillips:
Residual mercury content of amalgam restorations and its influence on compressive strength. J. Dent. Res. *35*:458-466, 1956.

35. Wilson, A.D., and R.F.Batchelor:
Dental silicate cements. II. Preparation and durability. J. Dent. Res. *46*:1425-1432, 1967.

Chapter 13

Practice Management

Just as negative influences in the dental experience start long before the patient ever sees the dentist (past, unpleasant experiences in other medical and dental practices, peer or parent negative comments, etc.) some positive forces are initiated long before the patient actually meets the dentist. Some of these perceptions depend on the receptionist and other auxiliary personnel as well as on the general office atmosphere.

An office run in a disorderly, disorganized manner is wasteful and reduces the quantity and probably the quality of service provided. Good practice management increases productivity and quality of care while reducing stress to the dentist and the staff. To achieve this, a variety of physiologic and psychologic factors for each individual dentist must be taken into consideration with the intent of organizing working conditions to achieve optimum efficiency. Constant re-evaluation, reassessment, and creativity also are required,

Efficiency is possible if several factors are analyzed carefully in the organization of an office. These include the personal make-up of the dentist (size, range of reaching ability, method of working), type of work required, type and quantity of auxiliary personnel available, and their spheres of activity.

A patient should be greeted by name (or nickname if he prefers) but not as "honey", "dear", or other indefinite words. The child should feel that he is the center of personal attention and is identified as an individual, not as an object.

Promptness of keeping appointments is of paramount importance, particularly with children who are not able to dispel fears (even in a waiting room equipped with toys). The time of day chosen and the length of an appointment depends on the temperament, age and health of the child. While some children are most cooperative in the morning, some are better after their naps, and still others do not mind coming into the office after regular school or nursery activities. The length of the appointment also depends on treatment requirements. While individual differences must always be kept in mind, there seems to be no significant difference in a child's behavior for longer or shorter appointments[8].

The type of attire the dentist and the auxiliary personnel wear has been discussed for many years. Studies indicate that the children are not influenced greatly by the dentist's clothes[2] even though many dentists feel informal dress is less frightening to children.

Basic floor plans and traffic patterns

The basic traffic patterns are important in the attainment of maximum efficiency in an office. It is essential to analyze the circulation patterns within the different areas of the of-

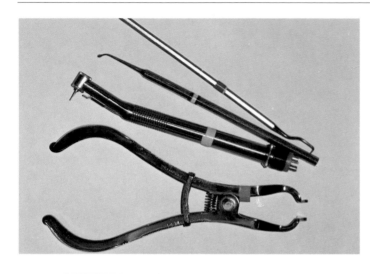

Fig. 13-1 Color coding of instruments allows easier sorting for different locations.

Fig. 13-2 Some of the many different arrangement possibilities (Courtesy of Dr. K. Kimmel).

fice as a whole as well as circulation patterns within each operatory so that proper work flow is achieved and traffic jams and bottlenecks are avoided. Discussions of floor plans for different types of practice are available[6] and dental suppliers and manufacturers are prepared to offer suggestions.

The number of operatories required is an individual matter and depends on the type of practice, the manner in which the dentist likes to work, and also on the number of professionals sharing the office. It is usually advisable to have more than one operatory for each dentist to reduce time wasted between patients and in resetting the operatory.

If more than one operatory is used by the dentist(s), color coding of the instruments to each room will permit easy identification (Fig. 13-1) and replacement after cleaning.

Equipment

The arrangement of equipment and its selection is a matter of personal preference and available space. New designs and technical developments are developed regularly and no attempt will be made here to catalog the various systems. Kimmel[7] has reviewed some modern commercial units and dental office designs (Fig. 13-2).

The equipment should be such as to give the child a sense of security and to allow the dentist to restrain the patient if necessary. If a large adult chair is being used, special types of inserts may be necessary to accomplish this. The chair selected for at least one operatory should permit easy wheel chair transfer of patients so that handicapped children can be treated. Doorways wide enough for wheelchairs should be provided.

Technical, functional, and safety criteria, however, also must be analyzed. The equipment should be functional, with good technical performance, as simple as possible, and have high safety standards. It must also be easy to service and to clean and maintain properly. Hygienic considerations should play an important part in equipment selection.

It is a matter of personal preference whether to have a working table with a retracting arm in front of the patient or an instrument area behind the child. The major advantage of the latter arrangement is that instruments will not "fly" from the working table because of

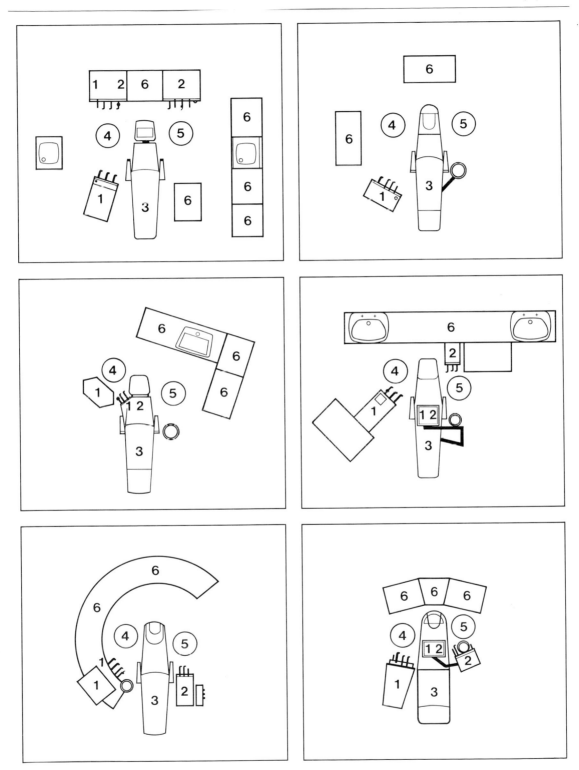

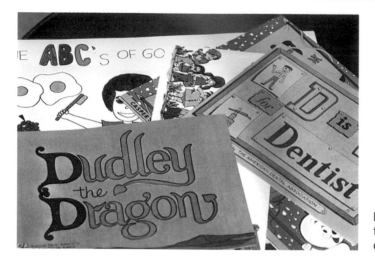

Fig. 13-3 Some of the many educational pamphlets available for patient distribution.

an unexpected patient movement. It is, however, important to remember to "tell, show, and do" if this arrangement is used as a child is entitled to know what is going to be done. The most comfortable position for the dentist depends on his physical characteristics and should allow good posture with a straight back to minimize the strain which results from forced, unnatural positions.

Much has been written about exposed hoses and retracting hose systems. Again, the simpler the system the more reliable and the easier to service. Children will understand and accept any equipment if they have become familiar with it.

Reception area

The manner of decorating a reception area depends on the type of practice. The decoration should be appealing, but should require little rearranging and reorganizing to minimize the work of the reception personnel. Light should be good enough to permit reading but safe and firmly fastened to avoid accidents. If a central point of interest such

as a fish tank is used, it should be enclosed to avoid damage by small children. If a bulletin board for children's efforts is provided, it should be updated regularly. A dental assistant or the receptionist should be able to adequately overlook the reception area and keep it neat and attractive. It is not necessary to decorate a reception area as a nursery, but it should have some objects that interest the child who is waiting. Toys or books that can easily soil or break are inappropriate because cleanliness and safety are important. Toys available in the reception area should be neat, clean, and frequently changed.

Patient education material such as that prepared by the American Dental Association can be displayed (Fig. 13-3) in the reception area to be read while waiting or to be taken home.

Business area

This is a major area of activity and as such must be planned to enhance efficiency and to prevent patient interference. It should give the impression of efficiency, be neat and uncluttered, have ample storage facilities, and carefully selected lighting. The working area must be adequate for all the people who need to use it.

Laboratory and radiograph processing area

The size of this area varies with the needs of the office and the type of machine used (panoramic, cephalostat, etc.). Modern equipment has greatly reduced the space and equipment needed for developing films. Some offices even have small developing units in the master operatory.

Some laboratory space is necessary in every office to allow for pouring of models and their preparation, but the size of the area depends directly on the amount of such work done. A good storage area for models and a good retrieval system also are important.

Private office and consultation room

This area is reserved for the dentist and is used for discussion of treatment plans with patients and their parents. It should be pleasant and quiet with a view box for demonstration of radiographs. If educational films are provided for patient and parent instruction, a separate space is set aside for this purpose so that some patients and parents can be watching while other patients are being interviewed.

The auxiliary personnel

In all types of dental practice, the auxiliary personnel are a major consideration. They are the first persons to have contact with the

patient and his or her family. It is important that the assistants communicate well with parents and patients and that they are prepared to handle telephone calls and questions promptly and properly[1].

The efficient use of a chairside assistant can greatly improve the efficiency and conserve the energy of the dentist. If a full-time chairside assistant is used, a receptionist is needed to answer the telephone, make appointments, and do necessary paper work. Some offices employ more than one dental assistant so that a substitute is available in case of absence, and to help generally by providing an additional pair of hands without the loss of the chairside assistant. However, increased staff increases overhead, and the advantages and disadvantages need to be weighed.

The chairside dental assistant is invaluable in a pedodontic practice. A child should never be left alone in the operatory. If the dentist must leave, the assistant should remain with the child. The dental assistant should also know exactly what a dentist wants to do, why it is done, and to whom it will be done so that she may anticipate the dentist's needs, help the child, and answer questions accurately. The assistant should be attentive to the parent, as many times the parent will tell the assistant something which is not considered important by the parent but which may be helpful to the dentist in providing service.

Treatment plan

It is advisable to have a complete treatment plan outlined for each patient, even if the patient will be referred to another professional for some aspects of the treatment. A treatment plan should be outlined after a thorough examination and complete diagnosis, and then be presented to the parent with a full explanation of all needs. Treatment planning should include a complete and clear explanation of preventive programs to avoid future disease conditions. All comments about the presentation should be recorded to minimize future misunderstandings. Organizing the procedures will decrease preparation time and allow the dental assistant to know what to set up as well as to estimate the approximate time needed for scheduling purposes. Good treatment planning will permit maximum dentistry in a minimum number of visits – a goal of most patients and dentists.

Setting of fees and collection

Fee setting should be uniform for all patients, taking into consideration the different factors which affect fees: time of the professional, of the auxiliary personnel, supplies, and all aspects of overhead.

Many different systems of fee collection have been developed and in some parts of the country banks have developed automated systems for this purpose. Some offices have installed computer billing by using their own office computer[5, 9]. Before using any of the systems for automation of bookkeeping or for collection of bills by a bank or other collection agent, it is important that the dentist evaluate carefully the type of contract, to avoid any practice that may adversely affect the dentist's image[12].

Record keeping

Efficient methods of records management, retrieval, billing and control are of vital importance in a dental office. As turnover of personnel is inevitable, the system of information retrieval must be workable and easily manageable. With the large number of pa-

tients treated daily, a smooth and efficient management of the business side of dentistry is essential[10].

Many business practice systems which are commercially available may be useful and can be adapted to an individual practice according to its size, type, the number of professionals, and the number of auxiliary personnel (hygienists, chairside assistants, secretaries, receptionist, laboratory technicians) employed. It is important that the system selected should not become too cumbersome if enlarged. The system should not require extensive training or expenditure of too much time for execution of tasks such as billing, recall, etc.[11]. Many printed forms should be evaluated; each manufacturer has some forms which are acceptable to a given situation and others that are not. Photographs on charts may be desirable and actually have many benefits. They provide a "before" and "after" record of treatment and may be particularly useful if malocclusion has to be evaluated at regular intervals. Photographing patients is easy and inexpensive, considering the amount of information provided and the ease of storage. With the development of cameras that develop film immediately and special attachments which permit a photo record as close as 5 inches, adequate close-ups are available with no delay. Only a few minutes are needed for the entire procedure and the resulting permanent record can be attached to the chart. The size and type of the appointment book varies with the size of the office. Daily schedule forms are commercially available to duplicate the appointment book according to operatories. A copy of the day's activities should be available in each operatory and each work area to avoid frequent disruptive trips to the central desk for appointment verification. The receptionist can make these copies as soon as the daily appointments are confirmed. These daily schedules include the name of the patient, the length of time reserved for him, and the type of work expected to be performed. In a pedodontic practice, it also indicates how many members of the family are in treatment at the same time. Allotment of time for emergencies is convenient and allows an easier flow of the patients regularly scheduled.

Business data are indispensable as part of a patient record. These data include: all cancellations and the reason for each cancellation, and whether or not the appointment had been confirmed (in cases of illness, the cause). The number of late arrivals, how late each was and the reason should be noted. Late arrivals and late cancellations are the source of much trouble for the practice and require close attention and supervision. The record should also include cost estimates, definite payment stipulations, and complete tabulation of payment progress. A ledger card as a financial record of the patient is essential and must be kept current[4].

Many practices with large numbers of child patients maintain a list of birthdays and regularly mail birthday greeting cards. Specially designed cards for this purpose are available from stationery catalogs for dental office use. Children enjoy receiving mail and this is an easy means of patient communication. A file can be maintained and cards sent out by the auxiliary personnel.

Appointment cards and excuse cards are also useful in getting cooperation for proper scheduling. Since most appointments are made long in advance, it is good practice management to call the day before the appointment and confirm the time and date with the parent. The number of broken appointments can be reduced in this manner.

It is common practice in many offices to have referral acknowledgement cards available because they demonstrate the appreciation of the dentist for a new referral. At the time of the first call, the auxiliary should ask the name of the person who referred the patient to the dentist. At that time, an acknowledgement card can be mailed to the referring patient or dentist and, if the patient was referred by another patient, a note can be placed in the referring patient's folder to allow a personal comment of appreciation at the next visit. This information, together with personal social data, promotes better communication and demonstrates personal interest.

Office communication system

The first telephone call of a parent to the office is often the first contact the parent has with the practice. It is important that the receptionist who answers the telephone does so promptly and pleasantly showing concern for the patient's needs. She should be trained to be efficient in obtaining and collecting information and determining whether an emergency appointment is necessary. She should also know how to screen calls so that the dentist will not interrupt treatment unnecessarily to answer a call that could be handled later, but she must know that the dentist is always available in case of a real emergency.

Accurate information should be obtained by the auxiliary from this initial telephone call, and more complete information when the patient arrives for the first visit. Several forms are available from different companies for initial telephone interview data; selection is a matter of individual preference. The form chosen should contain data about the patient's name, address, and age, who referred the patient, and the reason for the call. It is convenient to have a preprinted list of the most frequent reasons for an initial telephone call, such as tooth fracture, bleeding, swelling, and pain and its duration, to aid in the speedy recording of accurate data via the telephone. It is also important to know whether the patient has already visited other dentists and the reactions to these visits. A note of the apparent amount of concern of the parent is also helpful. A record card with more detailed information about problems and personal data will be completed when the patient arrives at the office.

The problem of telephone coverage during the lunch period and after office hours has to be analyzed carefully. In a large office with many auxiliaries it is often possible to alternate lunch hours to permit good telephone coverage. After office hours, answering services or electronic answering devices with a remote recall feature permit adequate continuity of service and good patient management.

The new sophisticated electronic telephone systems also permit evaluation of the efficiency of the lines and instruments in an office. It is possible for many telephone services to evaluate how long and how often a line is busy so that the dentist may consider either a change in personnel practices or the installation of extra instruments or lines.

An "intercom" system which relays information through signs or numbers rather than voice is highly desirable. Different colors or numbers can be used for each individual and combinations of lights, colors, and numbers can convey simple messages between treatment rooms, reception area, and private offices with a minimum of noise and a maximum of efficiency. An assistant can be summoned to any area where needed almost immediately, and learning the system is easy for newcomers to the staff.

Recall system

A good periodic recall system is the best method of maintaining good preventive programs and assuring adequate care of teeth and previous dental care. It is a means of educating patients and parents in maintaining good dental health and in periodic evaluation of dental conditions.

It is essential to evaluate preventive dentistry measures in children periodically. In this way interceptive orthodontics or treatment of any pathology may be instituted if necessary.

While regular return to the dental office is largely the responsibility of the patient and parents, it cannot be left entirely to them. It is an individual choice whether to make a future appointment for the patient, arrange such recalls by telephone, to mail a preprinted card with a reminder to call the office, or even to send a card with the proposed time of appointment. Because patients tend to move or leave the community, making an appointment without certainty of patient availability is risky and may lead to open spots in the appointment schedule. A telephone recall system has the disadvantage that there is a tendency for procrastination when the book is already heavily filled. The most widely used system is the mailing of cards, followed in some offices by a telephone call, as this prevents the patient from putting off making his own telephone call for the recall appointment.

References

1. Chambers, D. W.:
   Personnel management vs. managing a dental office. General Dent. *26*:66-71, 1978.

2. Cohen, S. D.:
   Children's attitudes toward dentist's attire. J. Dent. Child. *40*:285-287, 1973.

3. Deuben, C. J. and R. F. Geyer:
   Application of management skills in dental practice. Dent. Hygiene *50*:301-305, 1976.

4. Gerber, I. A.:
   Communication and record keeping in a large dental group practice. Dent. Survey, *50*:30-40, 1974.

5. Green, D.:
   Computer billing: are you ready or not? Dent. Manage. *15(6)*:31-42, 1975.

6. Kilpatrick, H. C.:
   Work simplification in dental practice; applied time and motion studies. 3rd Ed. Philadelphia, Saunders, 1974.

7. Kimmel, K. and R. O. Walker:
   Practicing dentistry. Ergonomic guidelines for the future. Berlin, Die Quintessenz, 1972.

8. Lenchner, V.:
   The effect of appointment length on behavior of the pedodontic patient and his attitude toward dentistry. J. Dent. Child. *33*:61-74, 1966.

9. Rens, R. D.:
   Data processing in the dental office. J. Calif. Dent. Assoc. *4(8)*:30-35, 1978.

10. Takavec, M. M.:
    From the operatory to the business office... Organization and management of a dental office. J. Calif. Dent. Assoc. *6*:48-52, 1978.

11. Tryon, A. F.:
    The problem oriented dental record. In Crandell, C. E., Comprehensive care in dentistry. Littleton, Ma., P. S. G. Publishing Co., 1979.

12. Walker, B. N.:
    We got out of the banking business. Dent. Econ. *65*:63-4, 66-8, 1975.

Chapter 14

Hospital Dentistry

While most children can be treated effectively in the dental office, certain patients require hospitalization for dental procedures. Children under the age of 3 seldom are good office patients if they require extensive treatment, and treatment given under general anesthesia is often the most efficient and successful method of providing appropriate dental procedures on patients who are unable to comprehend, cooperate or communicate. It is the preferred method for some mentally retarded, the emotionally disturbed, and for some patients with physical handicaps. However, not all physically and mentally handicapped children require hospitalization. Judicious use of general anesthesia can greatly relieve emotional stress in both patient and parent. Although some dentists administer general anesthesia in their private offices[1] this service is best performed in a hospital operating room supervised by trained anesthesiologists[2]. Many times a patient becomes more cooperative in the office after having initial care under general anesthesia, and future treatment in the dental office[14] then is feasible.

In summary, general anesthesia may be necessary in:

A. Patients retarded mentally to the degree that communication cannot be established
B. Children who are not amenable to behavior control by the usual guidance procedures or with acceptable degrees of restraint, premedication, or nitrous oxide
C. Patients with systemic disturbances that dictate the use of general anesthesia
D. Patients with emotional problems.

If the patient is ambulatory, a dental office visit should be scheduled and a dental examination made as complete as feasible. If possible, diagnostic radiographs should be obtained to permit development of a good treatment plan before hospital admission. A complete medical history, including history of past diseases and treatment as well as present systemic conditions and medication is sought. If dental radiographs cannot be made at the initial visit because of lack of cooperation, they should be made under general anesthesia before beginning treatment.

Systemic diseases

Diagnosis of cardiac disease is now being made at a much earlier age than in the past. It is advisable to start preventive dentistry measures early and to carefully monitor the cardiac patient during examination of the dental condition. If extraction becomes necessary, the cardiologist, the anesthesiologist, and the dentist must decide jointly on the need for hospitalization and the need for prophylactic antibiotic coverage.

Patients with hematologic disorders are also best treated jointly by the anesthesiologist, physician, and dentist to avoid emergencies particularly during extractions. Scheduling for these patients should be coordinated so that various procedures involving different specialties can be done simultaneously, thus reducing patient discomfort. For example, bone marrow biopsy can be performed when the patient is under anesthesia for dental treatment.

Psychological considerations

The psychological aspects of hospitalization of a child are very important, and must particularly be considered in hospitals that do not permit a parent to remain with the child. The child should be given an honest and truthful explanation of what to expect, especially when the hospital requires an overnight stay. This can be a traumatic experience for the young patient who has never been separated from his familiar surroundings. Certain hospitals have organized pre-admission visits and special activity programs with playrooms containing educational material to familiarize the child with the hospital and to permit better communication with the child[9].

Parents should receive an explanation of procedures and some background information about the treatment. If this is the child's first hospitalization, it may be a traumatic experience for the parents as well as for the child, especially if the child is very young. Parents must be reassured of the procedures because children are quick to sense insecurity. It is essential that no incorrect ideas be given to the child, that he is reassured and that separation fear be controlled. In some hospitals it is possible for the mother to stay with the child overnight, but this must be determined before making promises that cannot be kept. Some hospitals require the presence of a parent, particularly if there are behavior problems[11].

Hospital procedures

It is usually the responsibility of the dentist to make the initial admission arrangements with the hospital and to make sure that required work-up and laboratory tests are done. An examination by a physician on the hospital staff must be arranged, and the drugs that are to be administered to the child during the hospital stay ordered.

Each hospital has a protocol of established admission procedures. Specific laboratory work is required to provide information on the patient's well being. Laboratory test results must be available to the anesthesiologist and the dentist before anesthesia is administered. These tests usually include complete blood counts, chest X-rays, and urinalysis.

Special clinical laboratory tests may be indicated for some patients, such as prothrombin time (PT) and partial thromboplastin time (PTT)[3]. For black patients, special tests for sickle cell anemia are indicated.

If the hemoglobin is 10 gm/100 ml or less and emergency general anesthesia is necessary, a blood transfusion might be indicated. If the urinalysis reveals kidney disease, the patient should be re-evaluated before any general anesthesia is administered. General anesthesia should not be administered in the presence of respiratory infections.

Patients with heart murmurs should be evaluated carefully before anesthesia to assure proper medication. Patients on adrenocortical therapy need careful attention and may require additional steroid coverage which should be instituted during the preoperative and postsurgical period. Special care must be provided in diabetic children and insulin therapy adjusted. Patients with cystic fibrosis (if they must be treated under general anesthesia) should not receive atropine. The heavy thick secretion problem in these children makes suction during anesthesia necessary. Hemophiliacs must be premedicated.

Patients are usually admitted the day before surgery. After admission the patient should be examined by the pediatrician. Appropriate laboratory tests must be ordered or, if previously done, placed in the chart. The anesthesiologist will usually evaluate the patient the evening before surgery and order the appropriate premedication. It is important that the stomach be empty prior to the induction of general anesthesia. Specific orders must be written to this effect. If a patient is admitted in the afternoon for early morning surgery the patient should take nothing by mouth (N.P.O.) after midnight. If the surgery is scheduled for the afternoon, the patient should be N.P.O. at least 6 hours before surgery.

Patients are premedicated to assure cooperation in the initial phases of anesthesia and to reduce secretions. The use of narcotics as premedication depends on the age of the child because some narcotics are contraindicated in very young patients. The drug most frequently used to control salivary secretion is atropine sulfate. It is given intermuscularly (0.1 mg/10 lb. to a maximum of 0.4 mg-0.6 mg) about one hour before surgery. Sometimes scopolamine is used as the anticholinergic drug but it has some undesirable side effects, such as restlessness. Although scopolamine may be superior as an antisialogue, atropine is usually preferred. It should be noted that patients with Down syndrome may be hypersensitive to atropine. Succinylcholine chloride is used to facilitate intubation by acting as a voluntary muscle relaxant and is administered either intravenously or intramuscularly immediately before endotracheal intubation.

The choice of anesthetic is at the discretion of the anesthesiologist who must choose a non-explosive agent when dental equipment will be used. A mixture of halothane/nitrous oxide/oxygen is frequently used. If halothane is used, the conjoint use of epinephrine is contraindicated. If epinephrine must be used as a hemostatic agent during the procedure, it must be given in carefully controlled amounts and only after consultation with the anesthesiologist. During general anesthesia, vital signs such as respiration, blood pressure, pulse rate, temperature, heart sound and skin appearance are monitored continuously just as in any other surgical procedure. Intravenous fluids are usually started early to guard against dehydration, and to establish a route if intravenous medication becomes necessary.

Many hospitals will allow a policy of clean but not sterile technique for dental rehabilitation. This means that all those participating in the treatment will wear scrub suits, caps, and masks but not necessarily sterile gowns or gloves. This is a matter of hospital policy and a preoperative surgical scrub may or may not be required.

After the induction period of anesthesia and proper protection of the patient's eyes, the head is draped. Eye protection is very important to avoid damage from tooth or restoration fragments. Also, the eyes must be protected from the head drape.

If it was impossible earlier to obtain adequate pre-treatment radiographs, they can be taken at this time (Fig. 14-1). Before initiating dental treatment but after the patient has been draped and the eyes shielded, a pharyngeal pack is introduced. It is usually made of a very long continuous roll of cotton gauze that has been moistened. Its function is to prevent debris from entering the throat. A rubber dam also is used together with a mouth prop to facilitate dental treatment.

The treatment plan for the lesions should be such that no additional general anesthesia

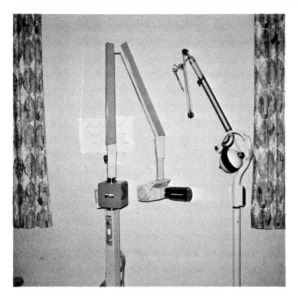

Fig.14-1   Mobile X-ray unit for use in operating room (Courtesy of Dr. S.W. Shore).

for dental purposes will be necessary in the immediate future. The decisions to perform pulp therapy, extractions, or restorations are influenced by the systemic condition present, the patient's and parent's ability to maintain adequate levels of oral hygiene, and the likelihood that future treatment may be accomplished without general anesthesia. Generally one quadrant is worked on at one time. If much tooth structure is destroyed, prefabricated stainless steel crowns are the treatment of choice, because they provide good coverage and can withstand severe chewing stress. It is advisable to perform extractions after other procedures are finished so that bleeding will not interfere with the restorative work.

Usually, the dentist provides the necessary dental instruments (Fig. 14-2). A well-trained chairside dental assistant (usually one who is familiar with the working habits of the dentist) should be available to assist during the treatment. It is desirable – and increases efficiency – to have a second dental assis-

tant help the chairside assistant. A mobile unit with high and low speed handpieces (Fig. 14-3) conveniently located, adequate work surfaces, and a good evacuation system are necessary.

The dentist customarily informs the anesthesiologist a few minutes before procedures are complete to allow adequate time for emergence from anesthetic. After all procedures have been performed satisfactorily and all debris suctioned to avoid danger of aspiration, the patient is extubated. After extubation the patient is taken to the recovery room and the vital signs are monitored. Following the stay in the recovery room the patient is returned to his hospital room. When it has been established that the patient's postoperative course is uneventful, he is discharged with appropriate discharge orders. The patient should be given a bland diet for a few days, and asked to return to the dental office in a week or 10 days for postoperative evaluation. Patients with major medical problems such as blood dys-

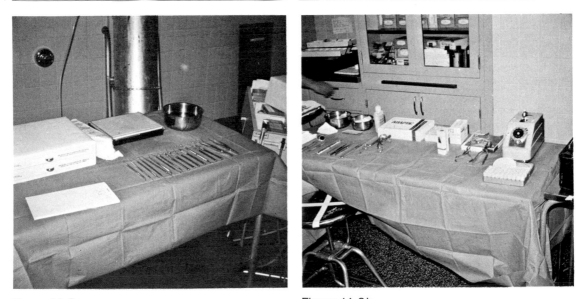

Figure 14-2a   Figure 14-2b

Fig. 14-2a and b   Dental instruments ready for use in operating room (Courtesy of Dr. S.W. Shore).

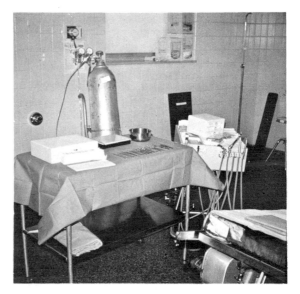

Fig. 14-3   Instrument table and mobile high and low speed unit for use in hospital dentistry (Courtesy of Dr. S.W. Shore).

crasias or heart disease may remain in the hospital until their condition has stabilized to the satisfaction of the physician in charge. The major disadvantages of hospital dentistry include:

1. postoperative side effects from drugs and physical agents used for anesthesia (sore throat, nausea, etc.),
2. cost of the hospitalization,
3. delays in planning (and postponement) because of operating room availability,
4. separation anxiety.

In addition to the potential complications from specific diseases requiring general anesthesia, potential complications from the anesthesia include aspiration following extubation, laryngeal edema, epistasis, stridor, pneumonia, etc. The danger of nose bleeds caused by the nasotracheal tube can be reduced but not eliminated by skillful placement of a well lubricated endotracheal tube. Care must also be taken in nasotracheal intubation to void damage to adenoid tissues which are often large in small children. To avoid aspiration, great care is taken in suctioning of debris and blood during treatment and before extubation.

Emesis sometimes occurs as a postoperative complication and patients may require an antiemetic. Laryngeal spasm may also occur. It is usually treated with oxygen in a humidified atmosphere. Succinylcholine chloride also may be administered for its voluntary muscle paralyzing properties. Above all, careful suctioning must be done before extubation since spasm may be caused by a foreign body in the larynx[7].

An important aspect of hospital dentistry is the completion of written orders. Each hospital has a set of directives which must be followed and which are supervised by an hospital records committee according to standards provided by the Joint Commission on Accreditation of Hospitals. The orders include[8]:

Admission orders:

These orders request the necessary laboratory examinations and request notification of the physician who will do the hospital admission physical examination and who will notify the anesthesiologist. They should state clearly that the patient must be N.P.O. for 6-8 hours before treatment.

Hospital charts:

Each hospital progress chart has several parts:

Admission note which includes:

1. a) a brief description of the physical condition of the patient.
   b) the immediate problem
   c) reason for admission.
2. Assessment (or impression)
   (a short report of the specific medical and/or dental problems).
3. Procedures that will be performed.

Operating room report includes:

1. surgical report
2. surgical findings and procedures
   (a dental chart may be included)
3. immediate postoperative condition of the patient
4. anesthesiologist's report.

Postoperative orders include

1. orders to the nurse to check for vital signs
2. medication required (including dimenhydrinate or prochlorperazine if necessary)
3. instructions for the patient
   (including ice if necessary)
4. diet restrictions
5. ice pack orders
6. high humidity tent

7. pain medication
8. Vaseline for dry lips.

Discharge note includes

1. final diagnosis
2. dental prognosis
3. discharge order – time.

The discharge note should include the patient's condition at the time of discharge, the medication and all the other instructions given to the patient and the date and location of the postoperative appointment.
Most hospitals require a *discharge summary* that is to be completed at, or shortly after, the patient's discharge from the hospital.

The hospitalized patient

With modern progress in medicine there has been a dramatic increase in quality and length of life of many patients who suffer from a wide spectrum of handicapping conditions. This has created the need for dentistry in a hospital setting to ensure proper care of these patients. At first many of these services were concerned only with the relief of pain by means of oral surgery. Today many services have undergone change and now place increasing emphasis on providing more complete dental health care for children who suffer from complicating medical conditions including good restorative and preventive care. In many of these conditons a close liaison between specialists in various other health disciplines is required. The dentist should be an integral part of the hospital team, providing a service that cannot be obtained from any other team member.
Because hospitalized, chronically ill patients require such a large amount of medical care, dental care often is given a low priority until a crisis arises. Many of the children who need dental care as hospital inpatients because of their medical disability require full medical and nursing surveillance. Patients should be evaluated for ability to practice oral hygiene procedures and must have these procedures performed for them if they are unable to do them alone. The principal responsibility of the dentist treating the chronically ill child is to provide relief of acute conditions and to maintain oral structures as normal as possible. The goal is to minimize or eliminate an oral problem that may also have aggravating effects on the systemic condition. The elimination of an oral infection, for example, will be benefical to the general condition.
Oral care for hospitalized patients should include:

1. examination of oral conditions, detection of pathology, and treatment planning,
2. teaching of effective oral hygiene methods and instituting oral hygiene procedures for patients who cannot perform these procedures themselves,
3. reduction, where possible, of oral manifestations of the systemic conditions and medication of the hospital patients, and
4. application of topical fluoride to increase tooth resistance to demineralization.

The physically and mentally handicapped are often unable to practice the personal oral hygiene essential in the prevention of dental disease. Consequently such patients are often more susceptible to oral diseases. If the patient is mentally alert enough to understand the reason for oral hygiene, the effects of dental plaque should be explained to him. A portable mirror with an illumination device is very helpful in these patients. Those too weak to sit up must be placed on one side when given oral hygiene. Suction is needed to avoid aspiration of water or saliva.
When certain medications that decrease saliva flow (such as atropine or scopolamine) are used, the oral mucosa must be observed for signs of dehydration. This is also a characteristic of mouth breathers.

Good dental care must be provided for patients who are to have radiation therapy of the head and neck region to avoid as much damage as possible. For the patient hospitalized for treatment of a malignancy in the head and neck region, which requires irradiation, a careful evaluation of the teeth, periodontal membrane and supporting alveolar bone is of great importance. Irradiation of the head and neck in the child interferes with growth, development, and eruption of teeth. The extent of the damage depends on the stage of development at the time of irradiation and the teeth may be completely absent or dwarfed[5,12]. There is also a danger of osteoradionecrosis but its incidence varies. Marciani and Plezia[10] found osteoradionecrosis in 10.5% of the 220 irradiated patients they studied, independent of the removal of teeth before initiation of irradiation therapy. However, Wescott et al.[15] demonstrated that a strict oral hygiene program and daily self treatment with 0.4% stannous fluoride gel can prevent dental caries development in the post-irradiation period. Initial reports[6,15] demonstrate that those patients who were willing to cooperate fully with a careful program of oral hygiene and fluoride application were able to avoid the development of post-irradiation dental caries. Irradiation therapy of the head and neck region often alters the structure of the salivary glands, with increased fibroblasts and decreased acinar cell structures. This may result in xerostomia, with a pronounced change in the normal microbial flora of the oral cavity[4].

The dentist working in a mental health facility has to be aware of the many problems of mental patients. Roth[13] lists some of the problems confronting these practitioners. The many possibilities for self-inflected injuries as well as injuries caused by others must be considered. Such patients may also suffer from intraoral lacerations caused by ingestion of foreign objects. Often a consultation with the ward attendant will disclose important information about the patient's habits.

References

1. Adelson, J.S.:
Clinical techniques for oral reconstruction with general anesthesia. I. Children. N.Y. State Dent. J. 36:339-343, 1970.

2. Album, M., C.L. Boyers, and R.I. Kaplan:
Hospital dentistry for the pedodontist: philosophy. J. Dent. Child. 35:153-160, 1968.

3. Braham, R.L.:
Clinical laboratory tests for patients hospitalized for dental procedures. J. Hosp. Dent. Pract. 12:117-122, 1978.

4. Brown, L.R., S. Dreizen, S. Handler and D.A. Johnston:
Effects of radiation-induced xerostomia on human oral microflora. J. Dent. Res. 54:740-750, 1975.

5. Burke, E.J. and J.W. Frame:
The effect of irradiation on developing teeth. Oral Surg. 47:11-13, 1979.

6. Caries prevention treatment saves patient's teeth after radiotherapy. J. Amer. Med. Assoc. 234.577-578, 1975.

7. Gaum, L.I.:
Laryngospasm in general anesthesia. Anesth. Progr. 18:69-71, 1971.

8. Kopel, H.M.:
Writing orders for the hospitalization of dental patients. J. Dent. Child. 35:405-409, 1968.

9. Macko, D.J. and F.A. Catalanotto.
Hospital dentistry for children: admission, management and discharge. J. Conn. State Dent. Assoc. 51:199-207, 1977.

10. Marciani, R.D. and R.A. Plezia:
Osteoradionecrosis of the mandible J. Oral Surg. 32:435-440, 1974.

11. McIntire, C.E.:
Complete dentistry for handicapped children under general anesthesia. J. Maine Med. Assoc. 62:221-222, 1971.

12. Pietrokovski, J. and J. Menczel:
Tooth dwarfism and root underdevelopment following irradiation. Oral Surg. 22:95-99, 1966.

13. Roth, H.:
The dental team in a mental hospital facility. J. Acad. Gen. Dent. 23(6):30-32, 1975.

14. Tocchini, J.J., T.C. Levitas and D.F. Redig:
The child patient and general anesthesia in the hospital. J. Dent. Child. 35:198-207, 1968.

15. Wescott, W.B., E.N. Starcke and I.L. Shannon:
Chemical protection against postirradiation dental caries. Oral Surg. 40:709-719, 1975.

Subject Index

307

quintessence
books

George E. White

Clinical Oral Pediatrics

Featuring an approach oriented to prevention, this textbook of pedodontics has been prepared by a large team of academics whose clinical experience provides useful insights into the practical problems faced by the dentist concerned with giving his child patients optimal dental care. Emphasis throughout is on practical technique and on motivation of the child-patient and the patient's parents.

The relationships between oral symptoms and systemic disease are given special attention; the social, emotional, and psychological problems associated with various dental disease states and malformations are considered in addition to physical health.

416 pages, 344 illustrations, of which 43 are four-colored, size 17.5 x 24.5 cm, linen bound with gold stamping and protective cover, ISBN 0-931386-32-2, price $68.00 plus handling and 6 % sales tax in Illinois/USA.

quintessence books

Kenneth A. Freedman

Management of the Geriatric Dental Patient

People are living longer; this is inevitably reflected in the composition of the dental practice population. Senior citizens have some oral health problems similar to those of the general population, and other problems that reflect their age and their general health status.

The dentist sees such patients in several settings: his office, homes for the elderly, and—occasionally—in the patient's own home. Each of the settings requires some adaptation if the older patient is to receive care under optimal conditions.

Management of the older patient requires some adjustment on the part of the dentist as well. He must be particularly careful to recognize dental problems associated with long-term use of certain drugs, and he must learn to understand that older patients require special attention. This book will help the concerned dentist to provide optimal care to a growing segment of the population, with minimal disruption of his normal routines.

148 pages, 80 illustrations (59 multi-colored),
17.7 x 24.5 cm, linen bound with gold stamping and dust
jacket, price $48.00, plus handling and 6 % sales tax in Illinois/USA.